Neurologic Differential
Diagnosis

Neurologic Differential Diagnosis

Second edition

Mark Mumenthaler, M.D.
Director (emeritus), Department of Neurology
Bern University
Bern, Switzerland

Translated and annotated by
Otto Appenzeller, M.D., Ph.D.
Visiting Scientist
Lovelace Medical Foundation
Albuquerque, New Mexico, USA

59 illustrations

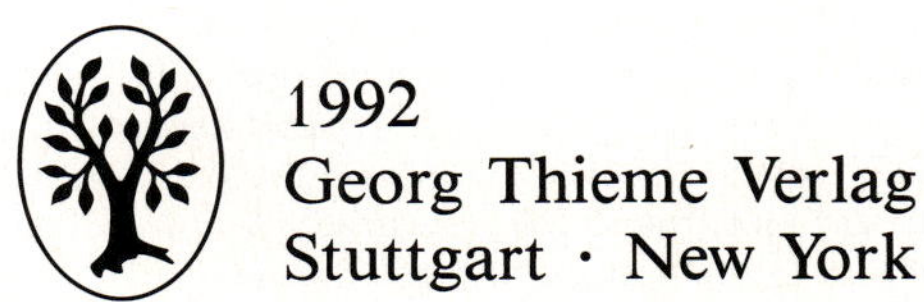

1992
Georg Thieme Verlag
Stuttgart · New York

Thieme Medical Publishers, Inc.
New York

Library of Congress Cataloging-in-Publication Data
Mumenthaler, Marco, 1925–
   [Neurologische Differentialdiagnostik, English]
   Neurologic differential diagnosis / Mark Mumenthaler; translated and annotated by Otto Appenzeller. — 2nd ed.
      p. cm.
   Translation of: Neurologische Differentialdiagnostik.
   Includes bibliographical references and index.
   1. Nervous system – Diseases – Diagnosis. 2. Diagnosis, Differential. I. Appenzeller, Otto. II. Title.
   [DNLM: 1. Diagnosis, Differential. 2. Nervous System Diseases – diagnosis, WL 141 M962n]
RC348.M9613 1992 616.6'0475 – dc20 DNLM/DLC for
Library of Congress 92-3211 CIP

Mark Mumenthaler, M.D.
Director (emeritus), Department of Neurology
Inselspital
Bern University
CH-3010 Bern, Switzerland

Otto Appenzeller, M.D., Ph.D.
Visiting Scientist, Lovelace Medical Foundation
2425 Ridgecrest Dr., SE
Albuquerque, NM 87108
USA

This book is an authorized translation of the German 3rd edition published and copyrighted 1988 by Georg Thieme Verlag, Stuttgart, Germany.
Title of the German edition: Neurologische Differentialdiagnostik.

© 1992 Georg Thieme Verlag,
Rüdigerstraße 14, 7000 Stuttgart 30, Germany
Thieme Medical Publishers, Inc., 381 Park Avenue South, New York, NY 10016

Typesetting by K+V Fotosatz GmbH
D-6124 Beerfelden
(Agfa MCS)

Printed in Germany by Gulde-Druck, GmbH,
D-7400 Tübingen

ISBN 3-13-665002-6 (GTV, Stuttgart)
ISBN 0-86577-432-3 (TMP, New York)

Preface to the Second Edition

The detonation of the first atomic bomb 47 years ago was among several profound changes in science that today directly affect and are a routine part of people's everyday lives. At about that time, neurodiagnostic tests became available, and clinical skills consequently were less sought after by trainees. Advances in medicine that would have been thought extraordinary 47 years ago are now taken for granted by the public, many of whom now have unrealistic expectations of what medicine can do for them. This is particularly true in neurology, where neurodiagnostic testing has been brought to the attention of the general public. Entrepreneurs and administrators, who for selfish reasons have exaggerated the benefits of the new technologies, are largely responsible for the public's misapprehensions, but neurologists themselves must take responsibility for technology's influence on the neuroscientific endeavor, whose objectivity has at times been tainted by faith in neurodiagnostic tests.

Nowhere is this lack of objectivity more apparent than in the recent literature on non-invasive diagnostic research, particularly magnetoencephalography, which has become notorious for its lack of scientific integrity. Among the most serious criticisms leveled at this work has been the failure to quantify the large uncertainties associated with estimates of nervous system function and physiology. MRI, PET, SPECT, and BEAM, as well as EMG, give highly speculative and approximate pictures of nervous system function only. The nervous system models used in the calculations and the appearance of the results in popular literature before exposure to the rigors of peer review has created a misplaced popular demand for these tests prior to and even instead of careful clinical neurologic examination. Partly fueled by this misguided popularity and by medical-legal considerations, some neurologists and other physicians have abandoned their well-honed clinical skills in favor of test reports, usually provided by others not involved in patient care. Inevitably, this has played into the hands of entrepreneurs, who have seized the opportunities for profit, and of administrators, who creatively try to reduce costs. All this has harmed patients and reduced the status of the profession.

Clinical neurologic diagnosis, with the recent judicious addition of noninvasive neurodiagnostic tests, together bring forth the best in neurologists, the most economical approach, and the very best in patient care.

The second English edition of Professor Mumenthaler's *Neurologic Differential Diagnosis* is in this respect a timely addition to the training of clinical neurologists, for it shows how best to arrive at a diagnosis and how judiciously to employ the support of neurodiagnostic investigations. The mastery of clinical neurology should remain the goal of neurologic training, and the second edition of *Neurologic Differential Diagnosis* will help achieve this mastery by those who aspire to enter the profession.

Albuquerque
January 1992

OTTO APPENZELLER
M.D., Ph.D.

Preface to the First Edition

A tortuous path connects the physician, his patient, and the final correct assessment of the patient's disease—and consequent appropriate therapy. This path encompasses several stages. The information gleaned from a careful history and physical examination is compared with the description of diseases in textbooks of medicine the physician reads during training and with information gathered from experience. From all this a correct diagnosis is eventually made.

The correspondence between patients' complaints and clinical findings and the description of disease, however, is not always close enough to assure the correctness of the diagnosis. In other cases, the correspondence between the findings and known disease patterns is not based on specific findings or on recalled or obligatory characteristics of diseases. In such cases the physician must reach an appropriate diagnosis by other means or must critically review the provisional diagnosis.

For both of these processes this book should be helpful.
- It is an aid for an overview of the characteristics of the most important neurologic syndromes, based on neuroanatomic and neurophysiologic considerations, and it helps in topical diagnostic considerations.
- It is also helpful in differential diagnosis of leading symptoms.

This book does not systematically discuss single diseases. It is restricted to differential diagnostic points of clinical importance that can be gleaned by the physician during his daily in-hospital and outpatient practices. It does not consider the results of complex investigations. Therefore this is not a textbook; it can be used to supplement a complete text on neurology but never to replace it. It is hoped that the book will help the practicing physician in differential diagnosis and in the correct assignment of the significance of neurologic symptoms and signs. This is not, however, a self-serving aim or intellectual game. It is a prerequisite for advancement of knowledge and clinical investigation and, most of all, a basis for appropriate therapy.

This book was made possible because of help and stimulation from many colleagues, to all of whom I extend my thanks. I am particularly grateful to Miss Elizabeth Stutz for secretarial help, and to Mr. Peter R. Schneider, University Artist, for his creative drawings. I am grateful to Dr. med. h.c. G. Hauff and his collaborators at Georg Thieme Verlag for careful production of this book.

Most of all, however, I am indepted to my patients. They have taught me to see and to differentiate.

MARK MUMENTHALER, M.D.

Contents

Introduction

The assumption is made that the reader is familiar with the fundamentals of neurology, can correctly interpret the history, is capable of a thorough neurologic examination, correctly interprets the meaning of important pathologic findings, and is familiar with neurologic diseases. The culling and ordering of all this information are usually sufficient for a correct diagnosis.

From the history and findings the disciplined physician will first decide where the lesion is: the localization of the pathologic process. After this, together with other information gleaned from the patient, an etiologic diagnosis is synthesized. Occasionally, however, there are doubts or a diagnostic impasse is reached. The present book will help the physician in checking the provisional diagnosis and in differential diagnostic considerations. It is therefore divided into two parts:

— In the first part, it is assumed that the physician has made a provisional diagnosis, that is, on the basis of the information obtained, has localized the process. In the first section of the book, *Syndromes: Topical and Symptomatic Aspects*, the characteristic syndromes are discussed according to their location in the nervous system. The neuroanatomic and neurophysiologic basis of the symptomatology and the etiologic processes responsible for such localization are described. This is important for a check on the correctness of the physician's topical diagnosis and is helpful in etiologic considerations.

— In the second part, *Leading Symptoms,* it is assumed that the physician is unable to localize the process on the basis of single findings. Help, therefore, is needed in interpreting the localizing value of the main findings or symptoms. In this part an attempt is made to help in the process that results in a diagnosis based on the correct interpretation of neurologic symptoms. Their importance is analyzed according to the origin of the symptoms, the involved body part, or other considerations. This allows an orderly classification of symptoms according to localization of lesions. This, in turn, facilitates the etiologic considerations of the significance of various leading symptoms. In some longer sections of this book, a "mirror" method is used as the basis for the differential diagnostic analysis of a particular leading symptom.

— An integral third part of the book is the subject index. This index is carefully and thoroughly constructed to facilitate the user's diagnostic efforts on the basis of various aspects of neurologic disease and other etiologic considerations.

The author has received valuable stimulation from a large number of publications—journal articles, monographs, textbooks, and atlases of anatomy. Of particular value were the following works: Robert Bing: *Compendium of the Brain and Spinal Cord Diagnosis,* Schwabe, Basel, 1945; Fritz Broser: *Topical and Clinical Diagnosis of Neurologic Disease,* Urban and Schwarzenberg, München, 1975; Joseph G. Chusid: *Correlative Neuroanatomy and Functional Neurology*, 16th ed. Lange, Los Altos, Cal., 1976; Elizabeth C. Crosby, Tryphena Humphrey, Edward W. Laner: *Correlative Anatomy of the Nervous System,* MacMillan, New York, 1962; A. Delmas: *Voies et centres nerveux,* Masson, Paris, 1970; Peter Duus: *Neurologische-topische Diagnostik*, Thieme, Stuttgart, 1976; Edgar A. Kahn, Robert C. Bassett, Richard C. Schneider, Elizabeth D. Crosby: *Correlative Neurosurgery,* Thomas, Springfield, Ill., 1955; John Patten: *Neurological Differential Diagnosis,* Springer, New York, 1977; Talmage L. Peele: *The Neuroanatomic Basis for Clinical Neurology,* 2nd ed., McGraw-Hill, New York, 1961; William D. Willis, Jr., Robert G. Grossman: *Medical Neurobiology,* 2nd ed., Mosby, St. Louis, 1977.

Some monographs or reviews that are important in neurologic practice are mentioned at the end of the book in the references. Journal articles that concern certain aspects of neurology can be gleaned from the more than 1,300 references in the author's textbook (M. Mumenthaler: *Neurology,* 3rd ed., Thieme, Stuttgart, 1990).

This book reflects the present state of knowledge and the experience of the author. It undoubtedly has many gaps, and it may be incomplete and may include mistakes. The author is grateful to all readers for hints, communications of personal experience, and constructive criticism.

1. Syndromes: Topical and Symptomatic Aspects

Circumscribed lesions of the nervous system, and especially of the neuromuscular system, cause a group of symptoms classifiable according to anatomic and neurophysiologic considerations. What follows is a description of such syndromes based on topical arrangements, site of the lesion, and neuroanatomic, neurophysiologic and etiologic considerations.

1.1 Cerebral Syndromes

Table 1 A lists symptoms and signs that indicate a localized process, disease, or dysfunction of the brain. None of these singly is, however, obligatory. The symptoms and signs listed in Table 1 B often accompany those in Table 1 A, but in themselves are not proof of localized dysfunction. (For the differential diagnosis of the symptoms and signs listed in Table 1 B, see the second part of this book.)

1.1.1 Syndromes of Hemispheric Motor and/or Sensory Pathways

When localized in the brain, a disorder of these pathways leads to hemisyndromes, that is, the symptoms are confined to one side of the body. This is to be distinguished from crossed symptoms (1.1.3.3; see Fig. 5) in which deficits of other systems can also be found on the opposite side of the body.

If only one system, for example the motor system (Fig. 1), is involved on one side of the body, it is considered evidence of cerebral dysfunction only if there is also paralysis of the face on the same side. This leads to a pure motor cerebral hemisyndrome, which is, however, very rare. When motor fibers for face, arm, and leg are close enough to be affected by a single process (internal capsule, peduncles, or pons), they are also in close

association with sensory pathways and other structures that are, as a rule, affected by the same pathologic process. When motor pathways are topographically isolated, they occupy a relatively large area, for example, in the centrum semiovale and in the cortex. In hemisyndromes due to lesions in these areas, a large part of the brain must be affected, and additional symptoms are the rule rather than the exception.

Because of these anatomic considerations, a pure motor cerebral hemisyndrome should prompt intensive search for additional clinical evidence, such as motor deficits of the face and other confirming symptoms and signs that the lesions are limited to the cerebral hemisphere (Table 2).

1.1.2 Cortical Syndromes

Lesions of the cerebral cortex give rise to local signs and eventually to psychopathologic syndromes, which are described in 2.1. Nevertheless, certain specific symptoms point to circumscribed cortical area dysfunction. Such "lobar syndromes" are summarized in Table 3 (and Fig. 2) and in Table 12 (and Fig. 18); they are fully described below.

1.1.2.1 Frontal Lobes

The frontal lobes occupy an extensive area, extending anteriorly from the central sulcus and comprising functional areas that, if diseased, may give rise to specific syndromes.

Lesions of the precentral region affect the pyramidal cells and, consequently, the motor representation of the body (*see* Fig. 20).

- Lesions of the precentral gyrus result in partial paralyses that are more circumscribed in the case of superficial lesions. For example, a facial or crural monoplegia may occur. The lesions may be so circumscribed that central paralysis of the extensor of the big toe may have to be differentiated from peroneal palsy. This is especially difficult since isolated lesions of the cortex do not cause spasticity. Thus, both central and peripheral extensor paralysis of the toe are flaccid.

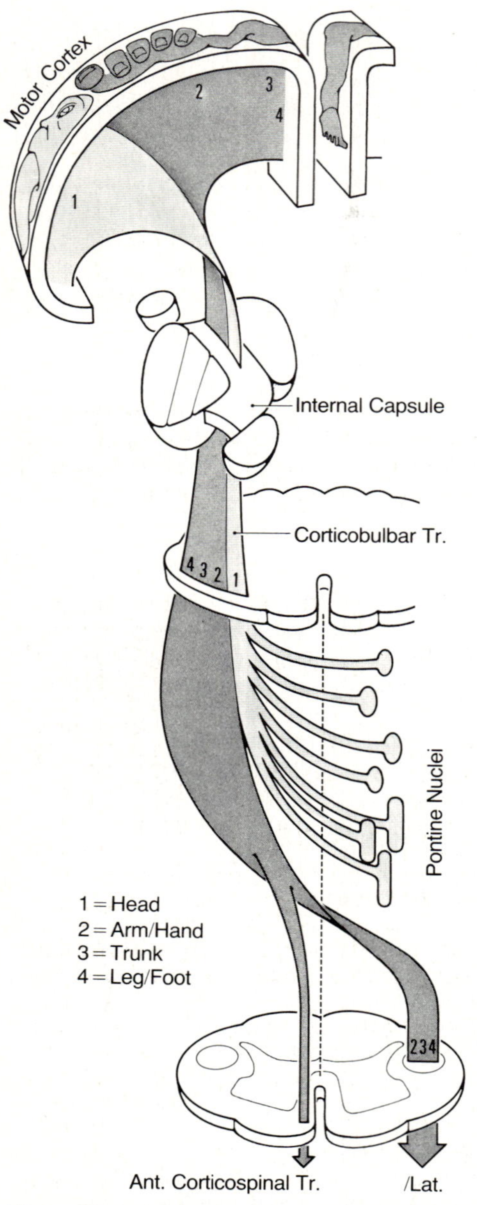

Fig. 1 Motor pathways from the precentral gyrus through the internal capsule and brain stem to the spinal cord

— Lesions of the second frontal convolution involving the corticovisual centers cause deviation of the eyes toward the side of the lesion (*see* 2.8.1).
— On occasion, irritative phenomena, differing from partial motor epileptic attacks, can occur (for details, *see* 2.3.1.1 and Fig. 20).

With lesions of the anterior convexity of the frontal lobes, particular modifications of motor function are found. They result from loss of cerebral inhibition, but are not specifically localizing. They are found in disturbances of cortical function associated with decreased attention and impaired consciousness.

— Grasping of hand and lips are early manifestations. The lips and jaw close reflexly on being touched. They may also turn toward the approaching object. An object placed in the hand may be forcefully handled, the hand following the outline in a magnetic reaction, or may be grasped reflexly. The signs are usually bilateral, but may be more prominent on the side opposite the lesion.
— Ataxia of the lower limb is particularly prominent when frontal pontocerebellar connections are interrupted. Walking is particularly affected, with incoordination of the side opposite the lesion, crossing of the leg, excessive abduction or adduction, and, occasionally, abasia.
— Involuntary resistance may be noted to passive movement of the limbs. This resistance is called gegenhalten and resembles catatonia. An assumed posture is maintained for an abnormally long period (posture perseveration). Passively executed movements may be actively continued by the patient (Kral's phenomenon). Observed postures may be imitated (echopraxia), and words or phrases repeated (echolalia).
— Lastly, there are psychopathologic abnormalities. Lack of initiative, spontaneity, and activity may lead to passive, inattentive, and disinterested behavior. Obsessive behavior may replace normal response to surroundings.
— Motor aphasia, due to a lesion of Broca's area, may result if the opercular of the posterior third frontal convulsion (which constitutes area 44) is involved (*see* 2.1).

Lesions of the orbital parts of the frontal lobes, particularly if bilateral, lead to impairment of affect and proper social behavior, which, in turn, leads to blunting of activities, disinhibition,

Table 1   Clinical symptoms and signs due to cerebral lesions or disease-related cerebral dysfunction

A: Proof of cerebral localization	B: Consistent with hemisphere disturbances
Epileptic attacks Disturbances of consciousness Organic psychosis Neuropsychologic dysfunction True homonymous hemianopia (Organic) paralysis of gaze (Organic) dystonias and other involuntary movements (Signs of increased intracranial pressure)	Headache Nystagmus Hemisymptomas Ataxia Disturbances of tone

primitive behavior, disintegration of social restraints, witzelsucht or moria, and, in severe cases, dementia.

Possible etiologic factors in frontal lobe disorders:

— Tumors (meningiomas with slowly progressive local symptoms, including focal epileptic attacks, psychiatric manifestations, longstanding nonprogressive, slowly advancing paralyses; rapidly progressive gliomas extending bilaterally in a butterfly fashion (butterfly gliomas) through the corpus callosum)

— Trauma, particularly frontal insults with frontal basal fractures (amnesia, anosmia, and eventually leakage of cerebrospinal fluid)
— Atrophic processes (particularly Pick's disease) and general paresis of the insane

1.1.2.2 Parietal Lobe

The parietal lobe is not easily delineated posteriorly from the temporal and occipital lobe (Fig. 2). Among its important parts are the postcentral gyrus, related to sensory function, the circumflex

Table 2   Accompanying symptoms of localizing value to cerebral hemispheres with motor hemisyndrome

Accompanying symptoms	Comments
Pronounced involvement of arm (face) in hemiparesis	There is a large cortical representation of the arm and face, giving rise to a large number of fibers that are widely distributed in the hemisphere, but caudally become closely associated with other motor fibers, including those serving the leg
Homolateral sensory disturbances without contralateral impairment of temperature or pain sensitivity in the extremities or contralateral cranial nerve deficits	The ascending posterior columns – after synapsing in the cuneate nucleus and nucleus gracilis in the inferior medulla oblongata – ascend in the medial lemniscus and, before their entry into the thalamus, approach the contralateral spinothalamic tract, which ascends in the spinal cord and serves pain and temperature sensation (*see* Fig. 52)
Definite paralysis of the face contralateral to the lesion	Corticobulbar fibers to the face cross to the facial nucleus at the midpons level (*see* Fig. 1)
Definite sensory impairment on the face contralateral to the brain lesion	The trigeminal lemniscus begins at about midpontine level and, together with the medial lemniscus, is responsible for sensation on the appropriate side of the body
Organic psychosis and neuropsychologic disturbances, epileptic attacks	These symptoms are proof of disturbances of cortical function
Homonymous hemianopia in the contralateral visual field	The postchiasmatic visual pathways are exclusively supratentorial

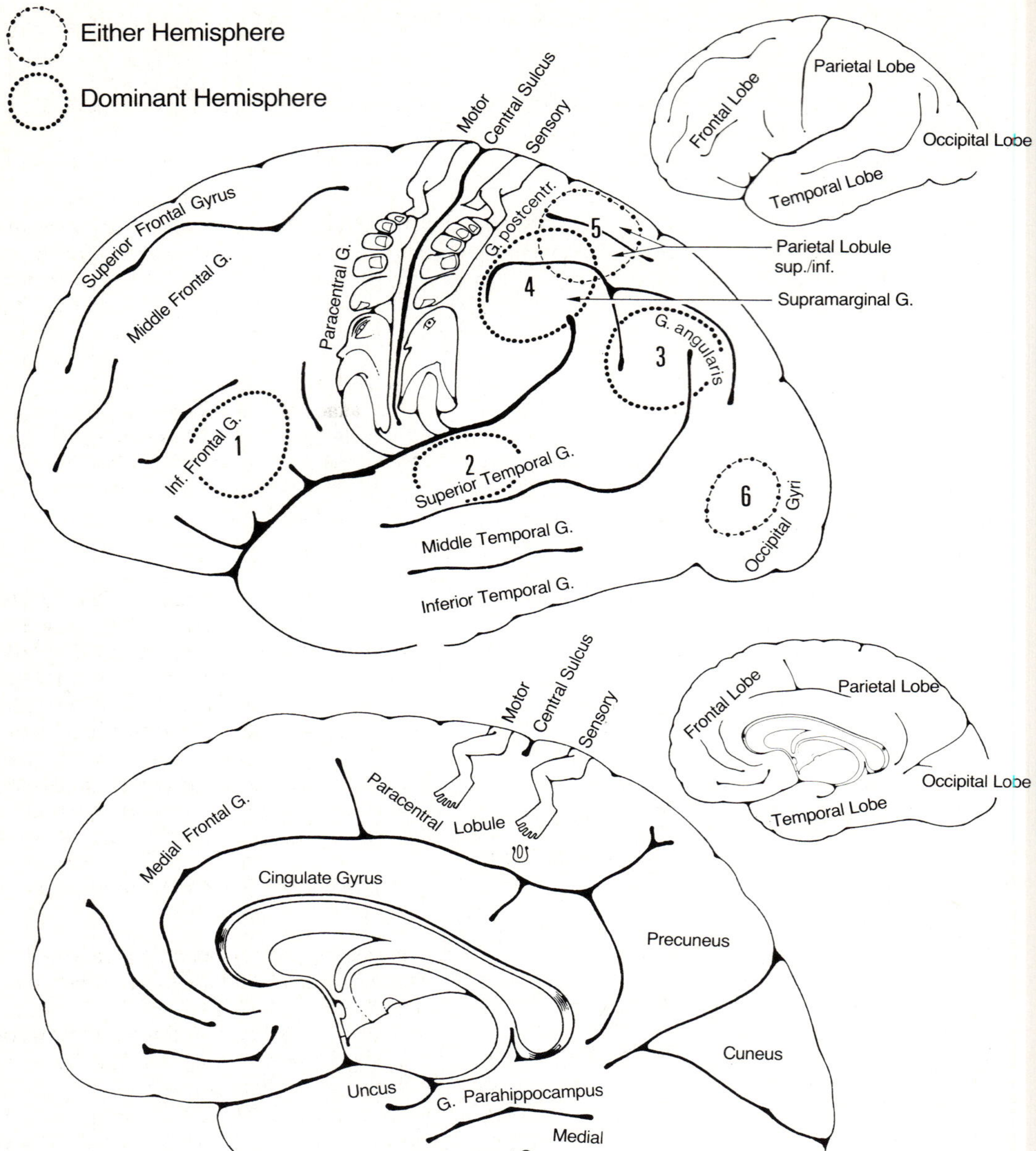

1 = Motor Aphasia   4 = Constructional Apraxia
2 = Sensory Aphasia   5 = Tactile Agnosia
3 = Alexia, Agraphia   6 = Visual Agnosia

Fig. 2   The four lobes of the cerebral cortex with their important neuropsychologic functions indicated or supramarginal gyrus, of great practical importance, and the angular gyrus, related to gnostic function.

Clinically, lesions of the parietal lobe involving the postcentral region and the upper part of the lobe give rise to

– Neurologic symptoms
  - sensory or sensory motor hemisymptoms
  - inferior homonymous quadrantanopia
  - hemianopic inattention on the contralateral side
  - impairment of optokinetic nystagmus, with the field moving in from the opposite visual field.
– Seizures
  Sensory jacksonian fits that may be followed by clonic attacks on the opposite side with deviation of the eyes, head, and trunk to the side opposite the lesion. A seizure focus in the paracentral lobule (situated on the medial part of the hemisphere) may cause paresthesias in the anogenital region with an urge to defecate and urinate.
– Neuropsychologic manifestations
  - disorientation in space and right/left confusion
  - tactile agnosia
  - constructional apraxia with lesions of the dominant hemisphere
  - amnesic aphasia and dyslexia

Etiological possibilities in lesions of the parietal lobe:

– Tumors, which initially are often manifest by epileptic attacks and increased intracranial pressure
– Trauma, particularly with lateral forces to the head
– Atrophic process (in these conditions, the neuropsychologic deficits are prominent)
– Disturbances in the territory of the posterior branches of the middle cerebral artery

1.1.2.3 Temporal Lobe

The temporal lobe cortex of the convexity of the hemisphere is related to language function (Wernicke area in the superior central gyrus) and serves as the central termination of pathways involved in hearing and smell. The basal region of the temporal cortex is related to the limbic system and is the termination of the sensory association pathways and vegetative afferents. In the inferior part of the temporal lobe white matter lie on the visual pathways originating in the inferior half of the retinas.

Lesions of the temporal lobe give rise to

– Neurologic symptoms including homonymous visual field defects, particularly upper quadrantanopias. A central disturbance of smell or hearing does not occur in unilateral lesions of the temporal lobe. Lesions deep in the lobe extending to the globus pallidus may give rise to movement disorders, including involuntary movement of the choreoathetotic variety.
– Epileptic attacks often characterized by psychomotor fits (*see* 2.3.3). Eventually these may become generalized; there are also episodic taste or smell sensations (uncinated fits). Occasionally, when Heschl's gyrus is involved, auditory hallucinations may be part of the seizures.
– Psychopathologic and neuropsycologic disturbances, manifest by disturbances of memory, particularly lesions involving the medial basal temporal lobes (hippocampus). Verbal memory is predominantly affected. Alterations of mood with depression and irritability and, occasionally, lack of inhibition and amnesic aphasic disturbances are other indications. Descriptions of impaired musical ability and time sense have also appeared.

Etiologic factors important in temporal lobe syndromes:

– Tumors, particularly glioblastomas and, more rarely, meningiomas such as sphenoidal meningiomas
– Trauma to the head, particularly contusions, due to frontal or occipital impact
– Vascular disturbances, including perinatal anoxia, to which the parahippocampal gyrus is particularly sensitive. These lesions may be latent for many years but eventually lead to temporal lobe seizures (psychomotor attacks) (*see* 2.3.3)
– Brain abscesses occurring after fractures of the petrous bone with the infection spreading into the temporal lobe
– Atrophic processes including Pick's disease, which may be largely localized to the temporal lobe

1.1.2.4 Occipital Lobe

Only a small part of the occipital lobe occupies the convexity of the hemisphere near the occipital pole. A larger part of the lobe is part of the medial surface of the hemisphere posteriorly. Here the visual pathway (the fourth neurons) terminates in the striate cortex in the region of the calcarine fissure. Also in this part are cortical areas 18 and 19, concerned with the processing of visual stimuli.

Lesions of the occipital lobe cause

— Neurologic visual disturbances, which are detailed in Chapter 2.5.2. Disturbances of gaze also occur. Lesions in areas 18 and 19 cause transient conjugate deviation of the eyes toward the side of the lesion with a gaze palsy to the opposite side. Pursuit movements of the eye remain impaired (whereas eye movements on commands arising in the frontal eye fields remain functional). These lesions most frequently cause disturbances in reading (dyslexia).

— Irritative phenomena, usually consisting of attacks of visual sensations. Those arising from area 17 are unformed flashes or sparks. Those arising in area 18 are often formed, and from area 19 there may be complex visual hallucinations. These positive phenomena may be combined with conjugate gaze and head turning to the side opposite the lesion. Generalized seizures may also occur.

— Neuropsychologic dysfunction, evident in visual spatial disorientation, color agnosia, and optic agnosia, including alexia.

Primary etiologic factors in occipital lobe syndromes

— Trauma, to the head, usually from the occipital or frontal direction

— Rarely, tumors; primary brain tumors and frequently metastases; meningiomas originating

Table 3   **Cerebral hemisphere (lobar) syndromes**

Neurologic deficits	Positive phenomena	Psychopathology and neuropsychology
Frontal lobe		
Paralysis (often circumscribed and localized)	Focal motor epileptic fits	Lack of initiative
Occasionally flaccid gaze paresis	Adversive fits	Flattening of affect
Grasping ataxia		Witzelsucht (moria)
		Motor aphasia
Parietal lobe		
Sensory hemisyndrome	Sensory jacksonian fits	Disorientation in space
Homonymous inferior quadrantopia		Tactile agnosia
Hemianopic neglect		Constructional ataxia
Decreased optokinetic nystagmus		Amnesic aphasia (dominant hemisphere)
		Dyslexia (dominant hemisphere)
Temporal lobe		
Homonymous visual field deficits, particularly upper quadrantanopia	Psychomotor attacks	Irritability
Impairment of movement coordination	Uncinate fits	Disinhibition
		Memory deficits
Occipital lobe		
Visual field deficits	Visual sensation and hallucinations	Color agnosia
Disturbances of optokinetic nystagmus		Disturbances of visual spatial orientation
Gaze paresis		Visual agnosia
Dyslexia		Alexia

from the posterior falx and superior sagittal sinus
- Disorders, which are frequent in the territory of the posterior cerebral or basilar artery and may give rise to bilateral symptoms

The cerebral lobe syndromes are summarized in Table 3 and illustrated in Figure 2.

1.1.3 Brain Stem Syndromes

The brain stem is composed of

- The diencephalon, which includes the thalamus and hypothalamus
- The mesencephalon, which includes the globus pallidus, the substantia nigra, and the red nucleus
- The pons
- The medulla oblongata.

In what follows, three common syndromes and their characteristic localizing features are delineated. The parts of the brainstem related to the basal ganglia will be considered as a functional entity belonging to the extrapyramidal system.

1.1.3.1 Basal Ganglia Syndromes (Extrapyramidal Syndromes)

The extrapyramidal system is composed of pathways and centers that, although not part of the corticospinal or corticobulbar systems, are important for motor function. The pathways belonging to this system are those fibers passing

- from the precentral, temporal, and parietal regions to the pons and cerebellum (the corticopontocerebellar fibers)
- from the cortex of the basal ganglia (the corpus striatum composed to the caudate and putamen), the red nucleus, the substantia nigra, and the reticular formation of the brain stem
- from neurons in the basal ganglia to the spinal cord (tectospinal, rubrospinal, vestibulospinal, and reticulospinal fibers) via interneurons (Fig. 3).
- In addition, functionally if not strictly anatomically related to the extrapyramidal system are fibers linking the various components of the basal ganglia and connecting them with the cortex. Finally in the extrapyramidal system are fibers arising in the cerebellum and thalamus, all of which form part of complex regulatory circuitry.

The extrapyramidal system is important in normal motor function.

- It influences muscle tone.
- It is instrumental in the reflexly polished movements of which we are capable.
- It allows for harmonious and economic motor activity with efficient interplay of movements. Closely involved in these functions are two neurotransmitters: dopamine and acetylcholine.

A disorder of the basal ganglia can give rise to an extrapyramidal syndrome with the following characteristics (for further details, *see* 2.12.1.2 and 2.14.1.8):

- Lesions of neurons of the globus pallidus and substantia nigra, which ordinarily inhibit muscle tone, cause an increase in tone. Lesions of the caudate, putamen, or subthalamic nucleus (nucleus of Luys) and the cerebellum result in a decrease in muscle tone.
- Motor function can be disturbed in two ways:
  - lesions of the pallidum and substantia nigra result in hypokinesia, a loss of primary automatic movements, and a decrease in associated movements (hypokinetic–hypertonic syndrome).
  - lesions of the neostriatum (putamen and caudate nucleus) cause involuntary hyperkinetic movements of different types most often associated with hypotonia. With lesions occurring in the perinatal and early postnatal period, athetoid and choreoathetoid movements are dominant. With lesions occurring at a later age, choreoathetoid movements are common. Ballismus is found with lesions of the subthalamic nucleus and outer pallidal layers. Lesions of the putamen or its connection with central thalamic nuclei usually give rise to dystonic syndromes and can even produce torsion dystonia.
- Psychologic disturbances are found in disorders of the basal ganglia and are manifest primarily in mood shifts, depression, obsessive activity, and repetitive thoughts. These are found in Parkinson's syndrome. In Sydenham's chorea, emotional lability and irritability are common, and dementia is characteristic of Huntington's chorea.

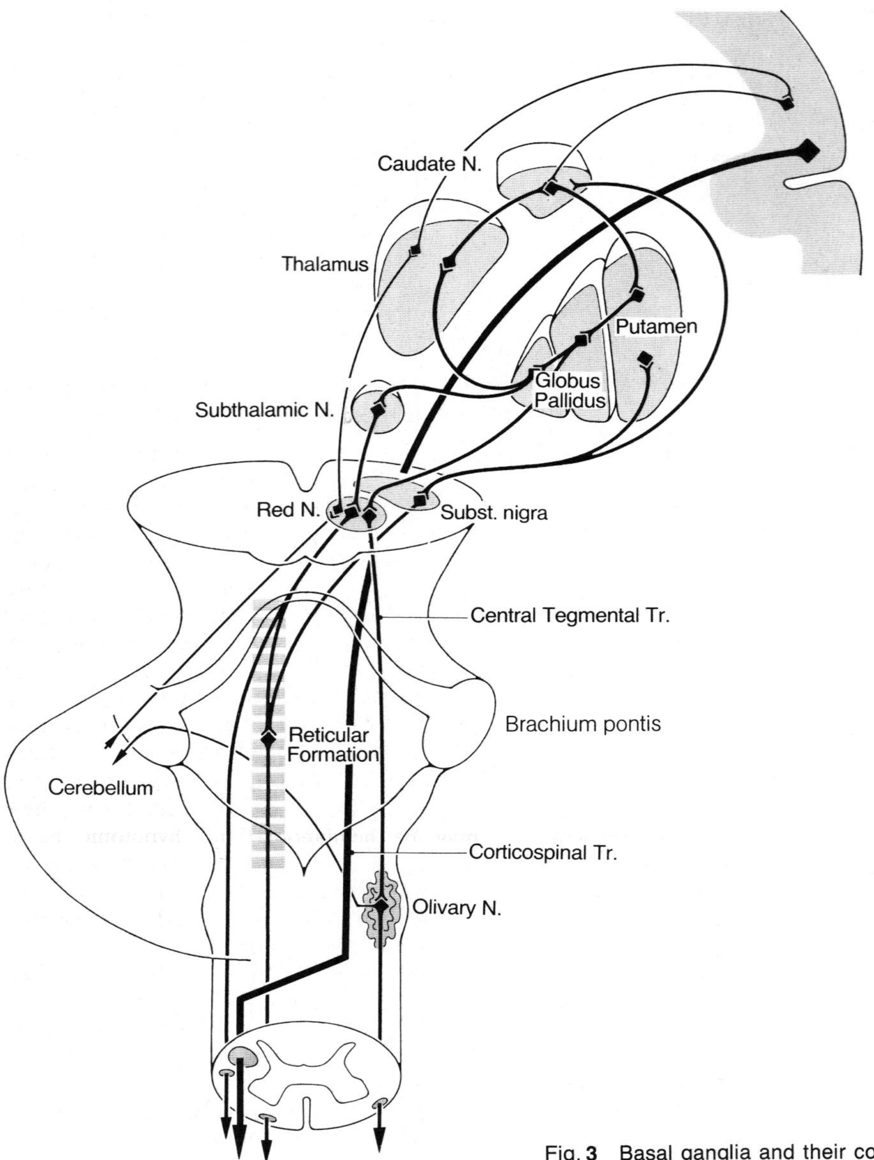

Fig. 3   Basal ganglia and their connections

The many disorders affecting the extrapyramidal system are
- Degenerative disorders, occasionally of a hereditary nature, among them Huntington's chorea and Parkinson's disease
- Metabolic disorders, including hepatolenticular degeneration (Wilson's disease)
- Genetic enzyme defects as found for example in olivopontocerebellar atrophy with symptoms of parkinsonism due to glutamate dehydrogenase deficiency
- Endocrine disturbances, for example, reversible parkinsonian-like states due to hypoparathyroidism
- Inflammatory diseases, including Sydenham's chorea
- Toxic states such as manganese intoxication and treatment with drugs including chlor-

promazine, both of which can produce parkinsonian symptoms
- Anoxic vascular insults, for example, torsion dystonia after perinatal brain injury
- Occasionally, tumors or other space-occupying lesions, which can present with hemiballisms when they involve the subthalamic nucleus of Luys

1.1.3.2 Diencephalic Syndromes

The anatomic parts of the diencephalon include

- The thalamus
- The epithalamus (including the habenular nuclei, the habenular commissure, the posterior commissure, and the pineal gland)
- The hypothalamus
- The subthalamic nucleus of Luys

The function of the diencephalon is complex.

- The thalamus is the penultimate way station of proprioception and exteroceptive sensitivity. In addition, impulses from the brain stem, the cerebellum, and hypothalamus also converge upon the thalamus. All of these afferent impulses are integrated and project primarily to the cerebral cortex to produce consciousness. Because the thalamus is part of the complex of extrapyramidal systems, its activity is important in mediating the effects of sensory and motor impulses from the cerebral cortex and in regulating their effect on movement.
- The epithalamus is important in the conduction of olfactory impulses and in the functioning of the light reflex.
- The hypothalamus, whose nuclei lie in the periventricular gray matter of the third ventricle, is related functionally to the posterior pituitary (neurohypophysis) and the mamillary bodies. The hypothalamus is the center of autonomic function. For example, the supraoptic and paraventricular nuclei of the hypothalamus produce antidiuretic hormone and oxytocin. These hormones reach the posterior pituitary through the supraopticohypophyseal tract, are released into the capillaries of the pituitary, and pass into the vascular system. This is an example of neurosecretion. Osmoreceptors situated in the supraoptic nucleus regulate antidiuretic hormone secretion and water and electrolyte homeostasis. Through numerous afferent and efferent connections the remaining nuclei of the hypothalamus are capable of influencing vegetative function of the body. Thus, exogenous and endogenous influences on olfactory and visceral function, sexual activity, sweating, temperature regulation, and affective behavioral aspects are manifest through the hypothalamic connections.
- The subthalamus comprises the subthalamic nucleus and belongs functionally to the extrapyramidal system (*see* 1.1.3.1 and 2.14.1.9).

Lesions of the diencephalon are generally classified as those affecting the thalamus and those affecting the hypothalamus. Nevertheless, there is often considerable overlap in the clinical manifestations produced by both kinds of dysfunction.

- Lesions of the thalamus cause contralateral impairment of sensation predominantly affecting deep sensibilities. Delayed perception, poor localization of touch, and unpleasant sensation in response to touching or even spontaneously on the affected side of the body (hyperpathia) are present. Motor manifestations include abnormal postures of the hand, characterized by flexion of the wrist and hyperextension of the interphalangeal joints (thalamus hand). Discrete involuntary choreoathetotic movements can also occur, and impairment of voluntary motions may be seen. Depending on the extent of the lesion, there may be hemianopia and hypotonic hemiparesis, which is often transient in nature.
- Lesions of the hypothalamus produce clinically severe disturbances of autonomic function and of impulsive behaviour.
  - Impairment of temperature regulation, sometimes leading to poikilothermia.
  - Impairment of water and electrolyte homeostasis, culminating in diabetes insipidus.
  - Disturbances of sleep-wakefulness cycles, hypersomnia, or sleeplessness.
  - Feeding disturbances, among them overeating associated with small genitalia and sometimes leading to adiposogenital dystrophy of Fröhlich, or, conversely, loss of appetite and cachexia (Russell syndrome).
  - Destruction of the hypothalamus can, because of its connection to the limbic system, result in abnormal sexual activity and aggression. On the other hand, destruction of the caudal hypothalamus may be associated with passive behavior and akinesia.

Etiologic considerations of lesions in this area include:

— Tumors in the suprasellar region (attention to field defects), particularly chromophobe adenomas, craniopharyngiomas, meningiomas of the tuberculum sellae, dermoid cysts, teratomas, pinealomas, gliomas of the optic nerve or of the hypothalamus

— Granulomatous conditions, for example, sarcoidosis
— Head trauma

1.1.3.3 Pontine and Medullary Syndromes

There are four main structures in the pons and medulla oblongata:

— The nuclei of cranial nerves III to XII
— Ganglion cells, some of which are diffusely distributed and give rise to the reticular formation extending up to the mesencephalon, and

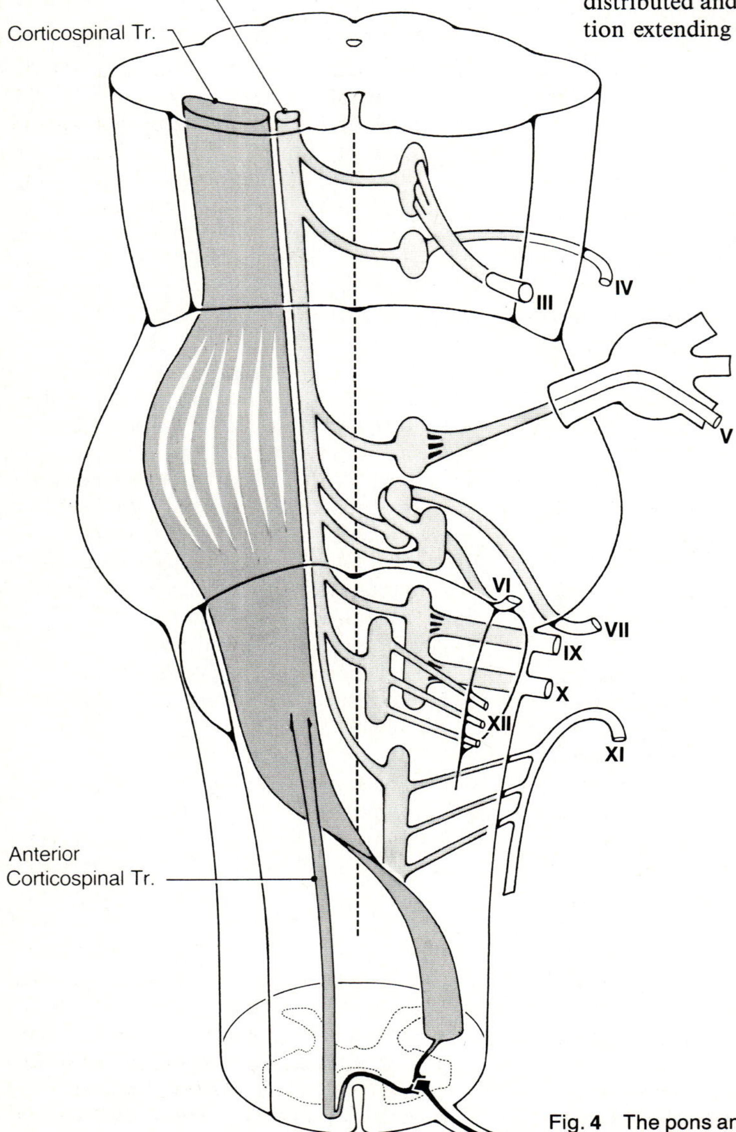

Fig. 4 The pons and medulla oblongata, showing the motor fibers and cranial nerve nuclei

olivary cells, which are connected to the red nucleus in the mesencephalon

- The connections of these nuclear masses with one another, with the cerebellum, the spinal cord, and brain
- Afferent and efferent fibers that connect the hemispheres, basal ganglia, and spinal cord and pass through without synapsing

These pontine and medullary structures are supplied by the vertebral and basilar arteries or their branches. The anatomic relationships of this area are illustrated in Figure 4.

Lesions of the pons or medulla result in syndromes with the following general characteristics:

- Motor deficits due to lesions of the cranial nerve nuclei can have the character of lower motor neuron paralyses (flaccidity with atrophy, possibly leading to fasciculations and exhibiting signs of denervation on electromyography). However, when lesions involve the passing pyramidal fibers, the paralyses assume a central spastic character. Because of the proximity of the nuclei of the cranial nerves and the pyramidal fibers, there are often bilateral pyramidal signs or unilateral lesions with crossed symptoms: (peripheral, nuclear) cranial nerve palsies on one side and (central) hemiparesis of extremities on the opposite side of the lesion (Fig. 5).
- Impaired ocular motility and nystagmus are frequent. Commonly there is a dissociated disturbance of ocular motility accompanied by double vision (lesions of oculomotor nuclei or

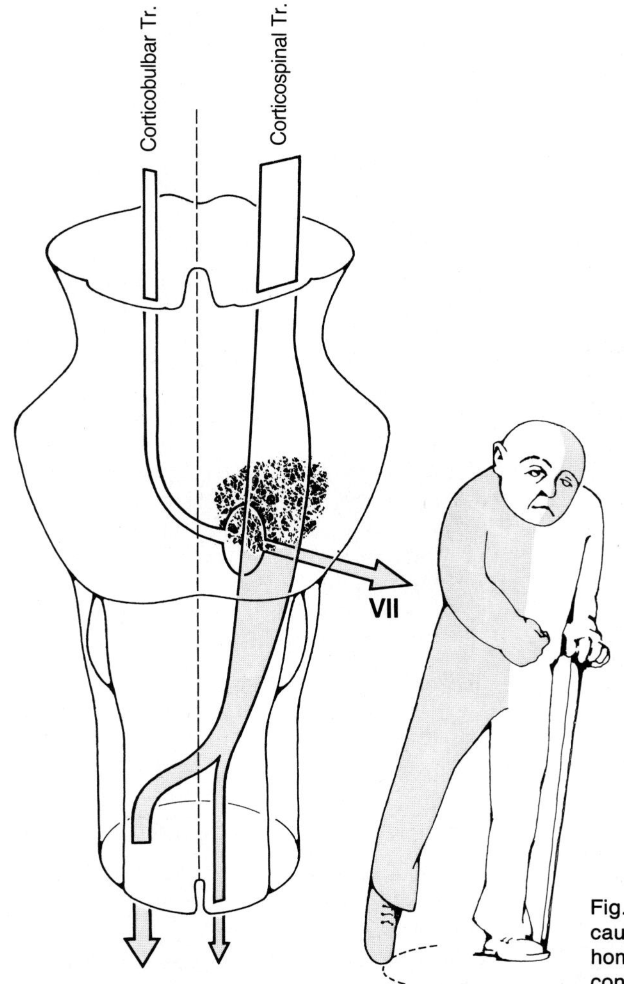

Fig. 5   Crossed paralysis due to a lesion in the caudal pons: Millard–Gubler syndrome with homolateral (peripheral) facial paralysis and contralateral spastic (central) hemiplegia

of the medial longitudinal fasciculus). Rarely, because of involvement of the para-abducens nucleus (the pontine gaze center situated at the level of the abducens nucleus in the caudal pontine region), there is a gaze palsy ipsilateral to the lesion. Nystagmus of the paretic gaze variety can occur with lesions of the vestibular nucleus or medial longitudinal fasciculus.

— Often there are ataxias or involuntary movements: for example, unilateral ataxia results from lesions of the ventral spino-cerebellar tracts or the superior cerebellar peduncles. Lesions of the dentate nucleus give rise to contralateral intention tremor. This may also be seen with disturbances of the efferent pathways from the dentate nucleus or with lesions of the red nucleus: contralateral hemiataxia or hemiasynergia occur with lesions of the red nucleus, and palatal myoclonus occurs with lesions of the central tegmental tract (or the dentate nucleus).

— Vertigo with rotatory components points to a brain stem lesion or a peripheral vestibular disorder.

— Sensory disturbances with dissociated sensory loss are characteristic of lesions of the medulla oblongata, because of the still separate anatomic course of the pain and temperature fibers in the lateral spinal thalamic tract and the other sensory afferents in the medial lemniscus.

— Impairment of consciousness, as in vegetative state, occurs with disturbances of the reticular formation, particularly its rostral portion.

— Seizure-like disturbances, the so-called tonic brain stem fits or paroxysmal dysarthria.

Common pathogenetic mechanisms are

— Ischemia in the vertebrobasilar territories
— Demyelinating lesions in multiple sclerosis
— Tumors, particularly brain stem gliomas
— Anoxia and brain stem herniations due to increased intracranial pressure of varied pathogenesis
— Systemic diseases

1.1.4 Cerebellar Syndromes

The cerebellum is anatomically close to the brain stem and is connected with brain stem structures by the three cerebellar peduncles.

— The cerebellum contains in its cortex and nuclei ganglion cells that are concerned with information processing and send efferent impulses to other structures.

— Information about position of limbs and muscle activity arrives in the cerebellum through the spinocerebellar pathways, in part via the inferior cerebellar peduncle (restiform body) and also through the superior cerebellar peduncle (brachium conjunctivum).

— Impulses from the vestibular structures concerned with position and movement of the head reach the cerebellum via the inferior cerebellar peduncle.

— Impulses from the brain synapse in the pontine nuclei and then pass through to the cerebellum along the medial cerebellar peduncle (brachium pontis).

— Efferent impulses from the cerebellar cortex pass to the cerebellar nuclei (and the olives) through the superior cerebellar peduncles to the red nucleus and the lateral ventral nucleus of the thalamus on the opposite side. This afferent information synapses in the thalamus and red nucleus and then passes onto the cerebral cortex rostrally via the rubrospinal tract and to the anterior horn cells of the spinal cord. The cerebellum is thus involved in the coordination of motor activity.

The cerebellar structures and their connections are illustrated in Figure 6. Continuous information on motor impulse traffic and movement is fed to the cerebellum, which then compares this input with actual motor activity and, through feedback mechanisms, influences and corrects any deviation from normal. There is a somatotopic representation of body regions in the cerebellar cortex. The cerebellum is supplied with blood from branches of the vertebral and basilar arteries (inferior posterior cerebellar artery, inferior anterior cerebellar artery, and superior cerebellar artery).

Certain general characteristics are found in syndromes due to lesions of the cerebellum:

— Reduction in muscle tone
— Lack of smoothness and grace in voluntary movements
— Changes in automatic movement sequences

Symptoms may include the following:

— Dyssynergia (impaired coordination of various muscles and muscle groups involved in a single movement)
— Dysmetria (impaired measure and extent as well as speed of an intended movement)

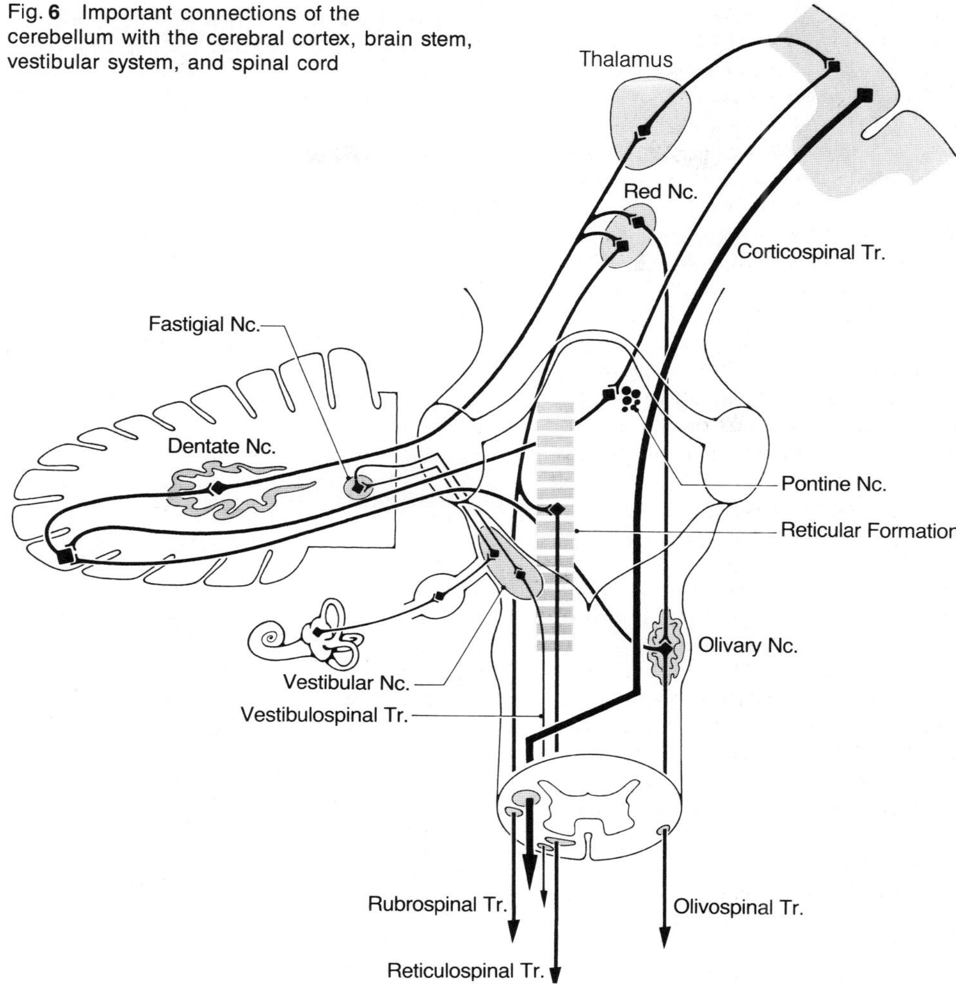

- Ataxia (disordered speed and trajectory of movements due to failure of muscular coordination in the attainment of a motor target)
- Intention tremor (increasing deviation from the ideal straight line of a movement as the target is approached)
- Pathologic rebound phenomenon (motions that overshoot their intended range because antagonist muscles are not immediately activated when the resistance to a movement is suddenly removed
- Dysdiadochokinesia (abrupt and jerky movements because the alternating activation of agonist and antagonist muscles is no longer quick and fluid enough)
- Hypotonia (apparent on passive movement, for example, by shaking of an extremity)

- Impairment of position sense, manifest by pastpointing in the Bárány pointing test ipsilateral to the lesion
- Impairment of stance in the Romberg test
- Ataxia of the trunk while sitting
- Unsteady, broad-based gait
- Nystagmus (particularly apparent when the gaze is fixated toward the side of the lesion)
- Dysarthria manifested by scanning and explosive speech

The most common causes of cerebellar syndromes are:

- Degenerative disorders, particularly system atrophies (cerebellar hereditary ataxia of Nonne—Marie, Holmes cerebellar atrophy, Menzel disease, late-onset cerebellar cortical

atrophy of Marie–Foix–Alajouanine, olivopontocerebellar atrophy)
- Genetic metabolic disorders (for example, ataxia-telangiectasia of Louis–Bar, Hartnup disease, hereditary paroxysmal ataxia, abetalipoproteinemia or Bassen–Kornzweig disease, GM_2 gangliosidosis with beta-hexosaminidase A deficiency
- Infectious diseases, for example, infectious mononucleosis; perhaps also acute cerebellar ataxia of childhood, kuru (slow virus infection)
- Acute intoxications, which can give rise to transient cerebellar symptoms (for example, intoxication with diphenylhydantoin)
- Acquired metabolic disorders, for example, hypercalcemia, cholestasis, ileal resection (with vitamin E deficiency)
- Symptomatic toxic cerebellar cortical atrophies (for example, alcohol, diphenylhydantoin, organic mercury poisoning)
- Malabsorption – for example, sprue – and paraproteinemias, or nonmetastatic malignant disorders (particularly carcinoma of the bronchus)
- Multiple sclerosis with lesions in the cerebellar white matter or cerebellar efferent fibers
- The rarer disturbances of blood supply of the cerebellum and cerebellar hemorrhage, cerebellar signs of sudden onset combined with hemiparesis due to softening at the border of the upper and middle third of the pons
- Tumors (medulloblastomas and spongioblastoma [cerebellar astrocytoma] in children; gliomas and cerebellopontine angle tumors)
- Abscesses
- Multiple sclerosis, in isolated cases, and in different members of the same family in familial episodic ataxia, can manifest intermittent disorders of cerebellar function

1.2 Spinal Cord Syndromes

The spinal cord consists of

- Neurons in the spinal cord gray, including
  - the anterior horn cells that innervate the striated muscle of the extremities and trunk
  - the secondary neurons of the autonomic nervous system in the lateral horn
  - interneurons

- The spinal cord white matter, which contains the afferent and efferent tracts that conduct impulses
  - from the cortex, brain stem, and cerebellum
  - to the brain stem and cerebellum

The structure and blood supply of the spinal cord and the relation of the spinal cord to its surroundings are assumed to be known to the reader, but Figures 7 and 8 depict an overview and summary of these relationships.

Syndromes due to lesions of the spinal cord depend on the site and extent of the damage. A combination of characteristic symptoms is summarized in Table 4 and described below.

1.2.1 Transverse Spinal Cord Lesions

Transverse lesions of the spinal cord are those that involve one or several segments and more or less disrupt the spinal cord. Inevitably such lesions interrupt afferent and efferent spinal cord tracts. The disruption of the spinal roots and anterior horns may occur in one or two segments and always in the background of the symptoms.

1.2.1.1 Complete Transection of the Spinal Cord

In complete transection of the cervical or thoracic spinal cord, the findings are

- Complete, eventually spastic, paralysis of all four extremities (tetraplegia) or of only the lower limbs (paraplegia), which in the case of complete lesions becomes paraplegia in flexion

- Complete loss of sensation below a certain level. The relationship of the spinal cord segments to the spinal column and to the sensory dermatomes are illustrated in Figure 9. Occasionally one finds a hyperalgesic border zone of sensory disturbance above the lesion (*see* 1.2.1.2)
- Disturbances of vasomotor function of (emotional) sweating and trophic disturbances (decubitus ulcers) due to interruption of the central sympathetic descending fibers situated in the lateral columns ventral to the corticospinal tracts (*see* Fig. 58)
- Paralysis of rectal and bladder function (*see* 2.18) and sexual disturbances in males (*see* 2.19)

- Segmental "flaccid" paralysis and muscle atrophy, the result of destruction (of one or several segments) of anterior horns

There are special characteristics of transverse lesions at the level of the lower spinal cord segments.

Syndrome of the epiconus (L4 to S2) is characterized by

- Preservation of hip flexion and knee extension
- Varying extent of the deficits of extension and external rotation of hips, knee flexion, and foot and toe movements
- Preservation of knee jerks
- Absence of ankle jerks
- Sensory impairment at and below L4 dermatomes
- Impairment of bladder and rectal function (autonomic bladder) (*see* 2.18).

Figure 10 shows examples of transverse lesions of the spinal cord with their motor deficits, reflex abnormalities, and sensory levels.

Syndrome of conus medullaris (S3 and distal to this segment) frequently occurs in traumatic lesions, tumors, or herniated discs and is accompanied by lesions of the roots that pass the damaged spinal cord segments (L3 and lower roots; *see* 1.3.1). Isolated conus lesions do not affect leg movement but give rise to

- Saddle anesthesia (Fig. 10; *see* Fig. 53)
- A flaccid bladder (with overflow incontinence), and paralysis of the anal sphincter (with incontinence of feces)
- Absence of anal and bulbocavernous reflexes with normal myotatic reflexes and absence of pyramidal signs.

1.2.1.2 Hemisyndromes of the Spinal Cord (Brown–Séquard Syndrome)

The characteristics of this syndrome depend on the anatomic relationships of the spinothalamic tract. This tract carries fibers for pain, temperature, and touch sensation from the body side opposite the lesion toward the brain.

The clinical characteristics of the Brown–Séquard syndrome and the anatomic relations that give rise to these characteristics are summarized in Figure 11. The following characteristic symptoms are evident below the lesions:

- Homolateral spastic paresis with hyperreflexia and pyramidal signs due to lesions of the lateral corticospinal tract

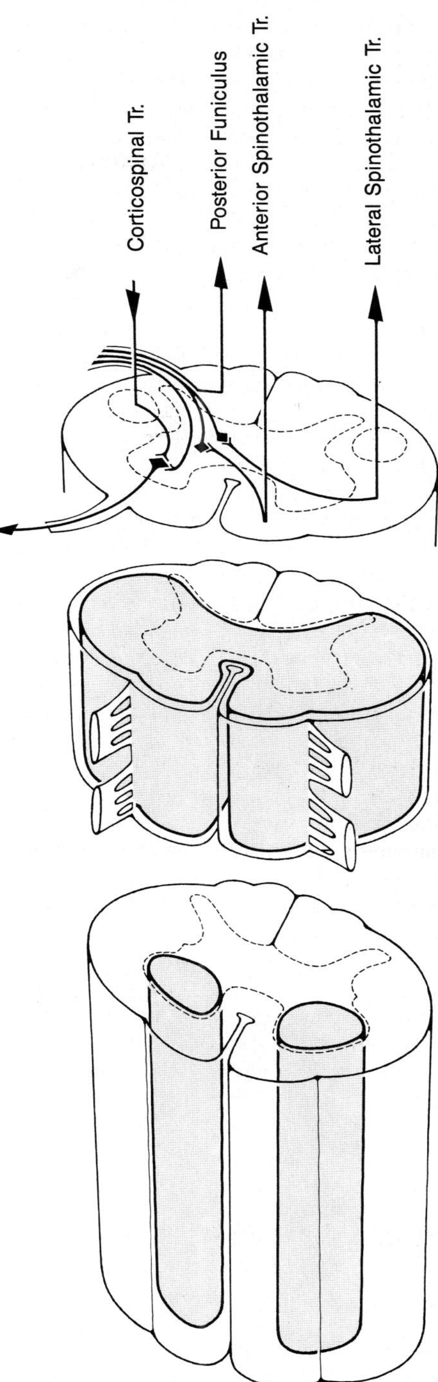

Fig. 7 Spinal cord and its important ascending and descending tracts. Localization of lesions due to anterior spinal artery syndrome (middle) and bilateral anterior horn lesions (bottom) (see also Table 4)

Table 4 **Symptoms as related to location of spinal cord lesions**

Location	Tone	Motor function	Touch	Deep sensibility	Temperature sensation	Sphincter function
Complete transverse syndrome	↑	Bilateral +	+	+	+	+
Brown–Séquard syndrome	= ↓	= +	x↓	= +	x +	no
Conus medullaris syndrome	no	no	Saddle anesthesia	Saddle anesthesia	Saddle anesthesia	Saddle anesthesia
Symmetric centro-medullary lesions	↑	Bilateral +	no	no	+	+
Lesions around central canal	↓	+	no	no	+	+
Anterior commissure lesions	no	no	Segment slight	no	Segment↓	no
Posterior column lesions	no	no	no	+	no	no
Corticospinal tract lesions	↑	+	no	no	no	no
Anterior horn lesions	↓	+	no	no	no	no

See also Figures 7 and 8.
no = normal; + = affected; ↑ = increased; ↓ = decreased; = = homolateral; x = contralateral; ⊘ = absent

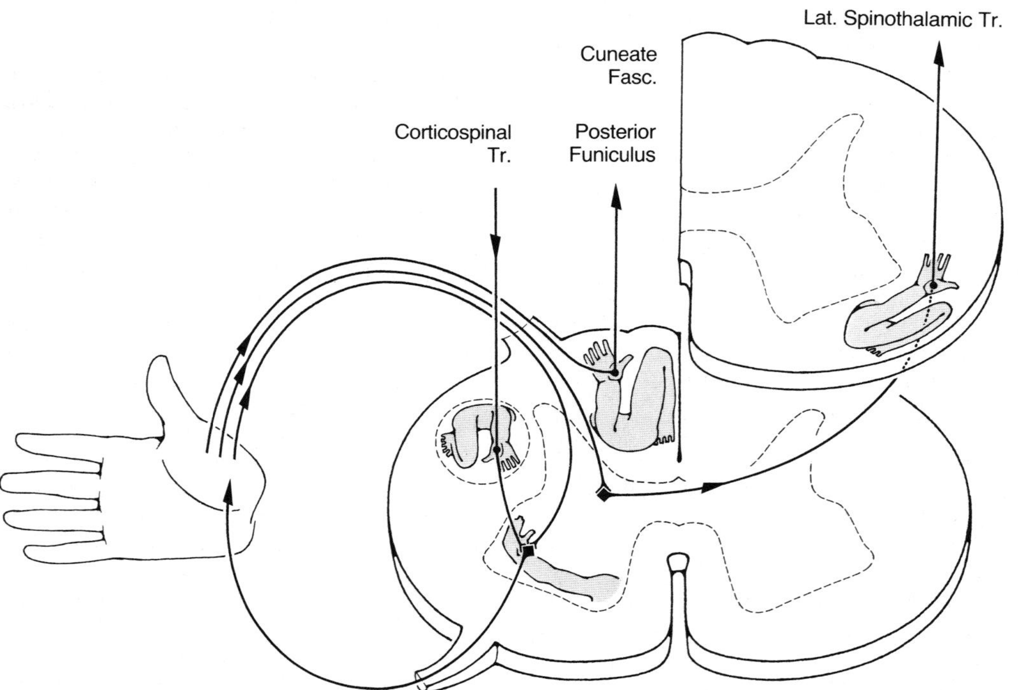

Fig. 8 Transverse section through the lower cervical cord illustrating somatotopic distribution of body parts within the corticospinal tracts, the posterior funiculus, the lateral spinothalamic tracts, and the motor neurons in the anterior horn

Vasomotor function	Muscle stretch reflexes	Pyramidal signs	Trophic muscles	Remarks
+	↑	+	Segmental ↓	
= +	= ↑	=	Segmental ↓	
no	no	∅	no	
+	↑	+	Segmental ↓	
+	∅	∞	↓	
no	no	∅	no	
no	no	∅	no	Ataxia
no	↑	+	no	
no	↓ to ∅	∅	↓↓	Fasciculations

- Homolateral impairment of vibration and position sense and of tactile discrimination due to lesions of the posterior columns, although touch and pressure senses are unimpaired because of preservation of the contralateral anterior spinothalamic tract
- Contralateral impairment of pain and temperature sensation which ascend in the crossed lateral spinothalamic tract
- Minor contralateral impairment of touch sensation due to a lesion of the crossed ascending fibers of the anterior spinothalamic tract
- Initially, homolateral hyperesthesia, perhaps due to "overloading" of the contralateral anterior spinothalamic tract with touch stimuli from the homolateral body side
- Homolateral vasodilatation with increased temperature and reddening of the body initially, later lower temperature and cyanosis on the affected side, the result of lesions of the descending sympathetic fibers in the lateral column
- Homolateral absence of emotional sweating due to lesions of the same structures − *see* above
- At the level of the involved spinal cord segment, homolateral total anaesthesia and "peripheral" flaccid paralysis with muscle atrophy (due to lesions of the anterior and posterior spinal roots and of the anterior horns of the affected segment)

A pure Brown−Séquard syndrome is very rare (it may occur with knife wounds to the spinal cord). Most often there are incomplete forms of the syndrome with varying combinations of the signs and symptoms described above and with symptoms and signs of involvement of the other half of the spinal cord as well. The most common causes of complete transverse and hemicord syndromes are

- Trauma with spinal contusion together with radiologically recognizable trauma to the vertebrae or direct injury to the spinal cord by penetrating trauma
- Tumors arising either in bony structures surrounding the spinal cord or, in the form of metastases or sarcomas, from soft tissues such as the nerves or the spinal coverings, which can give rise to gliomas, ependymomas, meningiomas, and neurinomas
- Nontumoral compressions (epidural hematomas or abscesses)
- Vascular processes (spinal angiomas, spontaneous or traumatic intramedullary hematomas, ischemia) (*see* 1.2.1.3)
- Myelits due to viral or parainfectious processes, heroin addiction, and after vaccination

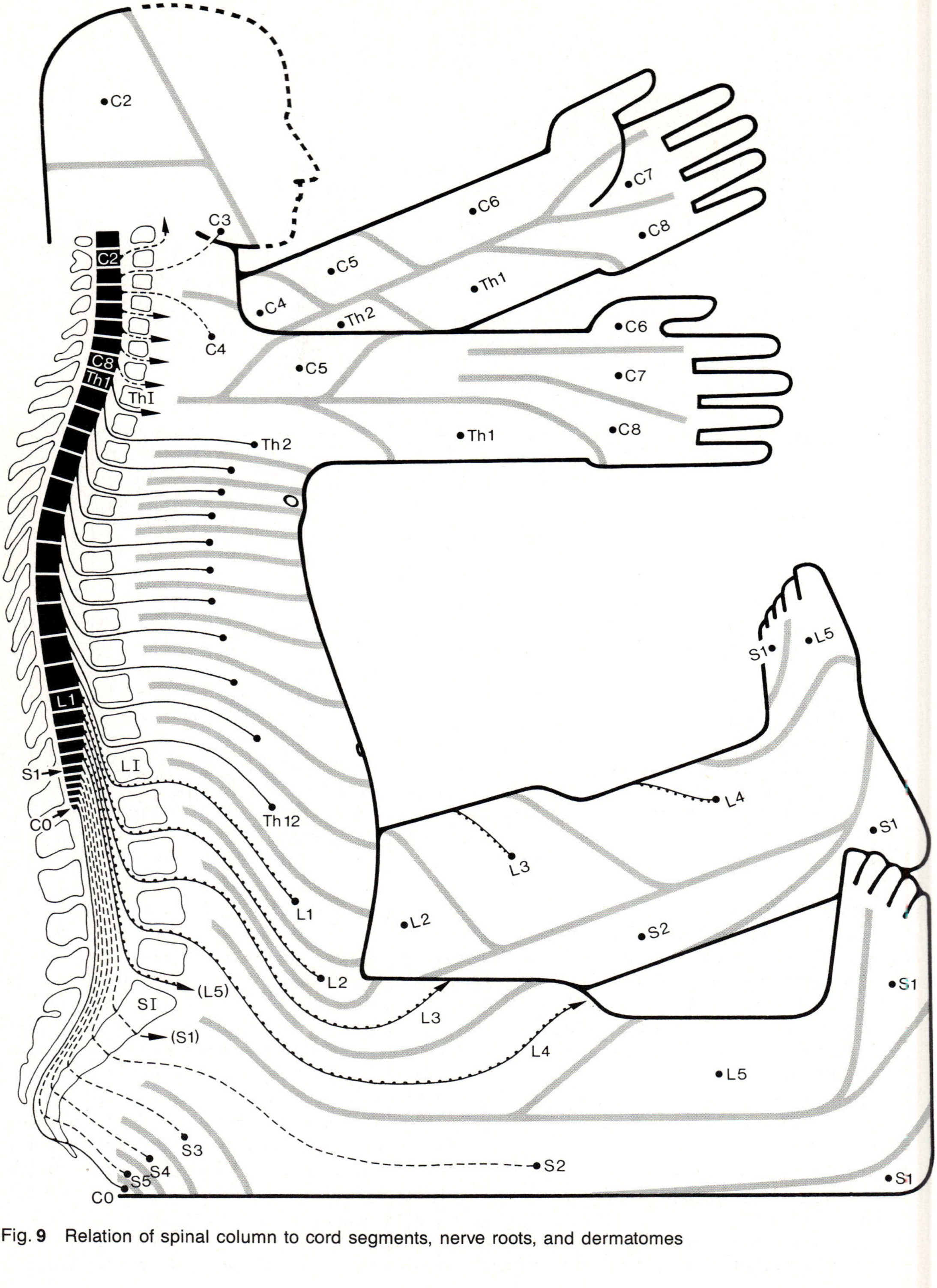

Fig. 9   Relation of spinal column to cord segments, nerve roots, and dermatomes

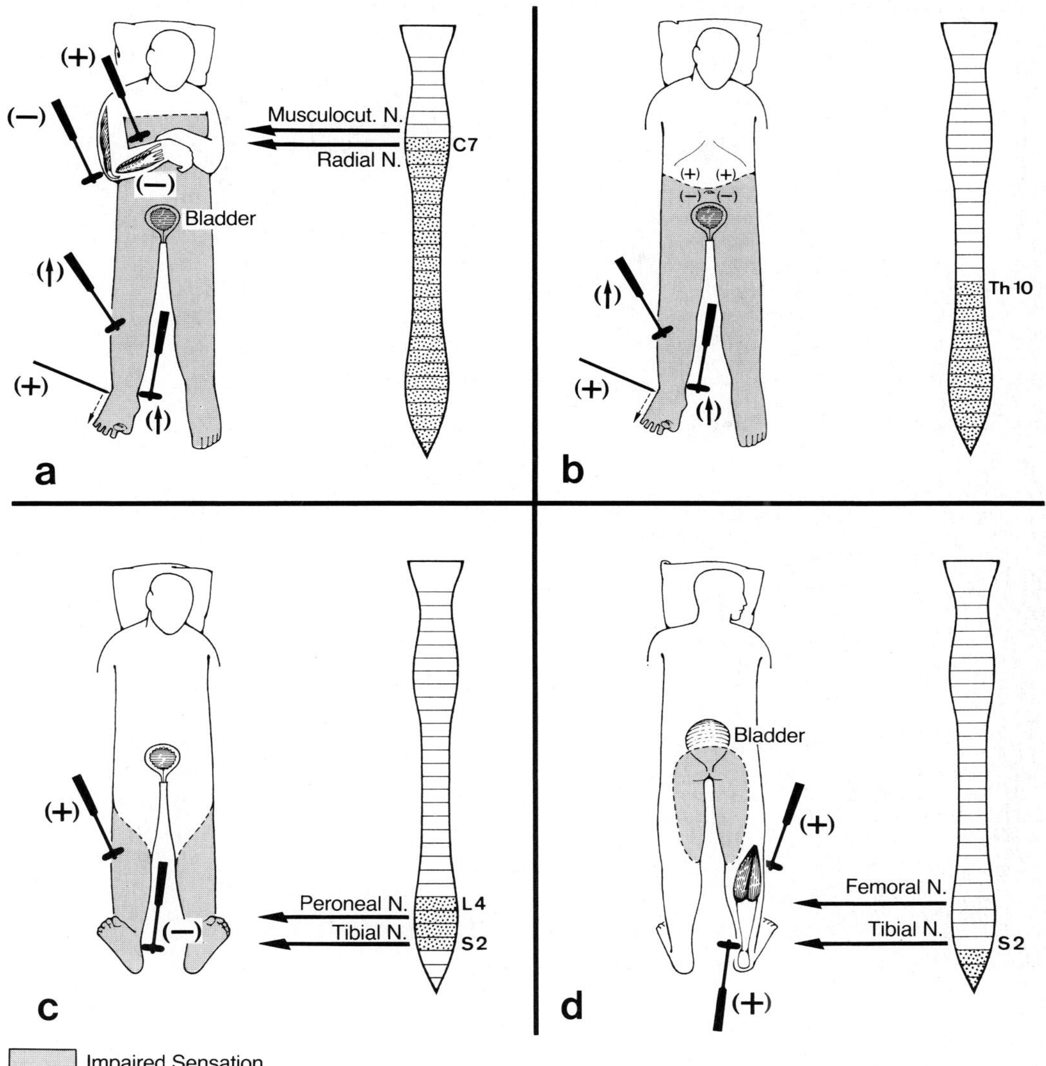

Fig. **10 a–d** Types of paralysis with transverse lesions of the spinal cord. **a** C 7-syndrome; **b** T 10 lesion; **c** epiconus syndrome; **d** conus syndrome

- demyelinating diseases (particularly multiple sclerosis)
- Radiation myelopathy after radiation therapy

1.2.1.3 Centromedullary and Other Partial Transverse Lesions of the Spinal Cord

Apart from transverse and hemilesions of the spinal cord, which have just been described, there are other possibilities of damage to the spinal cord with different anatomic distribution. Based on anatomic consideration, only the central part of the spinal cord may be involved; this part receives its blood supply through the anterior spinal artery and its penetrating parenchymal branches (the sulcocommissural arteries). The peripheral parts of the spinal cord and, in particular, the posterior columns are supplied by branches of the surrounding vascular plexus of the spinal cord

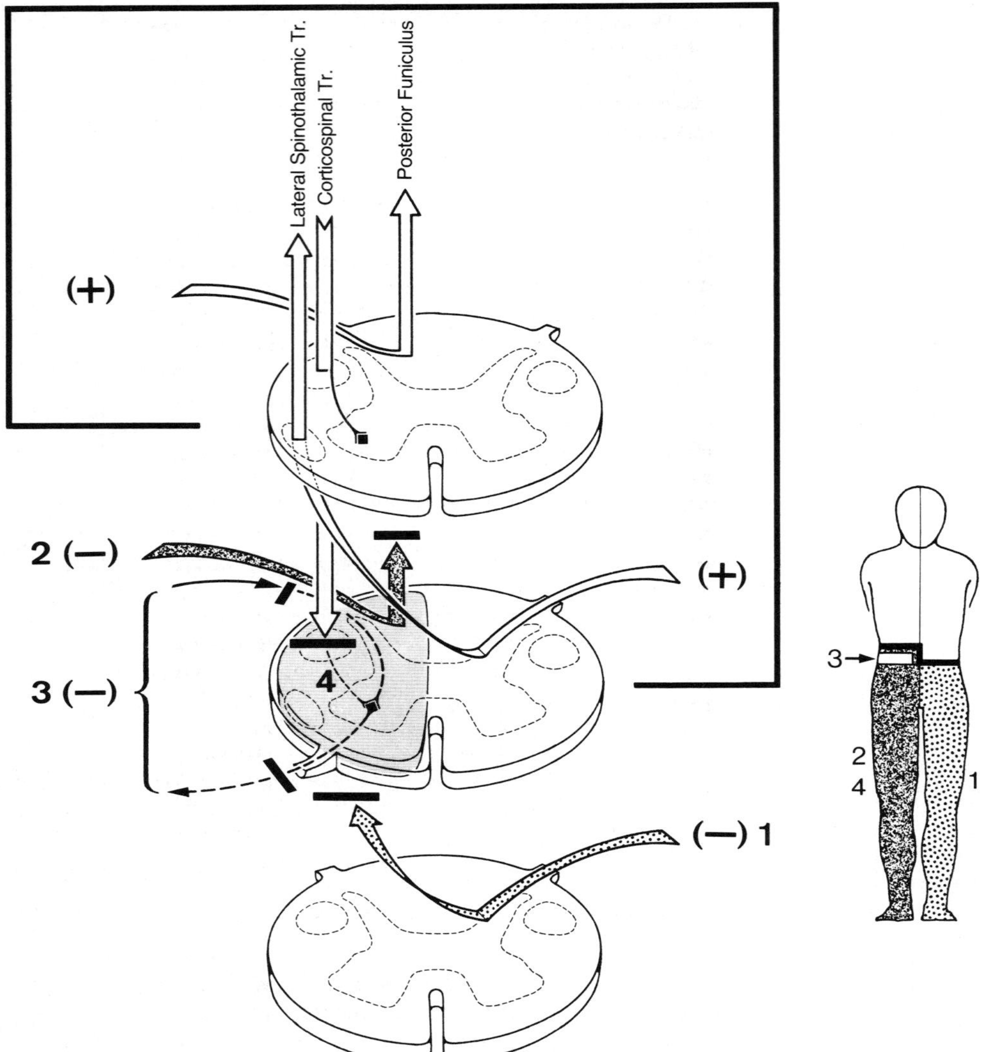

Fig. 11   Correlation of extent of spinal cord lesion in Brown–Séquard syndrome with resulting symptoms: **1** contralateral dissociated sensory loss for pain and temperature; **2** homolateral disturbance of deep sensibility position sense and touch; **3** segmental disturbance of all sensation as well as segmental flaccid paralysis; **4** homolateral spastic paralysis

surface and by the posterior spinal arteries (Fig. 12). Apart from vascular processes, there are other disorders that can affect parts of the central spinal cord or certain other areas of the cord (*see* below).

Provided the lesions involve both lateral spinothalamic tracts and corticospinal pathways, central spinal cord lesions exhibit the following clinical characteristics:

– Bilateral spastic paraparesis below the level of the lesions with increased reflexes and pyramidal signs in the legs. Such signs may be less pronounced distally when the lesions of the corticospinal tracts, whose peripheral component fibers are destined for the lower extremities, are less severely affected by the lesion.

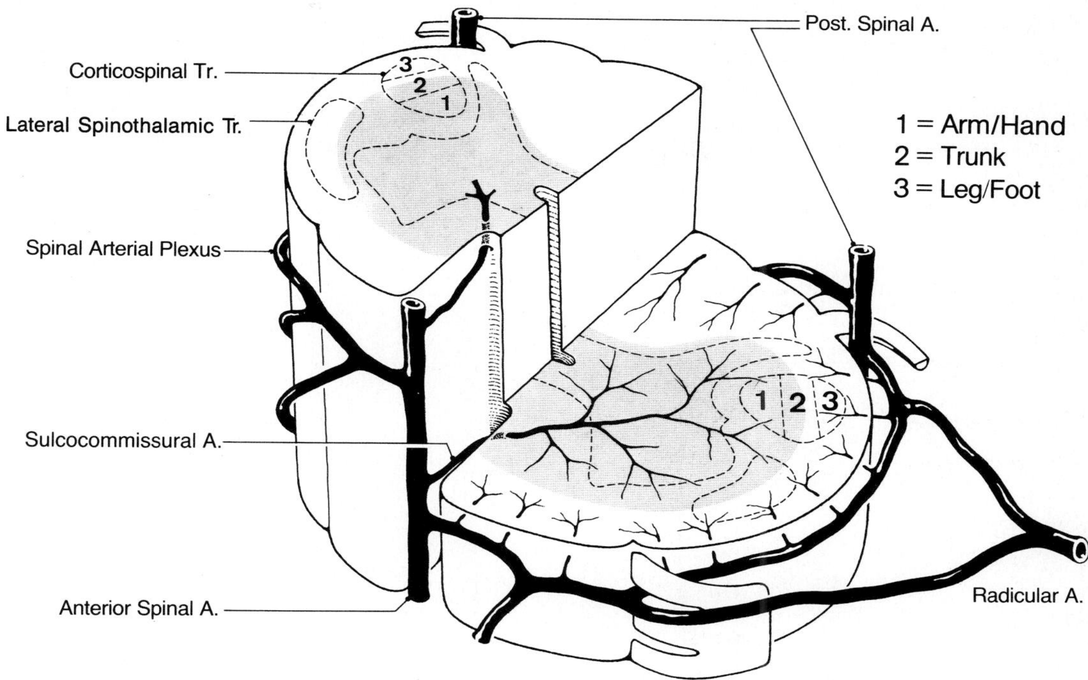

Fig. 12   Anterior spinal artery syndrome. Blood supply of the spinal cord; ventrolateral infarction

— Below the level of the lesion, bilateral dissociated disturbance of pain and temperature sensation with intact touch and deep sensibilities, due to lesions of the lateral spinothalamic tract but not the peripherally situated anterior spinothalamic tract and the posterior columns.
— Disturbances of bladder and bowel function (reflex bladder) and impotence, resulting from lesions of the central sympathetic pathways situated in the lateral columns.
— Bilateral vasomotor paralysis below the level of the lesion, accompanied initially by increased temperature and redness and later by cold and cyanosis, due to lesions of the central sympathetic pathways in the lateral columns of the spinal cord.

Vascular lesions causing ischemia that leads to varying degrees of softening of the spinal cord are diagrammatically represented in Figure 13. An acute transverse vascular lesion of the spinal cord also occurs with softening (*see* 1.2.1.1). If only the central part of the spinal cord is affected, the constellation of symptoms described above is usually found. With anterior spinal artery ischemia, a long central plug-like softening can extend into the lumbar region. Such a lesion modifies the above clinical symptoms somewhat. Below the level of the lesion, as defined by impairment of temperature and pain sensation, there is

— Flaccid (peripheral) paralysis without spastic paraplegia
— Absence of reflexes
— No pyramidal sign
— Atrophy of muscles, because of destruction of anterior horns and interruption of spinal reflex arcs at all levels below the upper limit of the lesion

Clinical symptoms due to other partial lesions of the spinal cord depend on their localization. Two examples are given (*see* 2.16.2.2 and Fig. 52).

A lesion involving the anterior commissure but sparing the lateral spinothalamic tract gives rise to

— Dissociated sensory loss occurring bilaterally but only in the segment containing the lesion. (Only fibers crossing to the other half of the spinal cord in the anterior commissure at the level of the lesion are involved, fibers being spared that have already crossed below the segment of the lesion to ascend in the lateral columns.)

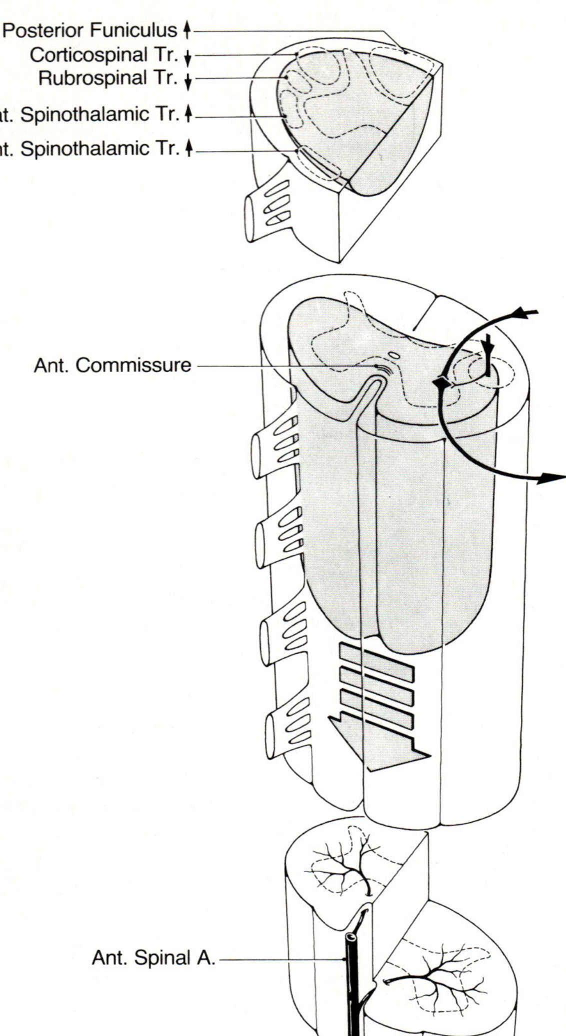

Fig. **13** Centromedullary infarction: segmental (above); extending over several cord segments caudally (middle); blood flow from the anterior spinal artery and the subcommissural arteries in the spinal cord (below)

– Impairment of coarse touch and pressure sensation for one to two segments below the lesion. (The fibers for these sensations ascend one or two segments in the cord before crossing in the anterior commissure to the opposite side.)

A lesion involving only one side of the central zone of the spinal cord produces the symptoms principally of a Brown–Séquard syndrome (*see* 1.2.1.2) but without impairment of homolateral deep sensitivity and only partial impairment of contralateral coarse touch and pressure sensation (the latter becomes markedly impaired with additional damage to the posterior columns).

The most common causes of centromedullary and partial transverse lesions of the spinal cord are

– Vascular disorders (ischemia in the territory of the anterior spinal artery, angiomas, plug-like traumatic and nontraumatic bleeding)
– Syringomyelia
– Intramedullary tumors (gliomas, ependymomas, metastases)
– Multiple sclerosis
– Trauma
– Myelitis

1.2.2 Lesions of the White Matter of the Spinal Cord

It is assumed that the reader is familiar with the topography of ascending and descending fibers in the white matter of the spinal cord (columns), summarized in Figures 8, 11, 12, and 52. Single afferent and efferent pathways can be involved in pathologic processes, and the resulting disturbance of function varies with the particular fiber tracts involved. Such dysfunction is evident below the highest level of the lesions and generally is bilateral. Certain diseases (*see* below) have a prediction for specific spinal cord tracts. Two clinical symptoms usually follow lesions of spinal cord columns:

- Disturbances of deep sensibility manifest as a loss of position and vibration sense in combination with ataxia, particularly with walking, and areflexia due to lesions of the posterior columns.
- Spasticity affecting the lower limbs with spastic paraparesis, due to lesions of the corticospinal tracts. Disturbances of sphincter function and hyperreflexia, including pyramidal signs, often do not appear.

These findings are frequently combined with symptoms of other lesions of the spinal cord or of other parts of the nervous system. Certain combinations of symptoms are characteristic for disorders of particular etiology.

The most common causes of systemic lesions of the spinal cord are

- Vitamin B_{12} deficiency, resulting in a combination of posterior column and pyramidal tract lesions, commonly associated with lesions of the optic nerve and the peripheral nerves
- Tabes dorsalis, yielding predominant posterior column symptoms and disturbances of posterior roots and optic nerves, disorder of pupillary function, and areflexia
- System disorders, many of them hereditary, for example:
  - Friedreich's ataxia, which results in disturbances of posterior column, spinocerebellar and corticospinal tract function and occasionally produces optic nerve dysfunction with nystagmus and typical deformities of feet, including a claw-like position of the large toes

- other types of spinocerebellar ataxia, in which posterior column dysfunction is minor in comparison to cerebellar atrophy
  - spastic (familial) spinal paralysis, resulting in pure dysfunction of the corticospinal tract
  - amyotrophic lateral sclerosis, marked by regeneration of corticospinal and corticobulbar tracts in combination with disappearance of anterior horn and bulbar motor cells
- Paraneoplastic column degeneration, particularly in carcinoma of the bronchus (occasionally combined with cerebellar atrophy, polyneuropathy, central pontine myelinolysis, or leukoencephalopathy)
- Various metabolic disorders and hereditary diseases with pyramidal tract dysfunction, including:
  - hyperglycemia
  - aminoaciduria
  - Sjögren-Larsson syndrome
  - ectodermal dysplasia of Bloch−Sulzberger (incontinentia pigmenti)

1.2.3 Lesions of the Anterior Horns

The anterior horns are anatomically in the ventral parts of the spinal cord gray matter. They contain, along with interneurons and inhibitory neurons, the motor neurons for the skeletal musculature. These structures are frequently affected in isolation. Isolated lesions of the anterior horns are clinically distinguished by pure motor deficits with the following additional characteristics:

- Flaccid, nuclear, "peripheral" paresis
- Atrophy
- Fasciculation (with chronic processes)
- Impairment or absence of tendon reflexes appropriate to the segments involved, with intact sensitivity and without trophic changes of the skin and nails

When structures adjacent to the anterior horns are also affected, as a result of processes that cause widespread damage, the clinical picture described above changes as follows:

- Additional lesions of the anterior commissure or of the lateral columns, particularly the lateral spinothalamic tract, cause further dissociated sensory loss. Such dysfunction must be carefully sought in patients with anterior horn disease.

— Impairment of corticospinal tract function (as in systemic disorders, amyotrophic lateral sclerosis, or the mechanical effect of centromedullary space-occupying lesions) add to the symptomatology a spastic element with increased tone, exaggerated reflexes, and pyramidal signs.

The most common causes of isolated or predominant lesions of the anterior horns are

— Infectious inflammatory diseases (poliomyelitis, due to poliovirus, or infection with other viruses, such as Coxsackievirus or echovirus)
— Degenerative system disorders
  ● various forms of spinal-muscular atrophy, including Werdnig—Hoffmann or Kugelberg—Welander
  ● amyotrophic lateral sclerosis, which produces lesions of the pyramidal tracts as well as anterior horn cells
— Ischemic lesions in chronic progressive myelopathies associated with atherosclerosis, usually combined with paraparesis
— Centromedullary space-occupying lesions (tumors, syringomyelia, hematomas). On careful examination, there is usually evidence of long-tract dysfunction, although pure disturbances of temperature sensations occur occasionally
— Rarely other afflictions, including
  ● diabetes mellitus
  ● lead poisoning
● mercury intoxication
● electrical trauma
● Creutzfeldt—Jacob disease
● peroneal muscular atrophy of the neuronal type (II)

1.3 Syndromes of Peripheral Nerve Lesions

Lesions of the nervous system lying outside the spinal cord will be discussed in this paragraph. This part of the nervous system consists of three main parts (Fig. 14):

— The mixed spinal nerve roots arising from motor and sensory roots.
— The anatomic reorganization of axons connected, the mixed roots in the cervical brachial and lumbosacral plexuses.
— The ramification of cords and nerves arising from these plexuses giving rise to mixed peripheral nerves and their final ramification into pure motor or sensory nerves. Damage to any of these parts of the peripheral nervous system gives rise to characteristic signs and symptoms that will be discussed under separate headings.

1.3.1 Root Syndromes

Each spinal root comprises

— Efferent motor fibers arising in the motor neurons of the anterior horns

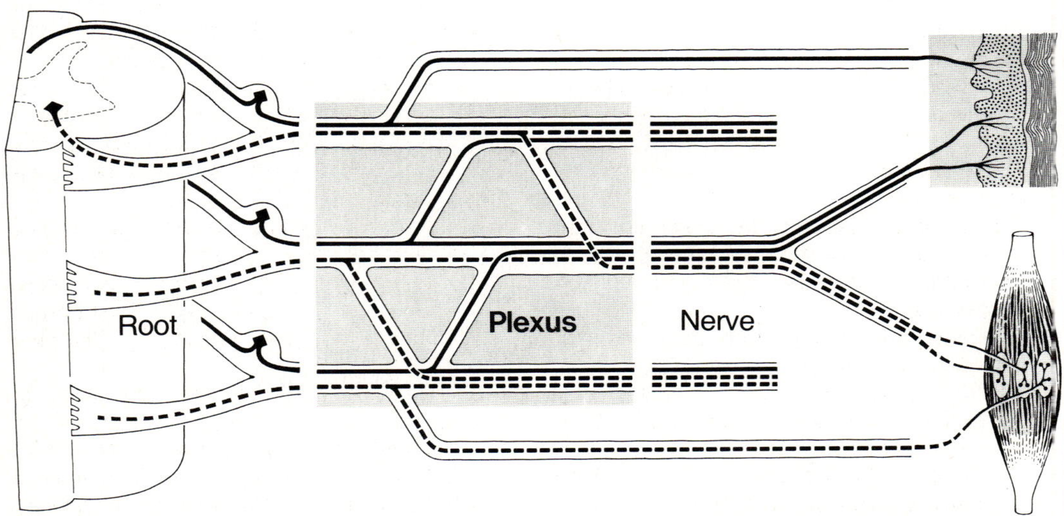

Fig. **14**   The three main subdivisions of the peripheral nervous system; roots—plexus—peripheral (mixed or pure motor or sensory) nerves

– Afferent sensory axons arising in postganglion cells of the posterior root ganglia

An isolated lesion of these separate axons in the roots is hardly ever found (exceptions: herpes zoster with unilateral lesions of a single sensory root; polyradiculitis, which occasionally gives rise to a pure motor disturbance symmetrically involving the motor roots). The rule is dysfunction of single or several mixed roots.

When a single mixed nerve root is affected, the following clinical symptoms arise:

– Pain or paresthesia arising in the appropriate sensory dermatome in the periphery
– Segmental sensory loss, which is more easily recognized by testing pain rather than touch sensations (*see* 2.16.2.1)
– Varying degrees of paresis of muscles that are innervated by the affected root, especially evident in muscles deriving their main motor innervation from the root (Table 5)
– Muscle atrophy, most marked in the small muscles of the hand when the caudal cervical roots are affected
– Rarely, fasciculations in affected muscles
– Impairment or absence of tendon reflexes, depending on the location of the lesion

Table 5 gives an overview of the most common (monoradicular) spinal root syndromes.

Table 6 gives a useful view of the paralyzed muscles in various root or brachial plexus lesions.

The most common causes of monoradicular mixed spinal syndromes are

– Disc herniation, particularly in the cervical region associated with spondylosis
– Trauma to the spinal column (lesions due to vertebral fractures, bleeding into root sleeves, vertebral luxation, traumatic ligamentous damage or rupture, or secondary trauma-induced spondylitic changes)
– Trauma to the shoulder (root avulsion with traction to the plexus, always associated with brachial plexus lesions)
– Herpes zoster
– Other viral infections (for example, tic radiculitis, often occurring in association with medullary or cerebral involvement)
– Root tumors (neurinoma, often in the form of hour-glass tumors)
– Tumors in the vicinity of roots (metastasis to the spinal column or, rarely, primary tumors such as bone sarcoma or sarcoma of soft tissues)

Clinical signs and symptoms in lesions of mixed spinal roots depend on the number and position of roots affected by the lesion.

If only a few roots are involved, then the symptoms enumerated in Table 5 are cumulative.

Involvement of many or of all spinal roots give a picture of polyradiculopathy (polyradiculitis), including

– Mixed flaccid paresis, usually symmetric
– Areflexia
– Later, atrophy of muscles
– Sensory disturbances, often circumscribed and occasionally totally absent
– Sphincter disturbances
– Occasional pain
– Sometimes, only after a 3-week period, the characteristic CSF findings of albuminocytologic dissociation

The symptoms and signs usually arise in a setting of polyradiculitis of the Guillain-Barré type (sometimes after an infectious disease or after immunization) or in patients with malignant meningeal infiltrations in which there are pleocytosis, pathologic cells in the CSF, and hypoglycorrhachia. For differentiation from polyneuropathy, *see* 1.3.5.

Affection of several roots below the second lumbar vertebra causes a cauda equina syndrome with the following characteristics:

– Impairment of all sensation in the saddle area (perianal, gluteal region, and back of the upper thigh) and the genital region. When the fourth and fifth lumbar roots and the first sacral root are involved, the sensory disturbance extends to the posterior part of the lower leg and to the medial aspect of the foot
– Absence of additional dissociated sensory loss (which would suggest lesions of the conus medullaris)
– In associated impairment of the fourth and fifth lumbar roots, paralysis of the small muscles of the foot, the long flexors and extensors of the foot and toes, and of knee flexors, extending to the gluteus maximus. The knee extensors remain intact
– Absence of ankle jerks with preservation of knee jerks
– Bladder and bowel sphincter disturbances with impotence (in complete cauda equina lesions)
– Atrophy of paralyzed muscles and a tendency to trophic ulcerations of the skin in analgesic areas

Table 5 **Important root syndromes**

Segment	Sensation	Characteristic motor deficits	Tendon reflexes	Remarks
C3 – C4	Pain or hyperalgesia in shoulder region (*see* Fig. 9)	Partial or total diaphragmatic paralysis	No changes in tendon reflexes	Partial diaphragmatic paralyses (C3 lesions) are ventral to those of C4 (dorsal part of diaphragm)
C5	Pain or hyperalgesia somewhat lateral to shoulder and extending partially over deltoid muscle region	Paresis of deltoid and biceps brachii	Impairment of biceps reflex	
C6	Dermatome extends on radial side of arm to thumb	Paralysis of biceps brachii muscles and of brachioradialis	Impairment or loss of biceps reflex	
C7	Dermatome extends laterally and dorsally from C6 dermatome to 2nd to 4th fingers	Paresis of triceps, pronator teres, and pectoralis major muscles and occasionally of finger flexors and ulnar finger extensor muscles, often with visible atrophy of the nar eminence	Impairment or loss of triceps reflex	Differential diagnosis from carpal tunnel syndrome is facilitated by loss of triceps reflex in root syndrome
C8	Dermatome is dorsal to that of C7 and extends down to 5th finger	Visible atrophy of small muscles of hand, particularly of hypothenar eminence	Impairment of triceps reflex	Differentiation from ulnar nerve paralysis by loss of triceps reflex
L3	Dermatome extends from greater trochanter across extensor surface to medial side of thigh across knee	Quadriceps and anterior tibial paresis	Loss of knee jerk	Distinguished from femoral nerve paralysis in that saphenous nerve distribution remains intact and adductors may be affected

Table 5   (continued)

Segment	Sensation	Characteristic motor deficits	Tendon reflexes	Remarks
L4	Dermatome extends from outer part of thigh across patella to anterior medial quadrant of lower leg and medial border of foot	Paralysis of the quadriceps and of the anterior tibial muscles	Diminution of knee jerk	Distinguished from femoral nerve paralysis, through associated anterior tibial muscle paresis
L5	Dermatome begins above knee over lateral condyle; it extends downward over anterior lateral quadrant of lower leg to big toe	Paresis and atrophy of extensor hallucis longus and often of extensor digitorum brevis muscles	Absence of posterior tibial reflexes (only useful in diagnosis when this reflex is unequivocally present on uninvolved side)	
S1	Dermatome extends from flexor side of thigh in posterior outer quadrant to lower leg over lateral malleolus to little toe	Paresis of peroneal muscles, occasionally also impaired innervation of the triceps surae and gluteal muscles	Absence of Achilles reflex	
Combination L4–L5	Dermatome of L4 and L5	Paresis of all lower leg extensors; impaired innervation of quadriceps muscles	Impairment of knee jerks and absence of posterior tibial reflexes	Differentiation from peroneal palsies through unimpaired function of peroneal muscles and impaired knee and posterior tibial reflexes
Combination L5–S1	Dermatome of L5 and S1	Paresis of coextensors and peroneal muscles; occasionally impaired innervation of triceps surae and gluteal muscles	Absence of posterior tibial reflexes and ankle jerks	Differentiation from peroneal palsy: lack of involvement of anterior tibial muscle and differing reflex changes

M. Mumenthaler, H. Schliack: Lesions of Peripheral Nerves, 6th ed. Thieme, Stuttgart, 1992

Table 6   Topographic diagnostic aids for motor impairment of radicular origin in the upper extremities *

Nerve roots shown as overlapping arches across the top (left to right): **C5, C6, C7, C8, D1**

C5	C6	C7	C7	C8	C8	D1
Rhomboids						
Trapezius						
Serratus anterior			II III IV V		Oppo-nens pollicis	Ab-ductor pollicis brevis
Postero-lateral part	Biceps	Pronator teres	Superficial flexor digitorum			
		Flexor carpi radialis	Palmaris longus			
Deltoids	Brachialis	Triceps		Flexor pollicis longus	Flexor pollicis brevis	Ad-ductor pollicis
anterior		Extensor carpi radialis	Extensor carpi ulnaris			Abductor digiti minimi
Supraspinatus	Brachioradialis	Extensor digitorum communis et proprii	Abductor pollicis longus / Extensor pollicis brevis			First dorsal interosseus
						Palmaris brevis
Infraspinatus	Supinator		Extensor pollicis longuss	Flexor II, III digitorum profundus IV, V		II – V dorsal interossei
			Flexor carpi ulnaris			
	Teres major	Latissimus dorsi				
Pectoralis major						

** The affected muscles can be designated as weak or the guidelines of the British Medical Research Council can be used, grading the weakness from 0 to 5.*

Grading (guidelines of the British Medical Research Council 1942)
0 = No muscle activity
1 = Visible contraction without movement
2 = Movement without gravity
3 = Movement against gravity
4 = Movement against moderate resistance
5 = Normal strength

— Preservation of sweating in analgesic parts — a symptom that helps differentiate these syndromes from those of plexus regions (*see* 2.20.1.2)
— Occasional subarachnoid block (Froin's syndrome)
— Many lesions causing cauda equina disturbances are associated with severe spreading pain during Valsalva's maneuver occurring with coughing, sneezing, and during changes of posture (Nafziger sign)

The most common causes of cauda equina syndromes are
— Trauma, usually associated with lumbosacral vertebral fractures or herniated lumbar intervertebral discs
— Tumors, particularly lipoma, dermoid tumor, ependymoma (occasionally with progression lasting over some years)
— (Congenital) spinal canal stenosis (with intermittent claudication of the cauda equina, *see* 2.15.5.1)

— There is probably also isolated "inflammation" of the caudal roots, the so-called Elsberg syndrome

1.3.2 Brachial Plexus Lesions

As a result of the complex anatomy of the brachial plexus the site of a lesion therein can be determined from motor and sensory deficits in the upper extremity. Figure 15 gives a schematic overview of the brachial plexus. More details can be found in appropriate textbooks.

The clinical symptoms of lesions of the brachial plexus are always mixed motor and sensory. Nevertheless, lesions of the upper plexus give rise to sensory disturbances that may be minimal or discrete. The clinical symptoms of circumscribed plexus lesions are given in Table 7, which is to be compared with the beginning of Table 8. Brachial plexus lesions can be differentiated from single cervical root lesions by one or more of the following features:

— Multiradicular sensory and motor deficits
— A history of trauma (dislocation of the shoulder) or anatomic abnormality (cervical rib)
— Circulatory disturbances in the supply territory of the subclavian artery or vein (particularly with compression syndromes of the thoracic outlet)
— Absence of cervical pain syndromes comparable to the typical root syndromes of the upper extremity detailed in Table 5. The distinguishing features of lesions of single peripheral nerve trunks of the upper extremity depend on characteristic weakness (Table 8)

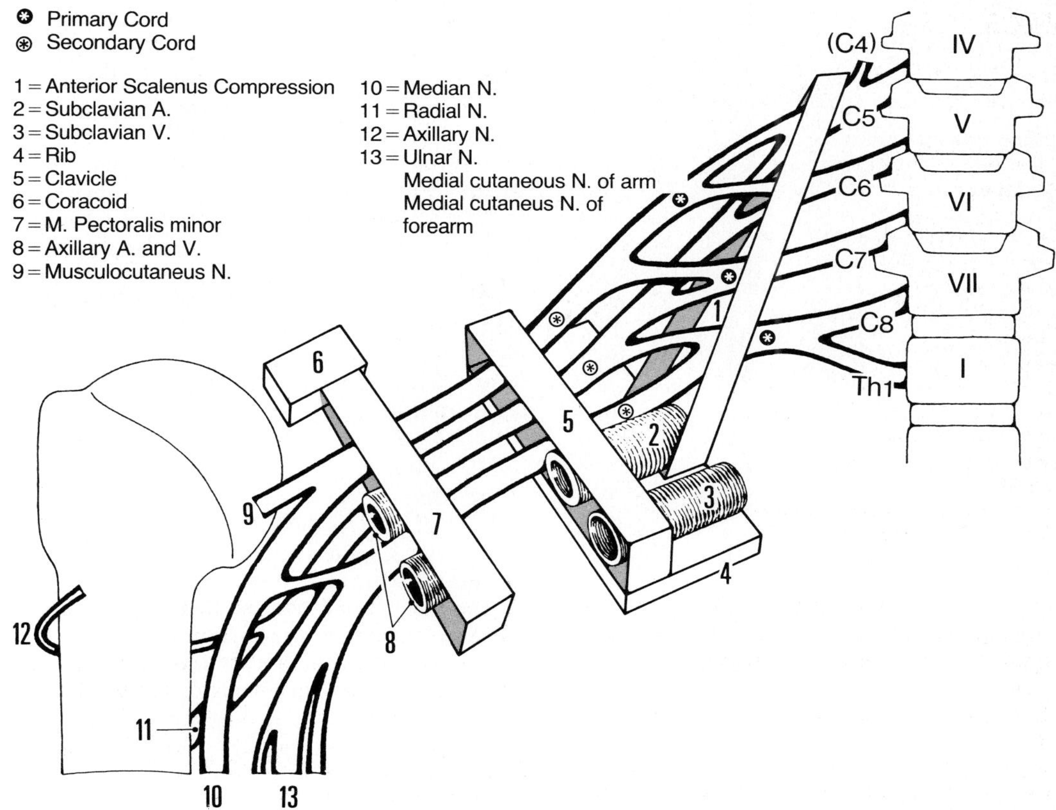

Fig. 15 The brachial plexus and the three likely sites of compression (scalenus anticus, costoclavicular passage, and insertion of the pectoralis minor in the coracoid process) (M. Mumenthaler: Shoulder-Arm Pain, 2nd ed. Huber, Bern, 1982)

Table 7   Symptoms of lesions of the brachial plexus*

Upper brachial plexus lesions
(Duchenne–Erb) Roots C5 – C6
Most common lesions
Abductors ⎫ of shoulder (hand rotated
External rotators ⎬ inwards during testing)
Elbow flexors
Supinator muscle (Triceps muscles)
(Hand extensors)
(and some additional scapular muscles)
(impaired sensation on lateral aspect of shoulder
  and radial forearm)

Lower brachial plexus lesions
(Dejerine–Klumpke) Roots C8 and T1
Small muscles of hand ⎫ Leads to claw-like
Long finger flexors ⎬ deformity of hand
(Hand flexors)
Impairment of sensation on the ulnar aspect of
  hand and ulnar forearm
(Horner syndrome)

C7 lesions
Triceps muscle
Pectoralis muscle
Long finger flexors
Impaired sensation of third finger

Dorsal fascicle lesions
(Posterior secondary cords)
Deltoid muscle
Triceps muscle
(Brachioradialis muscle)
Hand and finger extensors
Sensory disturbances of lateral aspect of upper
  arm and radial forearm

Lateral fascicle lesions
(Lateral secondary cord)
Biceps brachii muscle
Brachioradialis muscle
Pronator teres
(Hand and finger flexors)
Impaired sensation on radial forearm and radial
  aspect of hand

Medial fascicle lesions
Interossei and ulnar lumbrical muscles
Thenar muscles
Ulnar aspects of hand and deep finger flexors
Impaired sensation on ulnar border of hand

** See Fig. 15*

The most common causes of brachial plexus lesions are

– Trauma (direct to the shoulder, or traction to
  the arm)

– Compression in the anatomically narrow parts
  of the upper thoracic outlet (costoclavicular,
  scalenus anticus, and particularly with cervical
  ribs and subacromial compression)
– External pressure (as from prolonged carrying
  of a back pack or the Trendelenburg position
  during anesthesia)
– Neuralgic shoulder amyotrophy
– Tumors (sarcoma, Pancoast tumor, metastasis)
– Radiation damage

1.3.3 Lumbosacral Plexus Lesions

The anatomical arrangement of the lumbar plexus
(L1 to L4) and sacral plexus (L4 to S4) is similar
to that of the brachial plexus, and the roots are
rearranged into cords and peripheral nerves to the
lower extremity. In the leg the plexus gives rise
dorsally to the sciatic nerve (L4 to S3) and ventrally to the femoral nerve (L1 to L4). The sympathetic fibers that join the plexus leave the spinal
cord between the third thoracic and the second to
the third lumbar segments, but no further cauda-
ly than the third lumbar root. They reach the lumbar plexus via the paravertebral sympathetic
chain. This anatomic arrangement accounts for
the absence of autonomic, disturbances, particularly those of sweating, in lesions of the roots,
and the distinct involvement of autonomic function in lesions affecting the plexus. The lumbosacral plexus lies in the retroperitoneal space and is
therefore well protected from external injury. The
clinical symptoms of lesions of the lumbosacral
plexus – which are considerably rarer than other
lesions resulting in paralysis of the lower limb –
are as follows:
– Always mixed motor and sensory peripheral
  disturbances (with flaccid paresis and muscle
  atrophy)
– Loss of reflexes (loss of the knee jerk in lumbar plexus lesions and of the ankle jerk in lesions of the sacral plexus)
– Impairment of sweat secretion
– Frequent radiating pain into the leg
– Absence of disturbances of bladder function
  (except in the rare bilateral lesions of the "pudendal plexus" (S2 to S4) (*see* 2.18.1)

In the differential diagnosis of lesions of a lumbosacral root, the following findings are particularly significant:

– Extensive multiradicular disturbances
– Impairment of sweating (see above)

– A history compatible with anatomic lesions of the lumbosacral plexus
– Absence of a vertebral column syndrome such as back pain and impairment of movement of the lumbar spine
– Discovery of a palpable mass during abdominal, rectal, or gynecologic examination

For clinical manifestations of root syndromes of the lower limb, see Table 5. The clinical differentiation of lesions of single peripheral nerves of the lower extremity by their characteristic paralysis is also given in Table 9. The most common causes of lesions of the lumbosacral plexus are:

– Tumors and metastases in the retroperitoneal space (of the female genital organs) and particularly carcinoma of the colon, malignant lymphoma, carcinoma of the rectum, carcinoma of the prostate, and tumors arising from bone
– Retroperitoneal hematomas (particularly common in patients who have taken anticoagulants)
– Inflammatory conditions, such as tuberculous paravertebral abscesses
– Metabolic disorders such as diabetes mellitus with proximal asymmetric polyneuropathy, particularly with involvement of the femoral nerve
– Rare causes (these lesions include postradiation neuropathy, extension injuries to the nerves after prolonged squatting, and ischemia of the plexus in arteriosclerosis of the pelvic arteries)

1.3.4 Lesions of Single Peripheral Nerves

The anatomy and details of clinical symptoms due to lesions of single peripheral nerves are described in relevant texts. They are also summarized in Tables 8 and 9 for the upper and lower extremities. Below are listed general symptoms of lesions of the main peripheral nerve trunks:

– Motor and sensory deficits, typically flaccid peripheral palsies that vary with the anatomic characteristics of the affected nerve. Difficulties in differential diagnosis arise with lesions of pure motor branches such as the profundus branch of the radial nerve (causing paralysis of the supinator and of finger extensors) or the deep palmar branch of the ulnar motor nerve at the wrist (causing paralysis of interosseous muscles and atrophy) or pure sensory branches such as the lateral cutaneous nerve of the thigh in the region of the inguinal ligament (resulting in neuralgia paresthetica with sensory loss on the upper outer aspects of the thigh)
– Atrophy of affected muscles
– Denervation, demonstrated on electromyography of the affected muscle, and electrophysiologic evidence of delayed nerve conduction at the site of the lesion
– Impaired sweat secretion in the region of sensory loss
– A positive Tinel sign, a sign of eventual regeneration
– When a neuroma has formed, pain on pressure at the lesion site

The differential diagnosis from root or plexus lesions is based on exact anatomic analysis of the distribution of sensory and motor deficits. Hints for differential diagnosis are given in Tables 5 to 9.

Figure 16 gives an example of the differences between a root lesion, a plexus and a peripheral nerve lesion. The most common causes of lesions of single peripheral nerves are

– Direct trauma, including section or indirect trauma due to a fracture affecting the nerve
– Chronic compression syndromes, for example, the carpal tunnel syndrome with compression of the median nerve. These occur in areas of anatomically narrow canals
– Chronic mechanical damage with pathologic changes of surrounding structure, as when a fracture with involvement of the ulnar groove results in late ulnar paralysis
– Pressure from outside, which may be chronic or acute (for example, due to pressure in the upper arm, occurring with deep sleep and resulting in paralysis of the radial nerve or due to pressure on the nerve at the head of the fibula as a result of a cast or wearing an appliance, resulting in peroneal/pressure palsy)
– Tumors of nerves or of the neighboring structure (for example, neurinomas)
– Other space-occupying lesions such as retroperitoneal hematomas that compress the femoral nerve
– Ischemia most often manifest by mononeuritis multiplex as the initial symptom of a polyneuropathy, for example, in vasculitides such as periarteritis nodosa or in paraneoplastic conditions

Table 8   Clinical deficits caused by single peripheral nerve lesions of the upper extremity

Nerves	Affected muscles	Sensory impairment
Upper brachial plexus C5 – C6 Dorsal scapular nerve C4 – C5 Suprascapular nerve C5 – C6 (Axillary nerve, see below) (Long thoracic nerve, see below) (Musculocutaneous nerve, see below) (Radial nerve, see below)	Major rhomboids Minor rhomboids Supraspinatus Infraspinatus	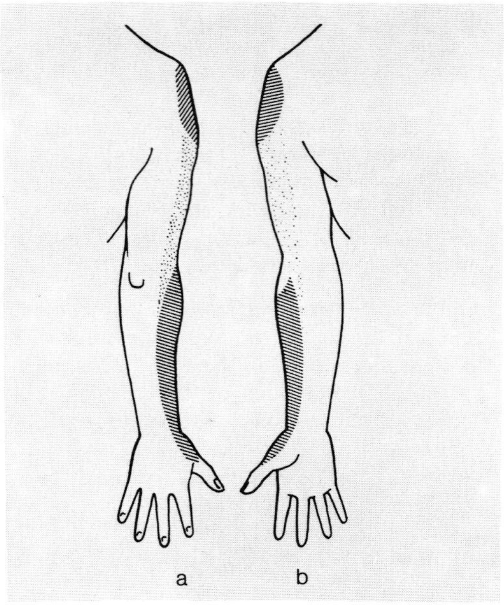 a b
Lower brachial plexus (C8) T1 Medial cutaneous nerve of arm C8 – T1 Medial cutaneous nerve of forearm C8 – T1 (Median nerve, see below) (Ulnar nerve, see below)	∅ ∅	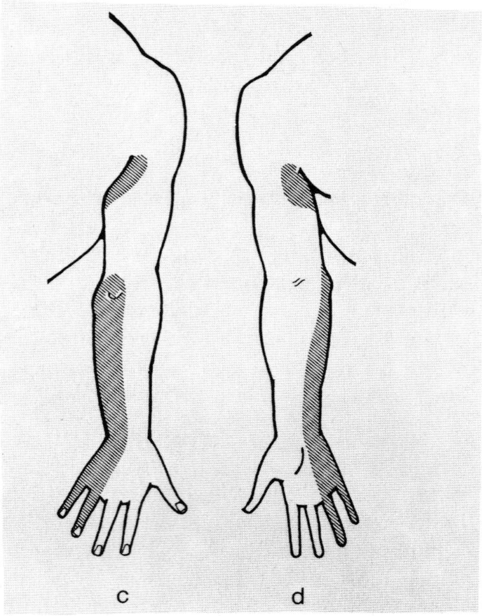 c d

Table 8   (continued)

Function	Special tests	Etiology	Remarks	Differential diagnosis
Abduction of scapula toward the spinal column	Standing with hands in hips, elbows pointed backward			
Abduction and external rotation of shoulder	Initial 15 degrees of shoulder abduction	Trauma (with or without shoulder dislocation)	Occurs in motorbike injuries	Tear of the rotator cuff; Root lesions (spondylosis, disc herniation, familial proximal neurogenic muscle atrophy)
Commonly involved in upper brachial plexus paresis are: abduction of the shoulder; flexion of elbow; supination of forearm (occasionally external rotation of shoulder)		Pack paralysis due to pressure on shoulder from carrying weights Neuralgic amyotrophy of shoulder serum neuritis Tumor infiltration	Long thoracic nerve is frequently involved One fourth of cases bilateral	Thrombosis of brachial vein Amyotropic lateral sclerosis
Adduction and abduction of finger; flexion of interphalangeal joints (flexion of wrist joints)		Trauma, birth trauma, scalenus anticus syndrome (with and without cervical rib), costoclavicular syndrome, "Pancoast tumor," infiltration with lymphomas, radiation therapy	In association with Horner syndrome Symptoms due to compression of subclavian arteries Early pain, and Horner syndrome	Root lesions, peripheral ulnar paralysis, amyotrophic lateral sclerosis, myopathies with distal muscle atrophy (e.g., myotonic dystrophy), syringomyelia

(continued)

Table 8   (continued)

Nerves	Affected muscles	Sensory impairment
Long thoracic nerve C5 – C7	Serratus anterior	
Axillary nerve C5 – C6	Deltoids	
	Teres minor	
Musculocutaneous nerve C5 – C7	Coracobrachialis	
	Biceps	
	Brachial (partially supplied by radial nerve)	
Radial nerve C5 – C8 (T1)	Triceps brachii and anconeus muscle	
	Brachioradialis	
	Brachialis (with musculocutaneous nerve)	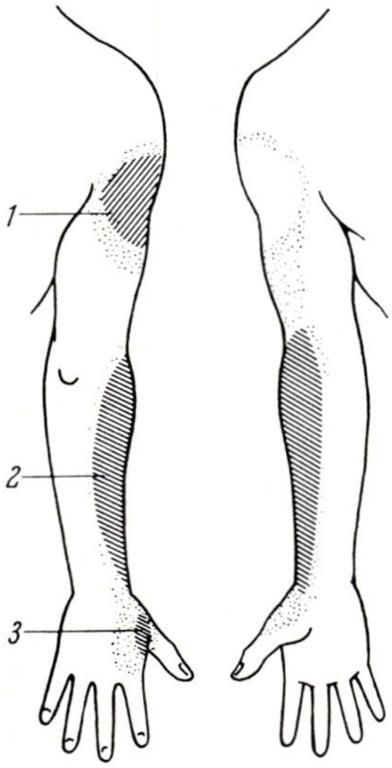
	Extensor carpi radialis brevis and longus	
	Supinator	
	Extensor digitorum	
	Extensor carpi ulnaris Extensor digiti minimi	
	Abductor pollicis longus	
	Extensor pollicis longus	
	Extensor pollicis brevis	
	Extensor indicis	

1 Axillary nerve
2 Lateral cutaneous branch (musculo-cutaneous nerve)
3 Superficial cutaneous branch of radial nerve

Table 8 (continued)

Function	Special tests	Etiology	Remarks	Differential diagnosis
Scapula pulled laterally and ventrally, lower part of scapula rotated	Pushing of extended arms against resistance (winging of scapula becomes evident)	Operative trauma in axilla / Lifting of heavy loads / Pressure palsies (pack paralysis) "inflammatory, allergic"	Part of neuralgic shoulder amyotrophy	Winging of the scapula (with the shoulder girdle variety) on progressive muscular dystrophy
Abduction at shoulder joint	Elevation of arms laterally above 15 degrees	Trauma (often with dislocation of the shoulder)		Muscular dystrophy
External rotation in shoulder joint				Tear of rotator cuff
Main suspending muscles of the shoulder joint (flexion and adduction of the upper arm); flexion of the upper arm and forearm; supination of forearm; flexion of upper arm	Flexion of elbows with supinated forearm	Trauma; rarely isolated with out trauma		Tear of long tendons of biceps muscle
Extension of the elbow				
Flexion of the elbow	In mid-position between pronation and supination			
Flexion of the elbow				
Extension (radial abduction) of metacarpophalangeal joints	With flexed finger joints	Fracture of upper arm	Triceps muscle spared	
Supination of forearms and hands	With extended elbow	Pressure palsy on upper arm	Spontaneous recovery	
Extension of phalangeal joints	Flexion of interphalangeal joints with flexed fingers	"Lead neuritis"	Often purely motor	
Extension and ulnar abduction of metacarpophalangeal joint		Isolated paralysis of deep branch at level of supinator muscle		
Small extensors of the fingers		Pressure palsy of sensory terminal branch, at thumb (cheiralgia paresthetica)		
Abduction of the proximal phalanx				
Extension of terminal phalanx of thumb				
Extension of proximal phalanx of thumb	Distal phalanx flexed			
Extension of index finger	Other fingers flexed			

(continued)

Table 8 (continued)

Nerves	Affected muscles	Sensory impairment
Median nerve C5–T1	Pronator teres and quadratus muscles Flexor carpi radialis Palmaris longus Superficial flexor digitorum Flexor digitorum profundus (II–III) Flexor pollicis longus Flexor pollicis brevis (superficial head) Abductor pollicis brevis Opponens pollicis Lumbrical muscles I–II	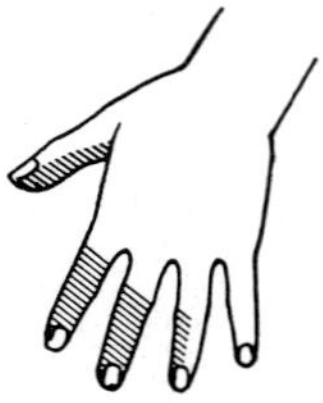 g 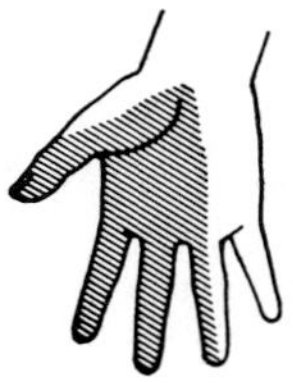 h
Ulnar nerve C8–T1	Flexor carpi ulnaris Flexor digitorum profundus (IV–V) Palmaris brevis Abductor digiti minimi Opponens digiti minimi Flexor digiti minimi brevis Lumbrical muscles III–IV Interossei Adductor pollicis Flexor pollicis brevis (deep head)	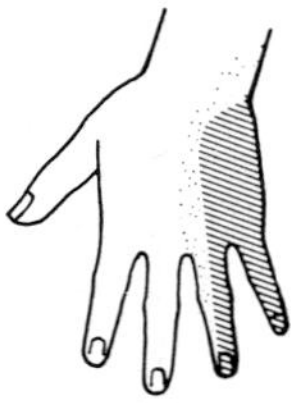 i 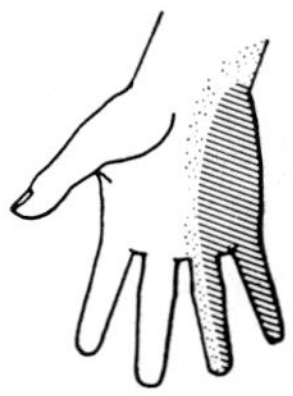 j

Table 8 (continued)

Function	Special tests	Etiology	Remarks	Differential diagnosis
Pronation of forearm Volar flexion of wrist radially Pure volar flexion of wrist Flexion of the middle phalanx of finger Flexion of terminal phalanges I and III Flexion of distal phalanx of thumb Flexion of proximal phalanx of thumb Abduction of metacarpal I Rotation of thumb Flexion of wrist joint, extension of inter-phalangeal joints II and III	Extension of thumb with grasping of an object (bottle sign) Touching of little finger with ter-minal phalanx of thumb	Traumatic, e.g. supracondylar fractures of humerus Pressure palsies of upper arm With supracon-dylar process of humerus Cutting injuries at wrist Carpal tunnel syndrome (professional) pressure palsies of hand	"Swearing Hand" with proximal paresis Good prognosis Complaints of brachial pain and paresthesia, mainly noctur-nal Often pure motor	Volkmann contrac-ture (Lower) plexus lesions Amyotrophic lateral sclerosis
Volar and ulnar flexion of the wrist Flexion of terminal phalanges IV and V "Skin muscle" of hypothenar eminence Abduction of little finger Opposition of little finger Flexion of little finger at proximal inter-phalangeal joint Flexion of proximal interphalangeal joint and exten-sion of inter-phalangeal joints III and IV Adduction and ab-duction of same Adduction of thumb Flexion of proximal interphalangeal joint of the thumb	Extension of fifth finger (with prominence of tendon) Wrinkling and retraction of skin on hypothenar eminence with abduction of fifth finger Lateral movement of little fingers Froment sign	Pressure at elbow Dislocation of the elbow with trauma to nerves Traumatic, due to fractures of the elbow Late paralysis after old elbow frac-ture Paresis with arthropathies and cartilage le-sions of elbow joint Pressure palsies at wrist Abnormally frequent flexion and extension of elbows	Professional Prolonged bed rest with or without addi-tional trauma, bilateral Particularly by medial epicon-dyle Particularly with lateral part of radial condyle Occasionally bilateral Mostly pure motor E.g., punch ma-chine operators or those handl-ing drills	Root lesions C8 Lower plexus lesions Medial epicondylitis Distal atrophy with muscle dystrophy (Dupuytren contrac-ture) Amyotrophic lateral sclerosis

M. Mumenthaler, H. Schliack: Lesions of Peripheral Nerves, 4th ed. Thieme, Stuttgart, 1982

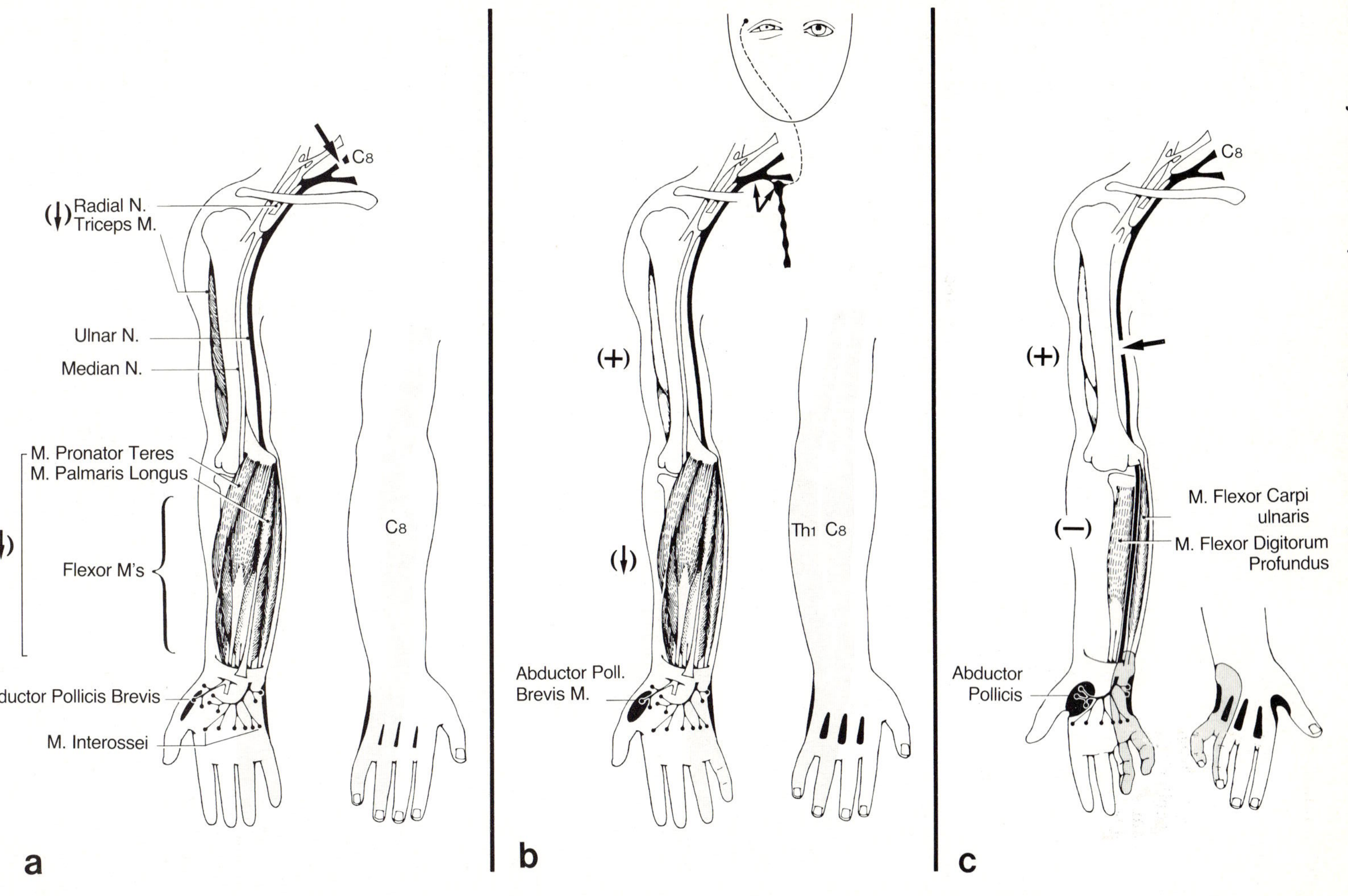

Fig. **16** Differentiation of C8 root lesion (**a**) from a lower brachial plexus lesion (**b**) and peripheral nerve (ulnar) paralysis (**c**)

1.3.5 Polyneuropathies

Because of the common anatomic and physiologic characteristics of all peripheral nerves, the consequences of hereditary anomalies, metabolic disturbances, and endogenous and exogenous toxic insults are similar. The result is a characteristic clinical picture of peripheral nerve diseases. The common clinical manifestation of polyneuropathies are

— Widespread symmetric distribution and slow to rapid progression of the symptoms
— Paresthesia of extremities, particularly the feet (often an initial symptom). Sometimes burning pain, similarly distributed, is also found
— Areflexias (usually and often ankle jerks) are absent before impairment of other reflexes
— Prominent distal sensory disturbances, often in the feet, with stocking and glove distribution that particularly affects vibration sense and epicritic sensory qualities
— Weakness, more prominent distally when manifest as weakness of dorsiflexion of the feet it eventually leads to steppage gait
— Eventual atrophy of muscles prominent distally. Rarely, disturbances of trophic function (skin, toes, fingernails, and bones) also occur
— The cranial nerves are not involved, except in rare cases such as ocular muscle palsies occurring with diabetes mellitus
— Electrophysiological evidence of denervation and marked disturbances of peripheral nerve conduction velocities
— The symptoms and signs are schematically shown in Figure 17.

Differentiation from polyradiculitis (*see* 1.3.1) is usually possible because of the distinguishing features of polyradiculitis:

— The course to maximum deficits is usually more rapid (days to weeks)
— Motor deficits are more prominent than sensory loss
— Proximal muscles can be prominently affected as well as distal function
— The upper extremity might be weaker than the lower extremity
— Cranial nerves may be involved, and bilateral facial paralysis may occur
— As determined electrophysiologically, conduction velocities are little affected, if at all (even though paralysis may be marked early in the course), whereas in polyneuropathy, sensory conduction is often affected at the beginning of the illness, and motor conduction velocities are markedly slowed throughout the course
— The CSF shows an increase in protein with normal cellular content about three weeks after the start of the illness.

For differentiation from myopathies, *see* 1.4.

The most common causes of polyneuropathy are

— Exogenous toxic insults (commonly alcohol, drugs, or solvents)
— Metabolic disturbances (often diabetes mellitus)
— Hereditary diseases, particularly those with known enzymatic defects (porphyria, Refsum's disease)
— Impaired absorption of vitamin B_{12}
— Collagen diseases (particularly periarteritis nodosa)
— Infectious diseases.

Table 10 shows in more detail the most common etiologic factors in polyneuropathy.

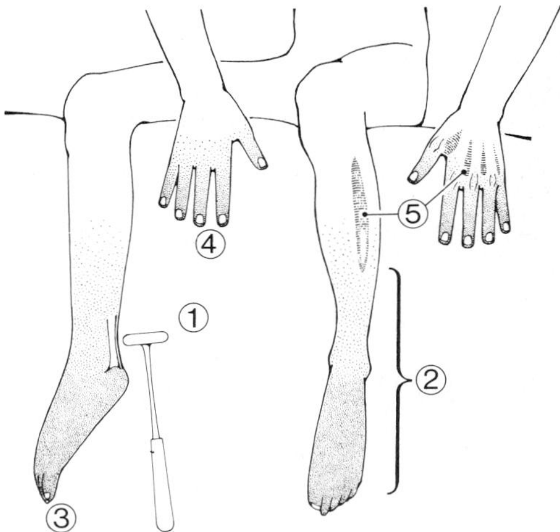

Fig. **17** Most common symptoms of polyneuropathy. **1** Absence of ankle jerks; **2** distal (stocking) sensory disturbance; **3** distal paralysis, particularly of dorsiflexor of the foot with footdrop; **4** distal (glove-like) sensory disturbance of hands; **5** atrophy of muscles (particularly in the anterior tibial compartment and interossei) (M. Mumenthaler: Minicourses for Continued Medical Education 28 [1978] 995–999)

Table 9   Overview of deficits due to lesions of single peripheral nerves of the lower extremity

Nerves	Affected muscles	Sensory impairment
Lumbar plexus L1 – L4	Prominently hip flexors (rotators of hip joint), adductors of thigh, extensors of knee	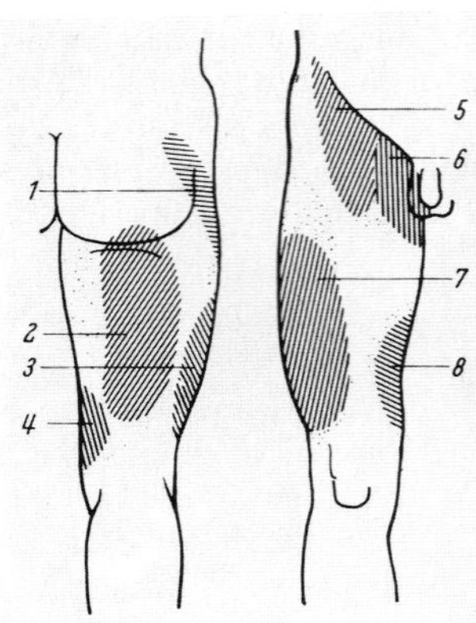 1 N. iliohypogastricus 2 N. cutaneus femoris posterior 3 N. cutaneus femoris lateralis 4 N. obturatorius 5 N. iliohypogastricus 6 N. ilioinguinalis 7 N. cutaneus femoris lateralis 8 N. obturatorius
Sacral plexus L5 – S3	Prominently gluteal muscles, ischiocrural group, dorsal extensors and plantar flexors of foot and toes	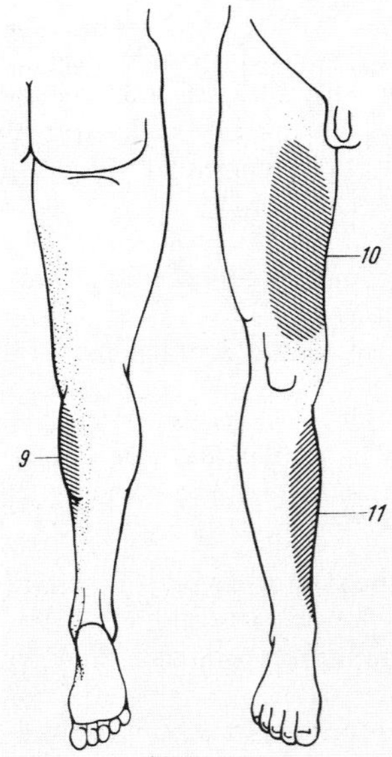
Femoral nerve L2 – L4	Iliac muscles Pectineus muscle Sartorius muscle Quadriceps femoris muscle	
Lateral cutaneous nerve of thigh L2 – L3	∅	
Ilioinguinal nerve L1(– L2)	∅	9 N. saphenus 10 R. cutaneus anterior n. femoralis 11 N. saphenus
Superior gluteal nerve L4 – S1	Gluteus medius muscle Gluteus minimus muscle Tensor fasciae latae	

Table 9   (continued)

Function	Special tests	Etiology	Remarks	Differential diagnosis
See Muscles		Traumatic, retroperitoneal processes (tumors), squatting, diabetes mellitus		
See Muscles		Tumors of pelvis, pregnancy and delivery, operative trauma		Multiple-root lesion, cauda equina syndrome, occlusion of pelvic arteries
Flexion and internal rotation of hip Flexion, adduction, external rotation of hip Extension of knee (and hip flexion)	Examination with patient sitting with calves hanging free	Operative trauma, injuries, overextension of hip, hemorrhage		High lumbar disc herniation, progressive muscular dystrophy (isolated affection of the thigh), muscle atrophy due to arthropathies of knee, femoral form of diabetic neuropathy, high lumbar disc herniation
Purely sensory	Pain on pressure immediately medial to anterior superior iliac spine	Chronic mechanical damage at passage through inguinal ligament	Meralgia paresthetica	
Mostly sensory	Difficulty on forced extension of hip joints Overextension of hip joint	Chronic mechanical damage at passage through abdominal muscles		Infection of hip joint
Internal rotation of hip with slight flexion Abduction of hip joint	Abduction of leg in lateral position Lowering of pelvis opposite lesion on walking (positive Trendelenburg test)	Traumatic, particularly intramuscular injection damage		Pelvic girdle and progressive muscular dystrophy

(continued)

Table 9   (continued)

Nerve	Affected muscles	Sensory impairment
Gluteus inferior L5–S2	Gluteus maximus	
Tibialis nerve L4–S3	Gastrocnemius Plantaris Soleus Popliteus Tibialis posterior Flexor digitorum longus Flexor hallucis longus Flexor digitorum brevis Flexor hallucis brevis Abductor hallucis Abductor digiti minimi Adductor hallucis Quadratus plantae Lumbricales Interossei	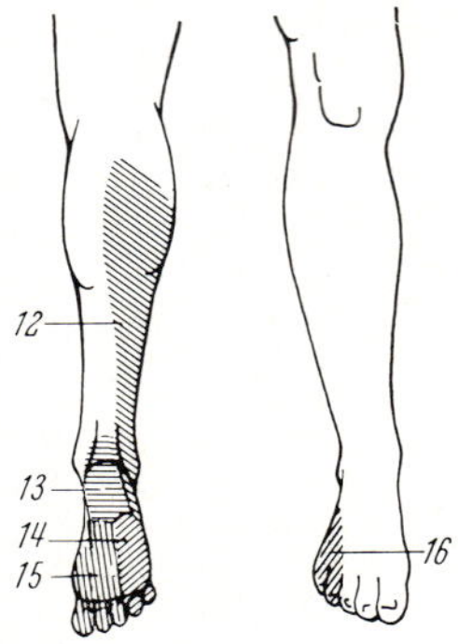 12 N. suralis 13 N. tibialis 14 N. plantaris lateralis 15 N. plantaris medialis 16 N. suralis
Common peroneal nerve L4–S2 Deep peroneal nerve Superficial peroneal nerve	Tibialis anterior Extensor digitorum longus Extensor hallucis longus Peroneus tertius Extensor digitorum brevis Extensor hallucis brevis Peroneus longus Peroneus brevis	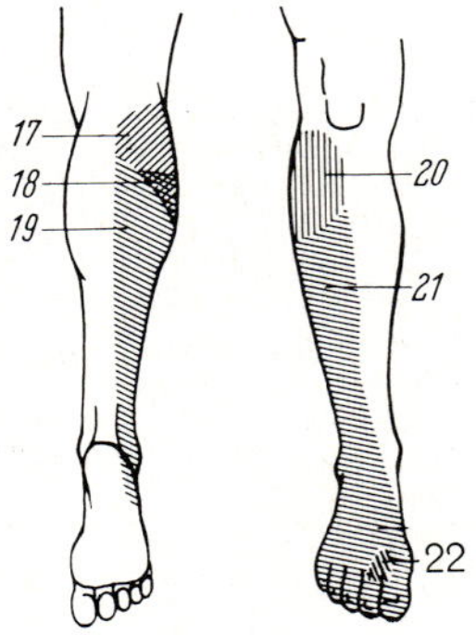 17 N. peronaeus communis 18 N. peronaeus superficialis 19 N. suralis 20 N. peronaeus communis 21 N. peronaeus superficialis 22 N. peronaeus profundus

Table 9   (continued)

Function	Special tests	Etiology	Remarks	Differential diagnosis
Extension of hip	Prone position, knee flexed 90 degrees, lift upper thigh from support			Muscular dystrophy
Plantar flexion of foot (and knee flexion)	Flexion of knees, initially 15 degrees	Injuries in posterior aspect of knee Occasionally, isolated lesions of sciatic nerve		Herniation of L5/S1 discs
Flexion of knee joint	90 degree flexion of knee Do not activate toe flexors			
Supination and plantar flexion of foot Flexion of terminal phalanges				
Flexion of middle phalanges				
Abduction of toes				
Dorsal extension of foot	Slapping gait	Direct trauma		Herniation of L4/L5, other root lesion, polyneuropathies, peroneal muscular atrophy, distal muscle atrophy in myopathies (Steinert) (vascular)-tibialis−anterior-syndrome
Extension of terminal phalanges of toes	Steppage gait	Fractures of fibula		
		Pressure palsy	Prognosis good	
Extension of first phalanges of toes		Paralysis due to injection of serum	Rare	
Eversion and plantar flexion of foot				

M. Mumenthaler, H. Schliack: Lesions of Peripheral Nerves 4th ed. Thieme, Stuttgart, 1982

**Table 10   Most common etiologic factors in poly-
neuropathy**

Genetic polyneuropathies
Hereditary and sensory neuropathies
● peroneal muscular atrophy of
    Charcot–Marie–Tooth
● neuronal type of peroneal muscular atrophy
● hypertrophic neuropathy of Déjerine–Sottas
● hereditary sensory neuropathy
Polyneuropathy in porphyria
Polyneuropathy in amyloidosis
Polyneuropathy in Refsum's disease
Polyneuropathy in metachromatic leukodystrophy
Polyneuropathy in metabolic disorders
Polyneuropathy in diabetes mellitus
● symmetric, predominantly distal form
● asymmetric, predominantly proximal form
● "mononeuropathy"
● amyotrophy or myelopathy
Polyneuropathy in uremia
Polyneuropathy in cirrhosis of liver
Polyneuropathy in malnutrition
Polyneuropathy in vitamin B_{12} deficiency
Polyneuropathy in paraproteinemias and
    monoclonal gammopathies
Polyneuropathy in infectious diseases
● leprosy
● parotitis
● mononucleosis
● typhus and paratyphus
● Rocky Mountain spotted fever
● diphtheria
● botulism
● tic paralysis
Polyneuropathy in collagen diseases
● periarteritis nodosa
Polyneuropathy in sprue and other malabsorption
    syndromes
Polyneuropathy due to exogenous toxic substances
● alcohol
● lead
● arsenic
● solvents (e.g., carbon disulfide poisoning)
● triarylphosphate
● thallium
● drug intoxication
    (isoniazid, thalidomide, nitrofurantoin)
● insecticides
Other polyneuropathies
● serum neuritis
● neoplastic
● sarcoid
● ischemic

*M. Mumenthaler: Neurology, 9th ed. Thieme, Stuttgart,
1990*

1.4 Myopathic Syndromes

Although myopathic syndromes primarily involve muscles they also include those internal diseases in which impairment of muscle function is a prominent symptom (Table 11). Not included, however, are neurogenic muscle atrophies — those disorders of peripheral nerves that produce muscle weakness because of involvement of peripheral motor neurons (anterior horn cells, peripheral nerve roots, or peripheral nerves). Muscle function depends on both the ultrastructure of the myofibrils, mitochondria, and other structural elements of the muscle fiber and the enzymatic metabolic processes that occur during muscle fiber contraction. The structure and metabolism of muscles can be disturbed by both inherited defects and acquired disorders.

In spite of numerous pathogenetic mechanisms, myopathies have certain common clinical features:

— Pure motor weakness
— Absence of sensory impairment
— Absence of fasciculations
— Symmetric distribution of symptoms (except in myasthenia)
— Weakness of a flaccid character (except in neuromyotonia, for example)
— Often impairment of reflexes
— Often accompanying atrophy
  ● in most cases a slowly progressive course, lasting for years
  ● in a few conditions (for example, polymyositis), rapid progression over months or weeks, or in the case of periodic hypokalemic paralysis or acute paroxysmal myoglobinuria, for example, hours
— Most often a proximal distribution of weakness
— Occasionally the weakness is more marked distally, as in myotonic dystrophy of Steinert. Or the weakness may vary in location and severity from hour to hour over the course of several days, for example, in myasthenia gravis
— Absence of external initiating factors. (Exceptions include the painful localized muscle weakness after exertion in phosphorylase deficiency or myasthenia and the generalized weakness on exposure to cold in paramyotonia congenita of Eulenburg)

Table 11   The myopathies

1. Dystrophic myopathies
   a. Progressive muscular dystrophy
   - type I (fascioscapulohumeral form)
   - type II (girdle form)
   - type III (X-linked pelvic girdle type)
     • malignant Duchenne type
     • benign Becker type
   b. Myotonic dystrophy (Curschmann–Steinert)
   c. Other dystrophic muscular processes
   - ocular muscular dystrophy
   - congenital muscular dystrophy
     distal forms
2. Myopathy with other congenital or early manifestations of structural defects
   a. Myotubular myopathy
   b. Ragged red fiber myopathy
   c. Nemalin myopathy
3. Syndromes with disturbances of muscle relaxation
   a. Myotonia congenita (Thomsen)
   b. Paramyotonia congenita (Eulenburg)
   c. Neuromyotonia with continuous muscle fiber activity
   d. Stiff-man syndrome
4. Myasthenia gravis
5. Myositides
   a. Polymyositis and dermatomyositis
   - idiopathic form
   - with collagen disease
   - in association with malignant disease
   - with other diseases
     • sarcoidosis
   b. Infectious myositides
6. Myopathic symptoms as manifestations of metabolic disturbances (with known metabolic abnormalities)
   a. Myopathies with known enzyme defect
   - glycogen storage diseases
   - acid maltase disease
   - phosphorylase deficiency (McArdle)
   - carnitine deficiency
   b. Myopathic symptoms with abnormalities of potassium metabolism
   - hypokalemic (familial) periodic paralysis
   - hyperkalemic paralysis (adynamia episodica hereditaria)
   - normokalemic paralysis
   - symptomatic hypokalemic paralysis
   c. Rhabdomyolysis (paroxysmal myoglobinuria)
7. Myopathic symptoms in association with other diseases (without known pathogenetic mechanisms)
   a. Myopathic symptoms with endocrinopathies
   - thyroid dysfunction
     • hyperthyroidism
     • hypothyroidism
   - Cushing's disease
   - acromegaly
   - hyperparathyroidism
   b. In association with malignant disease
   c. In association with collagen disease
   d. In association with infectious disease
     • botulism
     • tetanus
   e. Malnutrition
8. Myopathic symptoms with exogenous intoxication
   a. Alcohol intoxication
   b. Drug intoxication
   c. Other toxic substances
9. The remainder of muscle disorders and symptoms

M. Mumenthaler: Neurology, 3rd ed. Thieme, Stuttgart, 1990

— Absence of associated pain. (One exception is the exercise-induced pain in patients with phosphorylase deficiency, paroxysmal myoglobinuria, and neuromyasthenia)
— In summary, purely motor, most often symmetric, painless and usually slowly progressive symptoms that are more prominent proximally. Nevertheless, many forms of myopathy have other clinical characteristics.

It is necessary to differentiate myopathies from other diseases associated with weakness (*see* 2.13). They are most difficult to distinguish from chronic anterior horn cell disease, from polyradiculitis, from polyneuropathies, and occasionally from psychogenic pseudoparalysis (Fig. 17).

— Chronic anterior horn cell disease has the following distinguishing features:
  • fasciculations occasionally are evoked by percussion of muscles or by intravenous injection of 5 to 10 mg of edrophonium chloride (Tensilon)
  • bulbar muscles, particularly the tongue, may be involved
  • the corticospinal fibers or corticobulbar pathways may be involved, resulting in pyramidal signs or pseudobulbar symptoms
  • progression is often rapid — a matter of months. (However, in Kugelberg–Welander disease, it may extend over years)

Electromyography provides the easiest means of differentiating anterior horn disease from myopathies, and muscle biopsy findings are also often diagnostic.

- In patients with polyradiculitis or polyneuropathy, common findings are:
  - sensory loss (which may be discrete in certain polyradiculopathies)
  - predominantly distal muscle weakness
  - absence of reflexes, with minor weakness
  - a typical electrodiagnostic study
- The findings in psychogenic pseudoparesis are detailed in 2.13.3.

Table 11 is an overview of the numerous etiologic forms of myopathy and of myopathic symptoms due to other diseases.

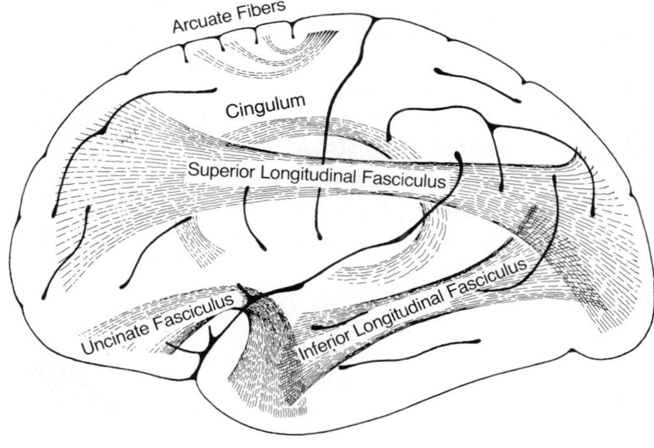

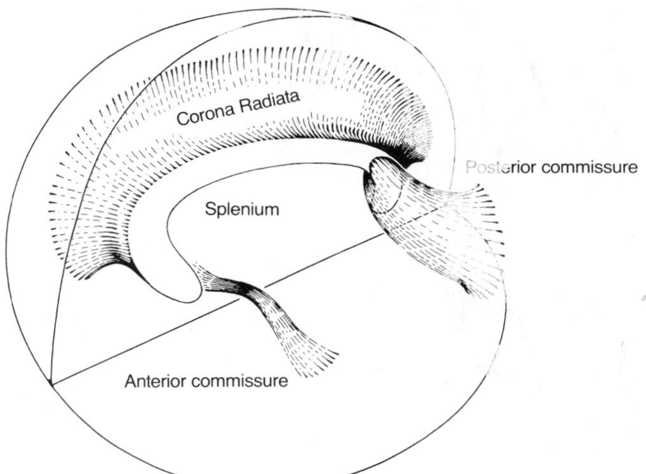

Fig. **18** Connections of major cortical areas

– Arteriosclerotic or other vascular dementias (for example, 'congophilic' angiopathy)
– Benign brain tumors (frontal meningiomas or colloid cysts of the third ventricle)
– Chronic encephalitis (particularly general paresis of the insane) and, rarely, Behçet's disease
– Metabolic disorders (storage diseases and leukodystrophies and hepatic encephalopathy with portocaval shunt and dialysis dementia)
– Endocrinopathies, particularly myxedema and hyper- and hypoparathyroidism
– Communicating hydrocephalus (abnormal gait, bladder dysfunction with antecedent history of subarachnoid hemorrhage or meningitis that could have lead to silting of extracerebral CSF pathways)
– Chronic intoxications (alcoholism and lead encephalopathy)

Dementia occurring without acute initiating disease, but progressing over weeks or months, with psychoorganic disturbances, suggests

– Malignant brain tumor or brain metastasis
– A variety of encephalopathies (for example, subacute sclerosing panencephalopathy or rapidly progressive paralysis of the insane [general paresis])
– Chronic subdural hematoma

- Internal hydrocephalus (particularly when due to disturbed reabsorption of CSF or noncommunicating hydrocephalus)
- Certain rapidly progressive metabolic disturbances and storage diseases
- Rapidly progressing vasculopathies

A psycho-organic disturbance with an acute initiating episode that rapidly stabilizes with little further progression suggests

- Skull-brain trauma
- Intracranial bleeding (from aneurysm, angioma)
- Ischemic events with encephalopathy
- Acute hydrocephalus (occurring in association with trauma, subarachnoid bleeding, or meningitis)

Neuropsychologic syndromes can hint at the localization of disorders, but not at their etiology (Table 12). Certain tests can clarify questions of etiology, and differential psychopathologic investigation does yield some information about etiologic factors in dementia.

- With senile dementia, the main features of psychopathology are impaired memory, lack of drive, disturbances of the sleep-wakefulness cycles, accentuation of previous behavioral peculiarities, which may degenerate into a caricature of the personality, and outbursts of unprovoked rage. As a rule, better days alternate with days of severely disturbed behavior. Initially the patient has some awareness of his condition
- In Alzheimer's disease the general signs of organic psychosyndromes are accompanied by disorders due to parietotemporal dysfunction: disturbances of geographic orientation, apraxias, and aphasias
- In Pick's disease, intellectual and memory function is preserved, while the personality becomes markedly disorganized, with blunting of affect, loss of ethical values, and social and sexual malfunction
- With general paralysis of the insane there is a predominant loss of critical values with marked self-aggrandizement and grandiose ideas
- A rare form of slowly progressive aphasia without other neuropsychologic deficits and without dementia is attributed to focal cortical atrophy

Organic neurologic symptoms and signs also differentiate and suggest the etiologic grouping of psycho-organic disturbances.

- Epileptic attacks are common with tumors of the brain, with atrophic processes (particularly Pick's disease), and with vascular lesions
- Focal neurologic and neuropsychologic symptoms limited to one hemisphere may, depending on their evolution and prominence and on their associated signs and symptoms, suggest the presence of a brain tumor, a subdural hematoma, a brain contusion, or an atrophic process
- Signs of increased intracranial pressure suggest a space-occupying lesion (tumor, chronic subdural hematoma) or obstructive hydrocephalus
- Primitive reflexes and instinctive movements (grasping, magnetic reactions, sucking reflexes, forced crying or laughing) or uninhibited sexuality are the hallmarks of atrophic brain processes due to degenerative or vascular disorders. Forced laughing or crying are also found in patients with amyotrophic lateral sclerosis. They may also be prodromes of epileptic fits
- The presence of rigidity, parkinsonian-like tremor, or choreoathetotic movements suggests a system degeneration such as parkinsonism-dementia complex, olivopontocerebellar atrophy, or Huntington's disease
- Ataxia and polyneuropathy are frequent accompaniments of toxic dementias

Table 13 links psycho-organic syndromes to their common etiologic forms by giving an overview of the characteristic symptoms and findings in these disorders.

2.2 Acute Confusional State and Coma

In the following section the discussion is limited to acute (transient) episodes of confusion and coma. The confusional states that occur in dementia (*see* 2.1) and accompanying losses of consciousness (*see* 2.3) are not covered in this chapter.

2.2.1 Acute Confusion and Disorientation, Amnesia

Patients are more or less disoriented to time and place. Their thoughts are not logical, critical, and properly ordered, and external circumstances do not govern their actions. The term *amnesia* refers to a hiatus in memory in conscious patients. When such a disturbance occurs acutely, it points to an organic disturbance of brain function.

The anatomic substrate of registration of sensory impressions, ecphoria, and memory are the hippocampus, the fornix, and the mamillary bodies, all parts of the limbic system. This system is very important in affective behavior, mood, and desires, and is therefore important in adapting and appropriately reacting to the social environment. Figure 19 shows these structures. This system is intercalated between the neocortex and the brain stem and is connected with both in an afferent and efferent fashion.

The hippocampus is connected to the mamillary bodies through the fornix, and the latter is linked with the anterior thalamic nucleus through the bundle of Vicq d'Azyr (the mamillothalamic tract). Impulses pass from the anterior thalamic nucleus via the thalamocingulate radiation to the cingulate gyrus where, after synapsing, they are redirected to the hippocampus via the Papez circuit. This circuit is connected through the mamillary bodies (which are not actually part of the limbic system) with the reticular formation of the brain stem through the medial forebrain bundle. Thus, the Papez circuit can influence activation or inhibition of the limbic system.

There are connections between amygdala via the ventral amygdalohypothalamic tract and hippocampus through fornices to the hypothalamus – a system of pathways that suggests interdependence of vegetative regulation with the limbic system. Impulses travel from the anterior thalamic nucleus (which is part of the Papez circuit) via association fibers to the neocortex, thus linking the limbic system with consciousness and memory. Stimulation of the amygdala causes oral automatism (licking, chewing, gagging, etc.) and affective outbursts. Excitation of the septal regions causes activation of genital vesical-anal reflexes. Hippocampal stimulation causes alterations in consciousness with twilight states and vegetative symptoms such as palpitation and sweating. Lesions of the horn of Ammon cause disorientation and impairment of memory, and bilateral resection of the temporal lobe in Rhesus monkeys results in the Klüver-Bucy syndrome. Bilateral damage to the mamillary bodies causes loss of memory and a confabulatory Korsakoff syndrome, while similar damage to the fornix causes only memory loss.

Episodes of organic, acute confusion and disorientation and of amnesia result from lesions of the above structures. These lesions often are functional (for example, toxic) in nature, but they can also be the result of gross anatomic lesions. Only if such lesions are present can neurologic examination disclose clinical deficits. Usually, however, only a detailed history obtained from relatives or friends will hint at the etiology of these disturbances. The following are possible causes of such disorders:

- Exogenous intoxication (alcoholism, Korsakoff's psychosis, Wernicke's disease), therapeutic use of narcotics and certain barbiturates – the most common cause
- Endogenous intoxication (metabolic disturbances such as hypoglycemia and uremia are the second most common cause
- Head trauma, often associated with neurologic deficits and, in late stages, with diabetes insipidus and bloody CSF
- 'Limbic encephalitis' – a component of a paraneoplastic syndrome or a result of herpes simplex infection
- Circulatory disturbances in the territory of both posterior cerebral arteries and of the posterior communicating arteries and their branches. The cause is a local arteriopathy, generalized hypoxemia, or migraine. An example of a specific symptom is total global amnesia (*see* 2.3.3)
- Electroshock therapy, which, after several treatments, can lead to episodes of retrograde amnesia and occasionally to permanent impairment of memory
- Epileptic twilight states (*see* 2.3.3)

2.2.2 Disturbances of Consciousness and Coma

Consciousness expresses itself, among other ways, in appropriate reactions to the surroundings. Clouding of consciousness is characterized by a disproportionately small response to stimuli or by delayed reaction to external stimuli. The disturbance can vary in degree from a dazed state through somnolence and stupor to coma. Coma itself can vary in intensity all the way to brain death. Normal consciousness requires intact functioning of the structures of the brain stem, particularly the rostral part of the reticular formation and its activating system, which extends from the cranial part of the pons rostrally, across the midbrain to the hypothalamus and the sensory thalamic nuclei. This reticular activating system projects to the entire cortex, and its functioning

Table 13 Dementia. Special aspects of history and findings in various etiologic forms

	History				Findings											Age	Remarks
	Sudden Onset	Slowly progressive *	Rapidly progressive **	Stationary	Epileptic Attacks	Focal symptoms	Visual disturbances	Increased intracranial pressure	Bilateral pyramidal signs	Neuropsycho-logic symptoms	Rigidity	Choreoatheto-tic movements	Primitive reflexes	Headache	Polyneuropathy		
Debility				+												0–	
Senile and prese-nile brain atrophy		+			(+)	(+)			(+)	+			+			50–	
Cerebral arterio-sclerosis		+							+		(+)		+			>50	
Vascular insults	+			+	+	+				+						60	Risk factors
Brain tumor and metastasis			+		+	+	+	+		+				+		40–	
Meningioma		+			+	+		(+)		+				(+)		40–	
Trauma	+	(+)			+	+				+				(+)		Any	Trauma usually prominent
Chronic subdural hematoma			+			(+)		+						+		Any	Changing levels of consciousness
Non-absorbent hydrocephalus		+	+						+					+		Any	History of trauma
Alcoholism		+			+										+	30–	
Bismuth therapy			+								+					Any	History
Chronic encephalitis			+		(+)	(+)			+	(+)	(+)	(+)		(+)		Any	
General paresis of insane		+			+	+			+	+				(+)		Any	Serology
Leukodystrophy		+			(+)		+		+		+				(+)	Any	
Storage diseases		+			+		+		+		+					Any	
Parkinson's dementia complex											+		(+)			50–	Occasionally with tremor and akinesia
Huntington's chorea		+										+				40–	
Epileptic dementia		+			++											Any	
Punch drunkenness		+			(+)				(+)								History of boxing
Supranuclear paralysis		+									+						Paralysis of upward gaze

Primary symptom.
* Months to years.
** Weeks to months.

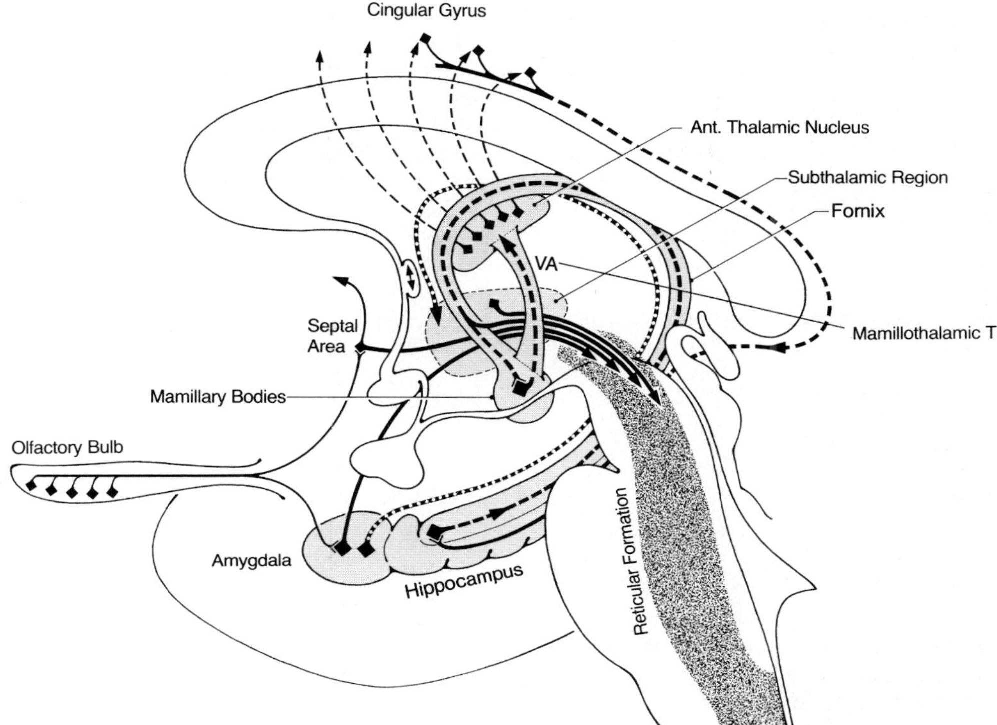

Fig. 19   Anatomic substrate of consciousness and affect

determines the alertness of the individual. Consciousness is impaired when metabolic or other causes disturb the function of cells in the rostral portion of the reticular formation.

The most important causes of disturbances of consciousness (up to coma) and the signs and symptoms commonly found are given below:

– Exogenous intoxication, most often caused by hypnotic drugs, tranquilizers, psychoactive medications, or alcohol. This cause should be considered in the absence of other apparent etiologic factors. A search for drug packages, interrogation of friends and family, determination of levels of drugs and poisons in the serum, and a check of beta activity in the electroencephalogram can all yield clues
– Endogenous intoxication resulting from metabolic disturbances such as diabetes mellitus, hypoglycemia, uremia. This possibility should be ruled out through appropriate laboratory investigations
– Ischemic cerebral vascular insults, stemming from extensive supratentorial infarction or marked basilar ischemia, and causing hemisyndromes, bilateral pyramidal signs, and cranial nerve dysfunction. In coma associated with bilateral paramedian thalamic infarcts there is spastic tetraplegia and horizontal gaze palsy initially; later there are serious memory deficits. Such vascular insults are more common in the older age groups and in the presence of risk factors
– Diffuse cerebral ischemia with anoxia, resulting from cardiovascular dysfunction (Stokes-Adams attacks, ventricular fibrillation), carbon monoxide intoxication, or strangulation. History is significant – clinical signs of cardiac insufficiency or electrocardiograms can be diagnostic
– Intracranial bleeding – for example, intracerebral or intracerebellar hematoma, subarachnoid bleeding, or subdural hematoma. One should be alert for signs of meningeal irritation, neurologic deficits, bloody lumbar puncture, fracture of the skull on skull roentgenogram, and eventually evidence on computed tomography (CT)

- Head trauma with contusion of the brain and brain edema. History, external injuries, lumbar puncture, the skull roentgenogram, and eventually CT, all can provide evidence of such injury
- Acute bacterial meningitis, meningismus, and fever with evidence from lumbar puncture. Signs of infection suggest this cause
- Encephalitis, with evidence to be found in signs of inflammation, lumbar puncture, and the electroencephalogram
- Intracranial space-occupying lesion, particularly brain tumor, brain metastasis, brain abscess, and intracranial hematoma. CT should be utilized. Search for signs of increased intracranial pressure and neurologic deficits. Most often, lumbar puncture is contraindicated
- Epileptic attacks (*see* 2.3). Attention to history, description of the attacks from witnesses, evidence of tongue biting, urinary incontinence, and slow awakening after 10 to 20 minutes of drowsiness with an intervening period of clouded consciousness, and eventually new attacks during hospitalization (status epilepticus)
- Orthostatic collapse, cardiac dysrhythmia, vasovagal syncope, swallowing syncope, micturition syncope, cough syncope, carotid sinus syndrome
- Breathholding attacks of childhood (always preceded by anger or crying, breathholding). Cyanosis or pallor occurs with attacks
- Other internal diseases, for example, cardiac failure or pneumonia. Signs of these diseases emerge from the general physical examination, electrocardiography, roentgenography of the chest
- Psychogenic 'coma.' Findings of neurologic and general examinations are normal. Fluttering of the lids and swallowing movements are evident; there is usually downward deviation of the eyes regardless of body position. When the oculocephalic reflex is tested, the patient may fix gaze on a distant point and the eyes move in the direction of head movement or the patient looks at the examiner. The EEG gives the impression of normal 'sleep' patterns; blood sugar and electrolyte status are normal

Diagnostic difficulties are usually found in two conditions involving or resembling a disturbance of consciousness:

- Coma vigil. The patient appears awake, with eyes open but not fixed, and is completely unresponsive to voice, and nearly so to other stimuli. Most often the cause is anoxia resulting from increased intracranial pressure and subarachnoid bleeding
- The 'locked-in' syndrome. Resembling a disturbance of consciousness, this syndrome is due to an infarction of the corticobulbar and corticospinal tracts at the level of the abducens nuclei in the mid portion of the pons. Patients are conscious, but can communicate only by means of lid movements or vertical eye movements. The most common causes are tumors, ischemia, and demyelination

2.3 Attack-like (Recurrent) Disturbances

The present chapter amplifies the preceding discussion of sudden disturbances of consciousness (*see* 2.2.1) and clouding of consciousness (*see* 2.2.2). Considered in this chapter are repeated attacks associated with disturbances of motor or sensory function and most often also with impairment of consciousness. This group of attacks is comprised predominantly of epileptic fits, but a number of other paroxysmal disorders are also included. Because such paroxysmal dysfunction must at one time or another occur for the first time, or without a previous history of attacks, the classification used in this chapter is arbitrary and differs from that in the previous chapter.

2.3.1 Attacks with Predominantly Motor Disturbances

Abnormal movements appearing suddenly or within several minutes

- Involuntary movements
- Inability to move

The underlying disturbance is usually due to a discharge of cortical motor neurons and rarely to discharges of other parts of the motor system. Attacks of paralysis, however, can result from functional disturbances of central motor tracts or muscles.

2.3.1.1 Attacks Characterized by Transient Episodes of Abnormal Movement and Abnormalities of Tone

Epilepsies:

- Classic grand mal epilepsy (always generalized fits with deep unconsciousness, cyanosis, foaming at the mouth, often tongue biting or urinary incontinence or both). Witnesses should be questioned; there may be history of an epileptogenic brain lesion. A search should be made for tongue biting and for soiled clothing. The EEG is always abnormal during an attack, but between seizures is abnormal in only 50%. All other types of epilepsy can be combined with grand mal attacks, and all types of focal epileptic attacks (see below) can combine with and end in a grand mal seizure with loss of consciousness
- Focal motor epilepsies (without loss of consciousness)
  - adversive attacks (tonic movement of the eyes, head, and arm to the side opposite the involvement)
  - Jacksonian fits (clonic movements starting in one part of the body, mostly the hand or face, often extending to the homolateral side in a 'march of convulsion')
  - partial motor epilepsy (clonic movement beginning on one side of the body without further extension often followed by hemiplegia, known as hemiconvulsive hemiplegia syndrome or Todd's paralysis)
  - epilepsia partialis continua of Koževnikov (continuous clonic movements of a circumscribed part of the body may be the manifestation of a focal motor status, but the EEG does not always show a focus in the appropriate contralateral motor cortex)
  - short twitching or myoclonic phenomena (found in myoclonic astatic petit mal of childhood and in myoclonus and myoclonus epilepsy).

Not strictly epileptic but often classified as such are convulsive syncopes, most frequently associated with tonic extension of the extremities

Figure 20 gives an overview of cortical areas from which focal epileptic attacks arise.

As *causes of epilepsy*, the following must be mentioned:

- Hereditary influences (particularly common in primary generalized attacks and also in grand mal and true petit mal)
- perinatal trauma (can give rise to all types of epileptic attacks, particularly temporal lobe epilepsy; indications of perinatal trauma are seizures or febrile convulsions in early childhood and sometimes other neurologic signs of perinatal brain damage, including lefthandedness, squint, and psychomotor retardation)
- Lesions of the brain acquired postnatally, such as traumatic; after meningitis or encephalitis; brain tumors; and vascular insults (can give rise to all forms of epilepsy, particularly focal types)
- Progressive disorders of the brain, particularly a tumor. Suggestive of this cause are the following elements:
  - late epilepsy, beginning after the 30th year of life
  - focal attacks or focal beginning in fits that become generalized
  - resistance to therapy
  - associated unusual headache
  - associated neurologic deficits
  - evidence of increased intracranial pressure
  - psychologic and behavioral disturbances

All these suggest pursuit of neuroradiologic and other investigations.

Tonic brain stem attacks ('brain-stem epilepsy') affect only half of the body, always occur ipsilateral to the lesion, and do not impair consciousness. Attacks are often provoked by changes in posture or by hyperventilation, cause painful contractures of all muscles of the hemibody lasting fractions of minutes, and are followed by a refractory period. The causes are mostly multiple sclerosis (younger patients) and vascular disorders (older individuals); a rare cause is tumor of the brain stem.

In familial paroxysmal choreoathetosis there are minute-long attacks of choreoathetosis beginning in distal parts of the body. The disorder is usually evident in childhood. Attacks culminate in a refractory period, as in tonic brain stem attacks.

Paroxysmal choreoathetosis in thyrotoxicosis has been described. Familial attacks of ataxia, nystagmus, and dysarthria have also been recognized. These may also sporadically occur in cases of multiple sclerosis and may include attacks of localized dystonias. Paroxysmal choreoathetosis has been described in patients with diabetes mellitus during recurring hypoglycemic episodes. Enzyme defects may give rise to episodic ataxia in combination with other encephalopathic symptoms as in carnitin-acetyltransferase deficiency.

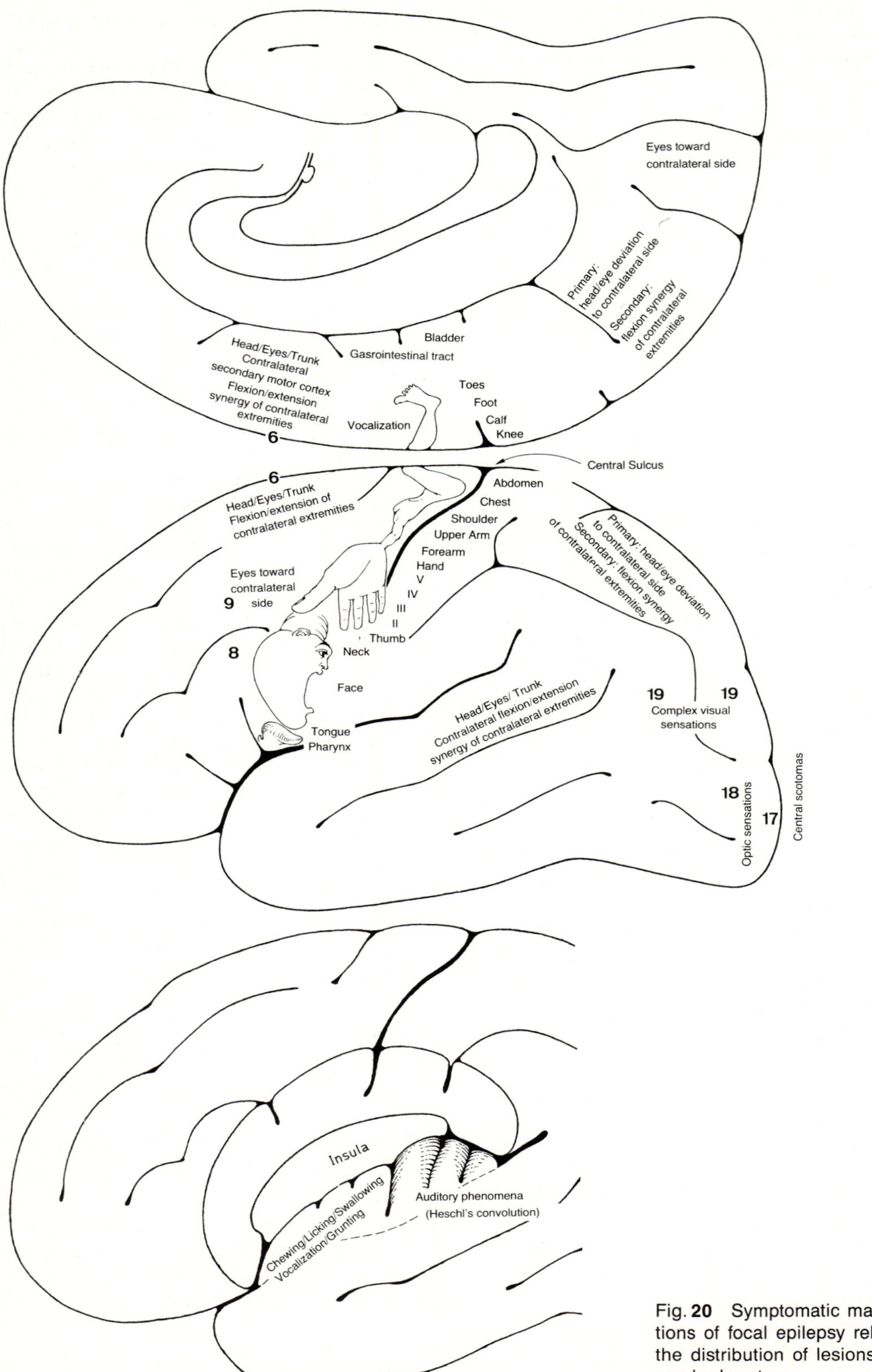

Fig. 20 Symptomatic manifestations of focal epilepsy related to the distribution of lesions in the cerebral cortex

Attacks of shivering ('startle disease') are seen in brain-damaged children. Disturbances of blood flow in the territory of the basilar artery have been associated with repeated attacks of transitory hemiballism. Segawa disease is accompanied by pronounced diurnal variations in the severity of focal dystonic movements which are manifest in childhood. A good response to L-Dopa is of diagnostic significance. Nocturnal paroxysms of dystonic movements occur in some patients with epilepsy and respond to carbamazepine.

2.3.1.2 Episodic Attacks of Motor Weakness

Transient dysfunction of central motor neurons can occur

- At the cerebral level (compare Fig. 1), as a manifestation of transitory blood flow disturbances
  Among these disturbances are
  - transient ischemic attacks (TIAs) with a local disorder of blood vessels, often associated with a generalized hemodynamic crisis or with emboli. TIAs are characterized by the sudden appearance of deficits lasting minutes to hours, subsequent attacks at the same site, the presence of risk factors, and sometimes, mostly in elderly subjects, bruits on auscultation of the extracranial blood vessels. TIAs can also occur in younger individuals with sources for emboli
  - migraine accompagnée: not always accompanied by a history of migraine, this dysfunction is most often associated with paresthesia and sensory disturbances, usually progressing over $\frac{1}{2}$ hour to 1 hour or longer, and rarely complete paralysis. Occasionally the opposite side is also involved during an attack. Such attacks are most often accompanied by contralateral headache (exception: migraine sans migraine) and generally occur in younger individuals or children
- At the level of the brain stem. Such disturbances in basilar blood flow can produce
  - so-called drop attacks, manifested by short hypotonia of the legs, leading to falls without loss of consciousness. Drop attacks are most often seen in older patients, and individuals with vascular risk factors or other signs of basilar artery insufficiency

- akinetic attacks, similar to drop attacks, and occurring in a context of myoclonic astatic petit mal. Such attacks are found in children with myoclonic jerks and other petit mal symptoms, and eventually short alterations of consciousness and appropriate EEG findings, and in adults as a manifestation of psychomotor epilepsy (see 2.3.3)
  - attacks probably localizable pathophysiologically to the brain stem and due to ischemia occur with loss of consciousness in laugh epilepsy and cough epilepsy
  - attacks of sleep paralysis, which occur with preservation of consciousness during wakefulness and last seconds to minutes as part of the narcoleptic syndrome (see 2.3.4)
  - the affective attacks of loss of tone (cataplexy)
  - unavoidable falls, usually forward, which can be early symptoms of Parkinson's syndrome
- At the level of the spinal cord. Such disturbances can include
  - habitual odontoid dislocation
  - transient paraplegia lasting minutes and dependent on head movement (commotio spinalis). Such paraplegia results from spinal column trauma; history is important.

Transient, more or less acute, dysfunction of muscle can also be due to abnormal metabolism of potassium, as in

- Hypokalemic periodic familial paralysis (hereditary, flaccid paralysis developing within hours into tetraplegia, without respiratory muscle involvement or participation of facial musculature; it often is induced by effort, cooling, or carbohydrate intake, and disappears immediately on the administration of potassium or within hours without treatment). Slowly appearing similar symptoms may be due to symptomatic hypokalemia with renal disease, abuse of laxatives, or primary aldosteronism
- Attacks of hyperkalemia with adynamia episodica hereditaria (Gamstorp) (hereditary and myotonic phenomena)

In some diseases of muscles, for example, myasthenia, paroxysmal myoglobinuria, and phosphorylase deficiency, rapid, but not really attack-like, weakness can occur (see 2.13.1.2)

2.3.2 Attacks Predominantly Characterized by Sensory Disturbances

Sensory disturbances include short-lived sensory positive phenomena (paresthesia, pain) and negative deficits (limbs going to sleep, loss of feeling). Some of the causes of these sensory attacks have already been described under the heading· of motor deficits.

With focal epilepsy in a setting of jacksonian fits, paresthesia can occur, sometimes followed by transient abnormalities in sensation. These are focal episodes, occurring mostly in one hand or starting in the face, and then spreading within minutes but remaining unilateral, except for those attacks that are secondarily generalized and eventually culminate in a grand mal seizure. Most such abnormalities in sensation, however, disappear within minutes without loss of consciousness. Occasionally they are accompanied by motor weakness.

Localized paroxysmal attacks of pain have also been described in epilepsy.

Tonic brain stem fits may be accompanied by pain in one-half of the body. Such pain may also be isolated, occurring without chronic muscle contraction.

The cause of such attacks in young individuals is practically always multiple sclerosis, which presumably is also responsible for localized attacks of pain lasting for minutes and for paroxysmal paresthesia.

In tetany, paresthesia occurs bilaterally ·in the hands and perioral region. Most often, younger individuals are affected, especially women. Anxiety, air hunger, and hyperventilation can trigger such attacks. Consciousness may eventually be disturbed, carpopedal spasms can occur, and a positive Chvostek sign is found. (For the similar symptoms of migraine accompagnée, *see* above.)

2.3.3 Attacks Predominantly Characterized by Impairment of Consciousness and Syncopes

The causes of sudden coma are described above (*see* 2.2.2), as are the sudden disturbances of consciousness associated with grand mal seizures and some other forms of epilepsy (*see* 2.3.1 and 2.3.2). In certain forms of epilepsy, however, the disturbances of consciousness are the primary manifestation:

- In absence epilepsy (pyknolepsy). This almost always occurs in children or begins in childhood, with frequent attacks — many every day — that last only seconds, characterized by staring, eventually some fingering of clothing or mouth movement, but not by falls
- In temporal lobe epilepsy (partial attacks with complex symptoms). Such twilight attacks last several minutes or hours and often are heralded and accompanied by chewing and other oral mechanisms. There is fingering of clothing and often purposeless and eventually abnormal activity, although actions sometimes appear useful and orderly. The patient does not remember the attacks. Temporal lobe epilepsy can manifest itself alone or in conjunction with attacks of disturbances of vegetative function and of mood (*see* 2.3.4)
- With temporal lobe status, hours to days of twilight states
- With petit mal status (status pyknolepticus) (epileptic-specific electroencephalogram is often the deciding diagnostic test)
- The differentiation of temporal lobe epilepsy from the disturbances of consciousness associated with hypoglycemia is sometimes difficult. Hypoglycemia most often occurs during fasting, but occasionally it occurs postprandially; it is associated with irritability and sweating. Blood sugar estimation and the immediate effect of intravenous glucose administration or of oral intake of sugar are factors in diagnosis. Hypoglycemia may be associated with insulin administration or islet cell tumors
- Also similar to temporal lobe epilepsy are attacks of beta-adrenergic hyperactivity, manifested by attacks of palpitation, a crushing feeling in the chest, anxiety, irritable behavior, and an immediate response to propranolol

Pseudoseizures are not rare in children (often imagined by mothers) and are frequently provoked by manipulations (attention to psychopathology of the mother, socioeconomic aspects and signs of trauma, particularly to the neck.)

Syncopes are defined as transient short-duration losses of consciousness accompanied by falls. The following causes should be considered:

- Cardiogenic (disturbances of cardiac rhythm, for example, Stokes-Adams syndrome, aortic stenosis)
- Vascular reflex syncope due to vagal activation and bradycardia (e.g., with severe pain)

- Vasovagal syncope (emotion, prolonged standing, with visual obscuration, dizziness and sweating)
- Swallowing syncope (after glossopharyngeal nerve injury; glossopharyngeal neuralgia)
- Pressor reflex syncope (post-Valsalva maneuver; e.g., caugh or gelastic; micturition or stretch syncope)
- Vestibular-cerebral syncope (always preceded by very short-duration dizziness)
- Impaired orthostatic vasomotor control; in this category are idiopathic vasomotor collapse of adolescence and also orthostatic hypotension (e.g., progressive autonomic failure, multiple system atrophy, Addison's disease, autonomic neuropathies, etc.)
- Focal arterial disease, e.g. vertebral and/or basilar pathology ('drop attacks') or aortic arch syndrome
- Rare causes of syncope, e.g., atonic brain-stem attacks, cataplexy as part of the cataplexy-narcolepsy syndrome, cryptogenic falls in women or falls in parkinsonism. All these attacks are in essence falls *without* loss of consciousness
- Many syncopes remain *etiologically unclear*

Vascular causes of sudden disturbances of consciousness (without coma) include

- Amnestic episodes (transient global amnesias, *ictus amnésique*). These occur rarely in migraineurs, more often without evidence of other vascular disease in middle life, with sudden loss of the capacity to remember and learn accompanied by more or less prolonged retrograde amnesia. Patients ask the same question over and over without remembering answers. The memory hiatus extends back over days or months. Activities remain orderly and complex. The attacks, which last one or several hours, are marked by disappearing retrograde amnesia up to the beginning of the episode and continuous amnesia for the duration of the attack itself. Rarely this occurs in younger individuals, induced by oxychinoline derivatives or in a setting of (basilar) migraine

Psychogenic disturbances of consciousness often have emotional affect. A psychogenic origin should be suspected when the motor components are atypical, when the attacks often occur in critical situations, when there are no pathologic laboratory findings, when the electroencephalogram is normal even during attacks and there is absence of postictal slowing of the electrogenesis of the brain.

2.3.4 Attacks of Disturbances of Vegetative Function

This group excludes those disturbances of vegetative function that occur in association with major diseases. It comprises disturbances of the sleep/wakefulness cycle, respiration, cardiac activity, nutrition, and sexuality. Hypersomnia and other disturbances of sleep are the leading symptoms in the following disorders:

- Narcolepsy (uncontrollable desire for sleep in inappropriate situations, lasting from 10 minutes to an hour. The subject can be awakened — for cataplectic attacks and sleep paralysis see 2.3.1.2.1; clinical examination and EEG are normal)
- Sleep-apnea syndrome due to upper-airway mechanical obstruction, neurologic disorders in the posterior fossa (e.g., syringobulbia, olivopontocerebellar atrophy; for symptoms, see Pickwickian syndrome)
- Pickwickian syndrome (obesity, episodic somnolence, confusion, loud snoring during sleep, difficulty in waking, long periods of apnea. Clinical examination is normal, but the EEG is pathologic)
- Kleine-Levin syndrome [found in young men and manifested by periods of sleep lasting several days, excessive eating (bulimia, polyphagia) and confusion]
- Nonepisodic, pathologic sleep, occurring in such conditions as encephalitis lethargica and trypanosomiasis and with organic processes in the posterior hypothalamus

Abnormal loss of weight is characteristic in

- Anorexia nervosa (occurs in young girls and women and is marked by decreased intake of food and by vomiting, often induced and secretive)
- Russell syndrome (tumor of the hypothalamus, mostly 3rd-ventricle, in young children, producing emaciation despite normal food intake and eventually associated with diabetes insipidus)

Acute episodic vegetative symptoms are sometimes seen in such disorders as

- Temporal lobe epilepsy, in which it can occur without twilight states (*see* 2.3.3). Characteristic symptoms are a sudden sensation in the epigastrium ascending to the throat, palpita-

tion dyspnea, air hunger, fear, a choking feeling lasting 10 minutes to hours
- Beta-adrenergic hyperactivity (spontaneous or induced by infusion of isoproterenol, and producing tachycardia, a feeling of pressure in the chest, fear, nervousness, dyspnea, and shivering, lasting for minutes to hours).

2.4 Disturbances of Smell

It is to be noted anatomically that the bipolar olfactory cells have a peripheral process in the olfactory epithelium. The process is found in a 2-cm square area of the olfactory mucosa, at the roof of both upper nasal passages. The central neurites of these neurons, gathered in bundles, penetrate the approximately 40 elements of the fila olfactoria and the lamina cribrosa, and terminate in the overlying bulbus olfactorius in the anterior fossa. These fibers synapse in the olfactory bulbs. Through the olfactory tract and the olfactory stria, most of the second-order neurons reach the amygdala, and pass on as tertiary neurons to the parahippocampal gyrus and finally to the cortical projection areas. Some of the second-order neurons reach the septal area and pass from there to the contralateral limbic system. The relations of these limbic system connections to the autonomic nuclei in the hypothalamus and to affective mechanisms have been discussed (*see* 2.2.1). Impairment of the sense of smell can be caused by lesions in the periphery up to and including the olfactory tract. This disturbance is always associated with an impairment of 'taste.' Abnormal olfactory sensations can occur with stimulation of the amygdala and of the hippocampus.

Simple impairment of smell (hyposmia) is difficult to assess without special apparatus. Most often it is caused by changes in the nasal mucous membranes and remains the domain of the ear, nose, and throat specialist.

Complete loss of the sense of smell (anosmia) is usually of concern to neurologists. It is associated with a subjective disturbance of taste (ageusia), which is due to the preservation of the four cardinal taste qualities without the capability of finally gauging flavor, for which smell is required.

The causes of anosmia are

- Changes in the nasal mucous membrane, particularly of the embedded sensory neurons. Such changes commonly occur in atrophic rhinitis, following acute viral infections with rhinitis, and unilateral or total absence of ventilation through the nose). In such cases, distortion of smell, often of an unpleasant character (parosmias), occurs
- Aplasia of the olfactory bulbs, producing total anosmia. This occurs in the Kallmann syndrome (hypogonadism with eunuchoid gigantism, absence of puberty, and occasionally color blindness)
- A number of generalized diseases such as diabetes mellitus, Sheehan syndrome, hypothyroidism, scleroderma, Paget's disease, zinc deficiency (for example, with histidine medication). Disturbances of smell and taste can also occur after laryngectomy or administration of penicillamine, L-dopa, phenindione, methimazole, betablockers, various antibiotics, antirheumatic drugs, antidiabetic drugs, hypotensive agents, clofibrate, amphetamine
- Contusion of the midbrain in the wall of the third ventricles, leading to a combination of anosmia and ageusia
- Severe head and brain trauma, resulting in tears of the olfactory fila or contusion of the olfactory bulbs or nerves. This is the most common cause of anosmia. Only a third of the cases are eventually reversible
- A tumor in the anterior fossa. With total anosmia without preceding trauma, an olfactory meningioma, which also causes psychopathologic changes, frontal signs, and epileptic attacks, should be suspected. Ancillary tests may be necessary for diagnosis

Spontaneous attacks of olfactory hallucinations must be distinguished from those changes in smell discussed above, which are disturbances in the response to actual smells. Olfactory hallucinations are almost always an expression of epileptic events. These sensations are paroxysmal, often unpleasant (cacosmias), and they are rarely due to activation of the olfactory bulbs. More often they result from activation of the uncus and the amygdala or the base of the temporal lobes. They sometimes accompany a complex of temporal epileptic symptoms or are the initial symptoms. Their cause can lie in scar tissue or in tumors of the temporal lobe, which result in so-called uncinate crisis. Rarely migrainous attacks may be accompanied by olfactory sensations together with the usual visual phenomena.

Disturbances of taste usually accompany those of smell (*see* above). Mostly, however, there is impairment of taste discrimination mediated by olfaction. True post-traumatic anosmia is accompanied by ageusia in only 5% of cases. Impairment of the sense of smell occurs after glossopharyngeal zoster. Disturbances of taste can occur as transient dysgeusia in elderly individuals, in case of psychosis, or after chemical damage to the mucosa of the tongue.

2.5 Visual Disturbances

To understand disturbances of vision, familiarity with the anatomy of the visual system is important. The visual stimuli impinging upon the retina initiate a photochemical reaction in the rods and cones (the first neuron of the visual pathways) which, in turn, activate the bipolar cells (second-order neuron) and the ganglion cells (third-order neuron). In the optic nerve the central projections of these neurons pass through the chiasm and the optic tract to the lateral geniculate body. There the synapse to the fourth-order neuron occurs. The central projections of the fourth-order neuron pass through the visual radiation to the cortical visual centers in the visual cortex, located around the calcarine fissure of the occipital lobe (Fig. 21). Certain fibers in the optic tract, however, reach the pretectal area, without synapsing in the geniculate body. In the pretectal area they synapse bilaterally to the parasympathetic Westphal-Edinger nucleus, which carries constrictor impulses to the sphincter pupillae via the ciliary ganglion, thus participating in the light reflex (*see* Fig. 36). Because of these anatomic arrangements and the topographic distribution of fibers in the visual pathways, it is possible to accurately localize the site of lesions. From the history it is also possible to draw conclusions about their cause.

2.5.1 Impairment of Vision (Decreased Acuity)

Purely ocular disturbances of vision are the province of the ophthalmologist, but must be considered by the neurologist in differential diagnosis.

2.5.1.1 Slowly Progressive Impairment of Vision (Unilateral or Bilateral)

Slowly progressive impairment of vision can have the following origins:

— Ocular, such as macular degeneration, familial Leber's optic atrophy, which is progressive over the course of years and is diagnosed by means of examination of the fundus
— Optic nerve compression (mostly unilateral visual impairment). One example is compression of the chiasm, marked by a pale optic nerve head, often by different visual field defects in both eyes, and eventually by headache. Its course is progressive over months or years. Causes of compression include tumor (meningioma, optic glioma in children, dermoids) aneurysm of the carotid artery (resulting in impairment of ocular motility), carotid calcification (eventually sellar enlargement)
— Chronic increase in intracranial pressure, manifested by papilledema, headache, enlargement of the blind spot, neurologic findings depending on the cause of increased cranial pressure, eventually by attacks of amblyopia (*see below*) and by a course progressing over weeks or months
— Toxic causes, e.g., some industrial solvents, probably also hydroxychinol derivatives
— Homonymous field defects. These, particularly when they appear gradually, may not be noticed by the patient (for example, in tumor of a hemisphere) and are often described as visual impairment

2.5.1.2 Sudden or Rapidly Progressive Visual Loss

Causes of unilateral disturbances:

— Fracture of the anterior fossa reaching into the optical canal. History and signs of head trauma, anosmia or external evidence of injury, paleness of the optic nerve head 3 weeks after injury, and appropriate radiologic studies all suggest this cause
— Vascular disturbances, for example
  ● arteriosclerotic ischemic optic atrophy, suggested by pseudopapilledema, eventually pale retinas, pallor of the optic nerve head, never complete blindness
  ● temporal arteritis, which often leads to complete blindness and occurs in elderly individuals. Nearly always patients com-

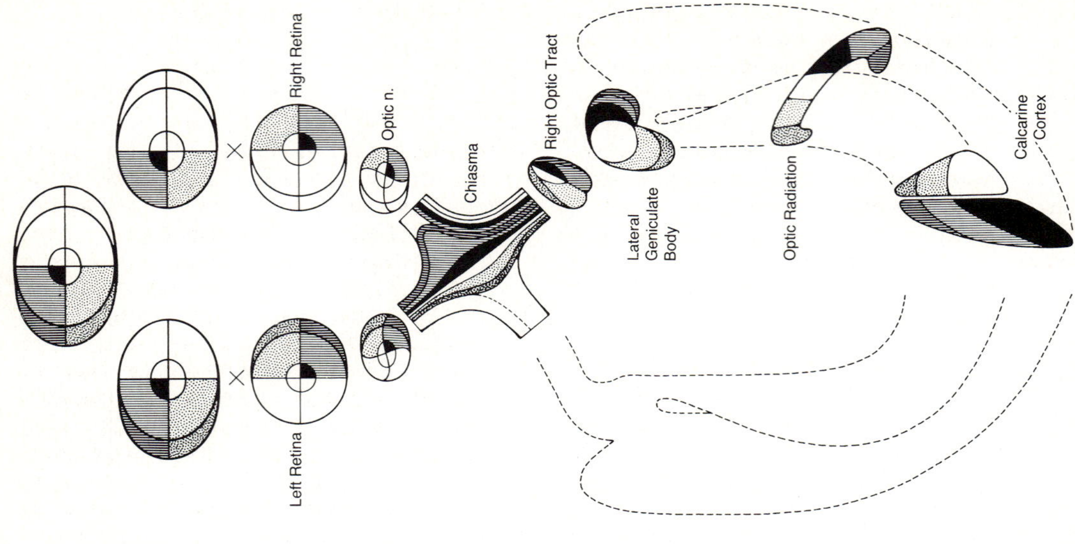

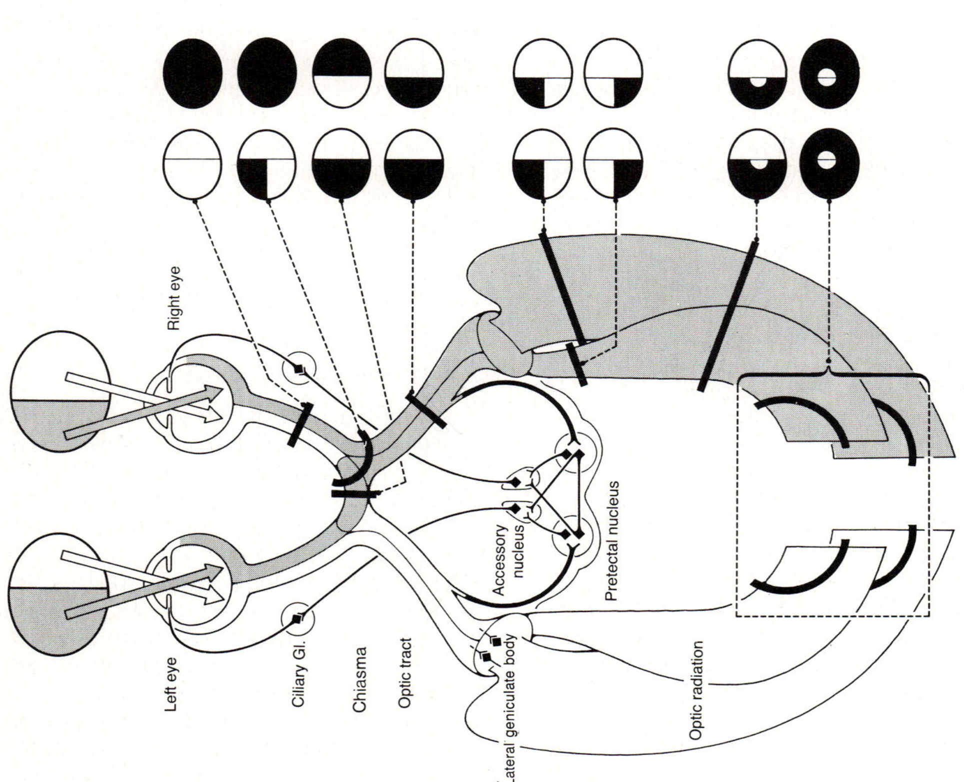

Fig. **21** Visual pathways; with lesions and appropriate visual field defects (left); with topical arrangements of fibers from the retina to the calcarine cortex (right)

plain of headache, and usually the sedimentation rate is increased. The temporal artery is most often pathologically involved

● amaurosis fugax with internal carotid stenosis (marked by bruits over the arteries and eventually by contralateral hemisymptoms) is another vascular cause of unilateral disturbance

— Retrobulbar neuritis, which reaches its maximum within a day or several days and occasionally produces pain in the eyes and flashing in the visual fields on eye movement, occurs mostly in younger individuals and never leads to complete blindness. At the beginning the fundus is normal, there is improvement within several days, and the disorder is seldom bilateral

— Attacks of amblyopia with papilledema (last only seconds; accompanied by evidence of increased intracranial pressure; also occur with pseudotumor cerebri)

Causes of bilateral sudden or rapidly progressive loss of vision:

— Vascular ischemia of the retina. Rarely bilateral retinal ischemia occurs with aortic arch syndrome, with sudden change from recumbent to upright posture

— Vascular bilateral visual cortex lesions, marked by impairment of basilar blood flow and sudden onset. Elderly individuals are especially at risk. Impairment of color vision precedes the onset of symptoms; pupillary reactions remain normal; differentiation from visual agnosia is necessary

— Intermittent compression of the posterior cerebral artery against the tentorium by supratentorial tumors causing displacement of the hemispheres may rarely cause similar symptoms

— Toxicity, for example, methyl alcohol (visual loss appears overnight; attention to history is important, later both optic discs appear pale); tobacco and ethyl alcohol (Tobacco-alcohol amblyopia progresses over days to weeks)

— Psychogenic blindness (pupillary reaction and fundus are normal; the patient does not behave like a newly blinded individual and has experienced none of the usual causes of blindness; opticokinetic nystagmus is preserved if the patient can be made to fix normal visual evoked potentials)

2.5.2 Impairment of Visual Fields

Field defects are rarely associated with changes in visual acuity. They are rarely noted by the patient, but when perceived, are often described as vague disturbances in vision. The field defect, determined instrumentally, allows localization of lesions in the visual system. This is shown diagrammatically in Figure 21. Horizontal field defects, which are not included in the figure, are of ocular (retinal) or optic nerve origin if unilateral. Bilateral horizontal field defects are sometimes due to lesions of the chiasma, but more often are due to a space-occupying or vascular disorder of the occipital lobe above or below the calcarine fissure. The etiology of field defects is not often apparent from the history alone because, as mentioned above, the visual field defect remains unnoticed by the subject. The principal causes of visual field defects follow:

— Intracranial supratentorial space-occupying lesions; including tumors, aneurysms, arteriovenous malformations, abscesses, and hematomas. Indications of such a lesion are a suggestive history, rapid progress, evidence of increased intracranial pressure, focal neurologic deficit, epileptic attack. Special investigations are often necessary for diagnosis

— Head trauma with contusion of the brain, indicated from history and neurologic deficits

— Cerebral vascular insults, most often with other longstanding deficits (*see* 2.3.1.2). Ischemia may be limited to the visual cortex on one side resulting in absence of other neurologic deficits, sparing of macular vision, and with only minor impairment of function

In bilateral ischemia of the visual cortex (*see* 2.5.1.2), ophthalmic migraine occupies a special position (*see below*).

— As a component of chiasmatic syndromes, in the form of bitemporal hemianopia and eventually binasal hemianopia (Fig. 21). In this setting, the following causes should be considered:

● chromophobe adenoma (secondary endocrine insufficiency)

● eosinophilic acromegalic adenoma of the pituitary, marked by enlargement of the sella turcica and by optic disc pallor

● craniopharyngioma, always found with endocrine symptoms, especially hypothalamic syndromes, for example, with diabetes insipidus (lack of drive); marked by destruction of the sella turcica with calcification

- meningioma of the tuberculum sellae showing hyperostosis on roentgenograms
- dermoid or teratoma, often found with hypothalamic syndromes
- aneurysm of the internal carotid artery, resulting in paralysis of extraocular muscles and often showing shell-like calcification on roentgenograms

When symptoms appear suddenly, hemorrhage in the chiasmatic region must be considered. Most often this results from a small vascular malformation or tumor. Sometimes associated with a monocular field defect is neglect of a visual field (which can be recognized only with simultaneous testing of both fields). This is a manifestation of a parietal lobe lesion.

2.5.3 Other Disturbances of Vision (without double vision, see 2.8.1)

To this category belong:

- Mouches volantes, harmless inclusions in the hyoloid body or local other changes in the refractive media or retina
- Scintillating scotomas, typically expressions of ophthalamic migraine accompanied by other manifestations of migraine, these are transient disorders with scintillation-enlarged homonymous scotomas, starting in the center of the visual field and progressing peripherally, the disorder progresses within 10 minutes and at the beginning is usually accompanied by contralateral hemicrania, except in migraine without headache. Most often found in children or young adults, they rarely leave residual permanent visual field defects
- With retinal anomalies, e.g., Moor's lines, recurrent stereotyped visual sensations have also been described
- Photophobia occurs in meningitis and migraine and can be associated with vascular lesion of the thalamus
- Unilateral visual loss in bright light can occur with homolateral carotid occlusion
- Primitive or complex formed visual hallucinations. Such hallucinations occur as the expression of an epileptic local phenomenon, with disorders of the visual cortex or visual association areas, or in a recently sustained hemi-

anopic field (as the product of autonomous discharges of cells that have been deafferented — so-called sensory-deprivation hallucinations)
- Palinopsia, that is, persistence or de novo perception of a previously perceived picture (occurs with occipital lobe lesions)
- Oscillopsia (rhythmic and constantly directed apparent movement of the surroundings found, for example, with nystagmus)
- Dysmorphopsia, in which objects are seen as smaller (micropsia) or larger (macropsia) than they actually are or as in some way deformed. This occurs with temporal lobe epilepsy, but also with migraine (the so-called Alice-in-Wonderland syndrome)
- Reading disabilities, for example, alexia (*see* 2.1), eye motility disturbances with dyslexia (*see* 2.1), ocular apraxia (*see* 2.8.2.2)
- Acquired disturbances of color vision and of color recognition (achromatopsia), often occurring with ischemia of the visual cortex (*see* 2.5.1.2) or with left-sided ischemic softening in the supply territory of the posterior cerebral artery (*see* 2.1)
- Seeing all subjects in one color (monochromatopsia), found bilaterally with digitalis intoxication, for example, in which all objects are yellow, and unilaterally with bleeding in the macular area (erythropsia).

2.6 Disturbances of Hearing

The anatomic basis of the sense of hearing comprises the conductive apparatus of the external and middle ear. The perceptive apparatus includes the cochlea with the organ of Corti, the auditory nerves (part of the eigth nerve and the vestibulo-cochlear nerve, also called the acoustic nerve), the central conduction of hearing from the cochlear nuclei, in part polysynaptic to the inferior colliculus, and the medial geniculate body. From the medial geniculate body the auditory input passes through the acoustic radiation through the posterior limb of the internal capsules to the cortical centers of hearing in the transverse temporal gyrus (Heschl gyrus). In the neighborhood of this gyrus are the secondary auditory cortical centers for analysis of acoustic signals, and dorsally adjacent to these structures in the sensory Wernicke speech area.

Most hearing disorders are in the province of the otologist. Nevertheless, some intracranial neurologic affections are associated with disturbances in hearing, and many patients with such disorders are referred either primarily or for additional consultation to the neurologist. For the neurologist it is important

— First, to distinguish between conductive and perceptive deafness
— To recognize the various causes of conductive deafness
— To partially interpret a number of other acoustic phenomena

2.6.1 Features Distinguishing Conductive from Perceptive Deafness

The differential diagnosis of the two types of deafness is made by means of the Rinne, Weber (Fig. 22), and Schwabach tests. Normally, air conduction is better than bone conduction, and this feature is used in the Rinne test:

The vibrating tuning fork (preferably 256 or 512 Hz) is first placed on the mastoid process. When the sound is no longer perceived, the fork is placed immediately in front of the ear of the patient. With normal hearing and with partial perceptive deafness, the fork should be heard for twice as long when it is at the ear as when it is vibrating on the mastoid (results of the Rinne test are normal). In conductive deafness, the fork is heard only, or predominantly, through the mastoid (results of the Rinne test are abnormal) (Fig. 22), indicating that air conduction is impaired or absent. With conductive deafness, bone conduction is better because the conductive apparatus between the drum and the oval window is damaged. The Weber test is carried out by placing the tuning fork in the midline on the forehead. With conductive deafness the sound is heard better on the impaired side, whereas with perceptive deafness the better ear hears the sound better (Fig. 22).

In the Schwabach test, used in bilateral deafness, a tuning fork is placed on the mastoid process of the patient, then on the mastoid of the examiner. In conductive deafness the patient hears the fork for a longer period than the examiner, whereas in perceptive deafness the patient hears the tuning fork for a shorter period or not at all.

2.6.2 Hearing Impairment or Deafness

Conductive deafness is in the province of the otologist. The neurologist is concerned with this type of deafness only as a consideration in differential diagnosis. However, perceptive deafness, often a cause of total hearing loss, and its pathogenesis are of concern to the neurologist.

Acute deafness or severe hearing impairment of sudden onset can be unilateral or bilateral. Possible causes are

— Virus infection, particularly mumps, without swelling of the parotid gland. Hearing loss is occasionally bilateral. Mumps in personal or family contacts and the complement fixation reaction suggest a viral cause. Herpes zoster, also without a skin eruption, can result in deafness. (Varicella titers increase with contact with chickenpox, other cranial nerve involvement)
— Meningitis (basal) due to a variety of infectious agents. Deafness most often occurs in seriously ill patients with meningismus, fever, CSF abnormalities and occasionally, though by no means always, involvement of other cranial nerves
— Disturbances of circulation, usually in the distribution of the internal auditory artery, manifest as cochlear apoplexy. These cause unilateral hearing loss, mostly in elderly individuals, and often show improvement of about 50%
— Trauma with fracture of the petrous temporal bone, suggested by history, appearance after a latent period, usually involvement of vestibular function, abnormalities on inspection of the drum such as rupture of the rim, hematoma, and roentgenograms of the pyramidal bone showing fractures
— Rupture of the oval or round window, often as a result of barotrauma associated with changes in atmospheric pressure during airplane flights

More or less rapidly progressive impairment of hearing (eventually leading to total deafness) can have the following causes:

— Intracranial tumors with involvement of the vestibular cochlear nerves. Hearing loss is unilateral [exception: the rare bilateral acoustic neurinomas with von Recklinghausen's disease], tinnitus is often present, and there is always involvement of the vestibular function as well. Sooner or later other cranial nerves,

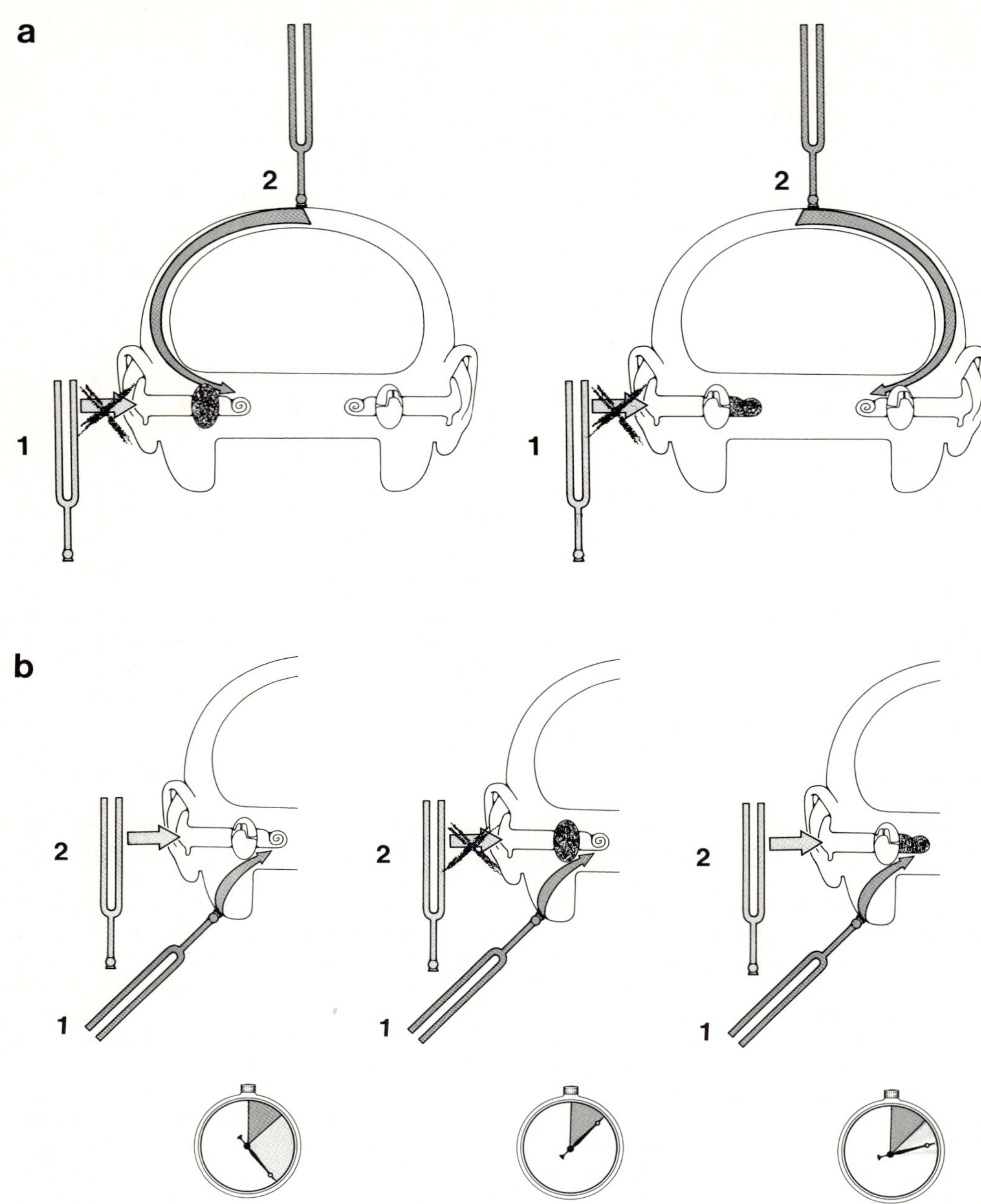

Fig. **22a** and **b**   Hearing tests. **a Weber test:** In right-sided conduction deafness (left diagram) the tuning fork is no longer audible in front of the ear, but the tuning fork placed on the forehead is audible on the deaf side. With right-sided perception deafness (right diagram) the sound is lateralized by the patient to the normally hearing ear. **b Rinne test:** With normal hearing (left diagram) the tuning fork is first placed on the mastoid; and when no longer audible there, the sound is still audible in front of the ear for about an equal time. With right-sided conduction deafness (middle diagram) the disappearance of the sound with a tuning fork on the mastoid (bone conduction) is also associated with failure to hear the sound with the tuning fork in front of the ear. With right-sided perception deafness (right diagram), the sound is perceived in front of the ear but with reduction in duration particularly the facial nerves, are affected, and later generalized symptoms associated with increased intracranial pressure appear; most often changes are noted in the CSF, which are due to the extra-axial location of the tumors. Such tumors must be differentiated from posterior fossa meningiomas, dermoids, arachnoid cysts, and cerebellar astrocytomas

- Other processes involving the subarachnoid space, including carcinomatous meningitis (*see* 2.9.2) and suppurative meningitis, leading to acute or subacute impairment of hearing (*see above*)
- Disease of bone and bone tumors. Among these are Paget's disease (marked by deformity of the extremities and a characteristic roentgenographic appearance of the skull), bone tumors or metastasis in the skull (commonly showing involvement of other cranial nerves and visible on plain films of the skull), glomus tumors (indicated by tinnitus, subjective and objective pulse synchronous bruits, involvement of other cranial nerves, increased intracranial pressure, and eventually a bluish tumor visible behind the drum)
- Genetic disorders associated with metabolic abnormalities, usually resulting in bilateral hearing loss and often showing other neurologic or neurocutaneous abnormalities. Examples are Refsum's disease (with symptoms of areflexia, hemeralopia, ataxia, increase in CSF protein content) and Niemann-Pick disease
- A variety of infectious diseases and internal disorders, including syphilis, particularly in the perinatal form, scarlet fever with otitis, measles, Cogan syndrome
- Multiple sclerosis with special sites of plaques. The deafness is rarely bilateral, but other sudden dysfunction of the nervous system and involvement of long tracts in the brainstem are noted
- Meniere's disease. Hearing loss ensues after many attacks, and there is concomitant loss of excitability of the vestibular apparatus, in the typical history (*see* 2.7.1)
- Drug-toxic causes, as after administration of streptomycin, neomycin, gentamicin, and transiently after quinine and acetylsalicylic acid
- Otologic causes – otosclerosis, chronic sound trauma (as in discotheques), presbyacusis, diseases of the middle ear, traumatic rupture of the oval window due to barotrauma, incurred during rapid descent from mountains or in aircraft

2.6.3 Abnormal Acoustic Phenomena

Tinnitus is in most cases a harmless phenomenon appearing, often bilaterally, in middle-aged or older individuals. It is always unpleasant and more bothersome in quiet surroundings, but it is not usually treatable. There is no accompanying deafness that could not be attributed to other causes, no other neurologic dysfunction, and no headache. Tinnitus can, however, also occur in polycythemia vera or with increased intracranial pressure; for example, it is found in one out of five patients with pseudotumor cerebri (*see* 2.7.1). Unilateral tinnitus is often etiologically identical to the bilateral phenomenon, but it can also be due to local processes with lesions of the vestibulocochlear nerves. Such lesions also produce homolateral impairment of hearing with eventual symptoms of posterior fossa dysfunction. Unilateral tinnitus also accompanies Meniere's disease (*see* 2.7.1).

Pulse-synchronous auditory noises. These are frequently perceived in bed when there is no surrounding noise, and they have no significance. If, however, such noises are heard continuously, they can be the result of stenosis of the carotid artery, arteriovenous malformation, or glomus tumor. In such cases, careful auscultation of head and neck and a thorough history to exclude epileptic attacks or neurologic deficits are indicated. Paracusia or acoustic hallucinations are usually manifestations of temporal lobe dysfunction. In one such hallucination, noises are perceived as abnormally loud or soft, but the former can also occur with paralysis of the stapedius muscle in connection with peripheral facial nerve paralysis. A sequence and occasionally a repetitive series of words (paliacusis) or true acoustic hallucinations (elementary or even complex word synthesis or melodies) are almost always due to temporal lobe dysfunction. They are occasionally part of a temporal lobe twilight state (*see* 2.3.3). Occasionally these are not recognized as hallucinatory in nature. The abnormal function usually arises in the upper lateral temporal lobe, the result of tumor, scar, arteriovenous malformation, or other cause.

2.7 Disorders of Equilibrium, Vertigo and Dizziness

Equilibrium is the capacity to move effectively and maintain balanced posture even under conditions of stress. This capacity depends on the normal cooperative functioning of a large number of structures in the nervous system, particularly

- The vestibular apparatus
- The visual system
- The proprioceptive mechanisms and
- The motor system

The vestibular apparatus, the visual system, and the proprioceptive mechanism represent the three columns or information channels upon which the motor system is dependent in executing the appropriate movements and necessary corrections in posture.

The anatomic substrate of this system is illustrated in Figure 23. Following is a summary of the activity of this system.

- Input from the vestibular apparatus (semicircular canals, sacculus and utricle):
  - reach the vestibular nuclei in the brain stem
  - from which pass impulses via the vestibular spinal tract to influence tone, the reflex activity, and with it the function of the truncal musculature
  - via the medial longitudinal fasciculus, impulses also reach the neck muscles and thus influence position of the head
  - through the vestibular spinal tract, connections are established with the vagus nuclei, which in turn can affect autonomic function (vomiting)
  - simultaneously the position of the eyes (nystagmus) is influenced through the medial longitudinal fasciculus, maintaining optical orientation in space
  - impulses also pass via vestibular cerebellar fibers to the nodulus and flocculus of the cerebellum and to the fastigial nuclei and red nucleus, through which a connection with the cerebellar regulatory system is established
  - the medial longitudinal fasciculus establishes connections with the thalamus from which impulses pass via thalamocortical fibers to the cortex. From the cortex, association fibers transmit the passage of impulses to the motor centers and the pyramidal pathways

  - at the same time, vestibular impulses also reach the dentatorubral pathways and the red nucleus through the cerebellum (fastigial nuclei and dentate nuclei) and pass again to the thalamus, where impulses after synapsing reach the extrapyramidal regulatory system, which governs tone and motor activity. (Compare with Fig. 3)
  - a cortical center for incoming vestibular impulses is found posterolateral to the temporal lobe near the sylvian fissure

- Sensory afferents pass from the periphery to the cerebellar nuclei through the dorsal spinocerebellar tracts (together with the vestibulocerebellar tracts), via the inferior cerebellar peduncle, and through the ventral spinocerebellar tract, via the brachium conjunctivum. In the cerebellum these fibers synapse to participate in the motor control of the cerebellar regulatory system
- Visual influences are mediated by the occipital cortex in the calcarine fissure, containing the visual association centers, in areas 18 and 19, where visual afferent input is compared with memory traces and interpreted and 'recognized.' From the visual association area, optomotor association fibers pass in the internal sagittal plane of the occipital and parietal lobes to the motor centers in the anterior, central, and precentral regions. Through this system, visual afferents are capable of influencing eye movement and the extrapyramidal regulatory activity

In the differential diagnosis of disturbances of equilibrium and dizziness it is necessary to consider dysfunction or lesions in the four systems (vestibular, visual, proprioceptive, and motor). A description of characteristic features of dysfunction in each of these systems is given below, together with the most common causes of such disturbances.

2.7.1 Dizziness with Vestibular Dysfunction

Dizziness with vestibular lesions. In the acute (initial) phase, dizziness of vestibular origin is always associated with a feeling of rotation — a merry-go-round-like sensation — along with inability to stand, nausea and eventual vomiting, sweating, and nystagmus. Later, after days or weeks, the acute symptoms subside, although disturbances of vestibular function may continue. Deficits that

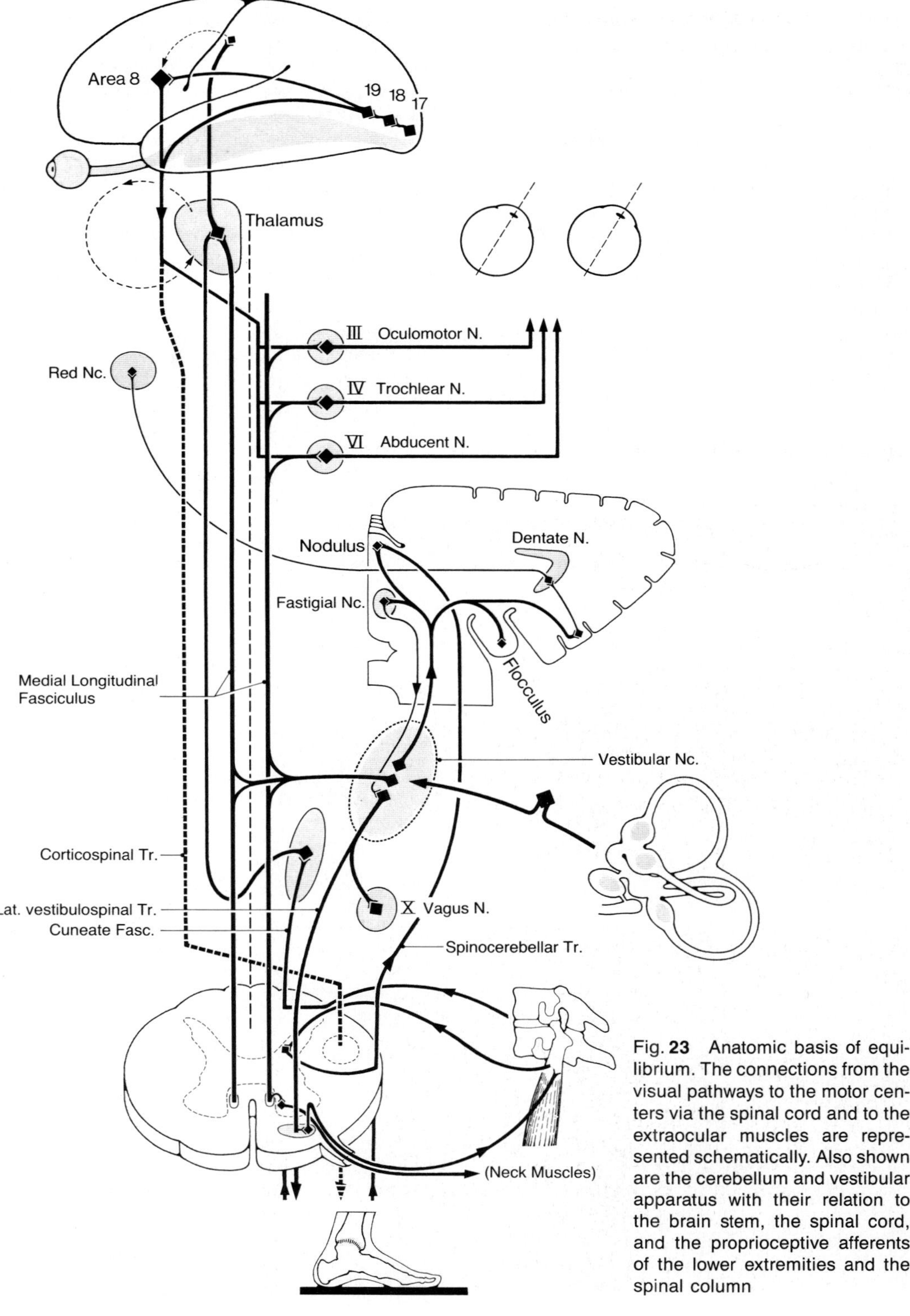

Fig. **23** Anatomic basis of equilibrium. The connections from the visual pathways to the motor centers via the spinal cord and to the extraocular muscles are represented schematically. Also shown are the cerebellum and vestibular apparatus with their relation to the brain stem, the spinal cord, and the proprioceptive afferents of the lower extremities and the spinal column persist are different in peripheral and central vestibular dysfunction. They are described in Table 14.

In unilateral vestibular dysfunction, there is usually complete functional restoration after several weeks: The patient is not severely incapacitated even in stressful situations. With bilateral loss of vestibular function (usually of peripheral, but occasionally of central origin), only the function of the proprioceptive and visual systems remains in control of equilibrium. The result is unsteadiness and a tendency to fall while walking on an uneven surface or soft ground (walking on a mattress is an effective test) and also during twilight or darkness.

Nystagmus is an important finding with both vestibular and cerebellar lesions. A gaze paretic nystagmus occurs with lesions of the supranuclear centers that are related to eye motility, although it also occurs, although rarely, in primary extraocular muscle weakness, for example, myasthenia gravis. Occasionally optokinetic nystagmus is also impaired.

Nystagmus can also occur with marked visual loss and can be of congenital origin. Congenital nystagmus disappears with lid closure, whereas nystagmus of vestibular origin continues. Certain individuals may produce voluntary nystagmus. In intoxication and some hereditary metabolic disorders, nystagmus may occur paroxysmally together with ataxia and, eventually, dysesthesia. Nystagmus also occurs in one fifth of patients with pseudotumor cerebri manifested by headache and evidence of increased intracranial pressure without focal neurologic deficits or space-occupying intracranial lesions. The characteristics of various forms of nystagmus are given in Table 15 and Figure 24. The direction of nystagmus is given according to its fast component.

The causes of vestibular dizziness or disturbances of equilibrium are

— Lesions of the peripheral vestibular apparatus:
  ● Meniere's disease (short rotatory attacks of dizziness lasting minutes to several hours, accompanied by tinnitus or other auditory

Table 14   Symptoms of peripheral and central lesions of the vestibular apparatus

	Peripheral vestibular apparatus	Central vestibulocochlear nerve	Central vestibular apparatus
Vertigo	Marked rotatory vertigo	Less intense	Marked
Duration of vertigo	Short	Continuously recurring	Longer
Vomiting	Marked	None	Marked
Nystagmus	Mostly horizontal	Rapid component to opposite side	Occasionally rotatory or dissociated vertigo
Hearing	Often involved	Tinnitus always occurs eventually	Not involved
Standing and walking	Veering toward affected side on walking		Always impairment of standing and walking
Vestibular tests impaired			Vestibular disharmony (contradiction in direction of labyrinthine symptoms
Remarks	No other neurologic dysfunction (except eventual hearing loss)	Mostly associated with other peripheral, cranial nerve, and cerebellopontine angle symptoms	Associated brain stem symptoms almost always apparent immediately or soon after onset

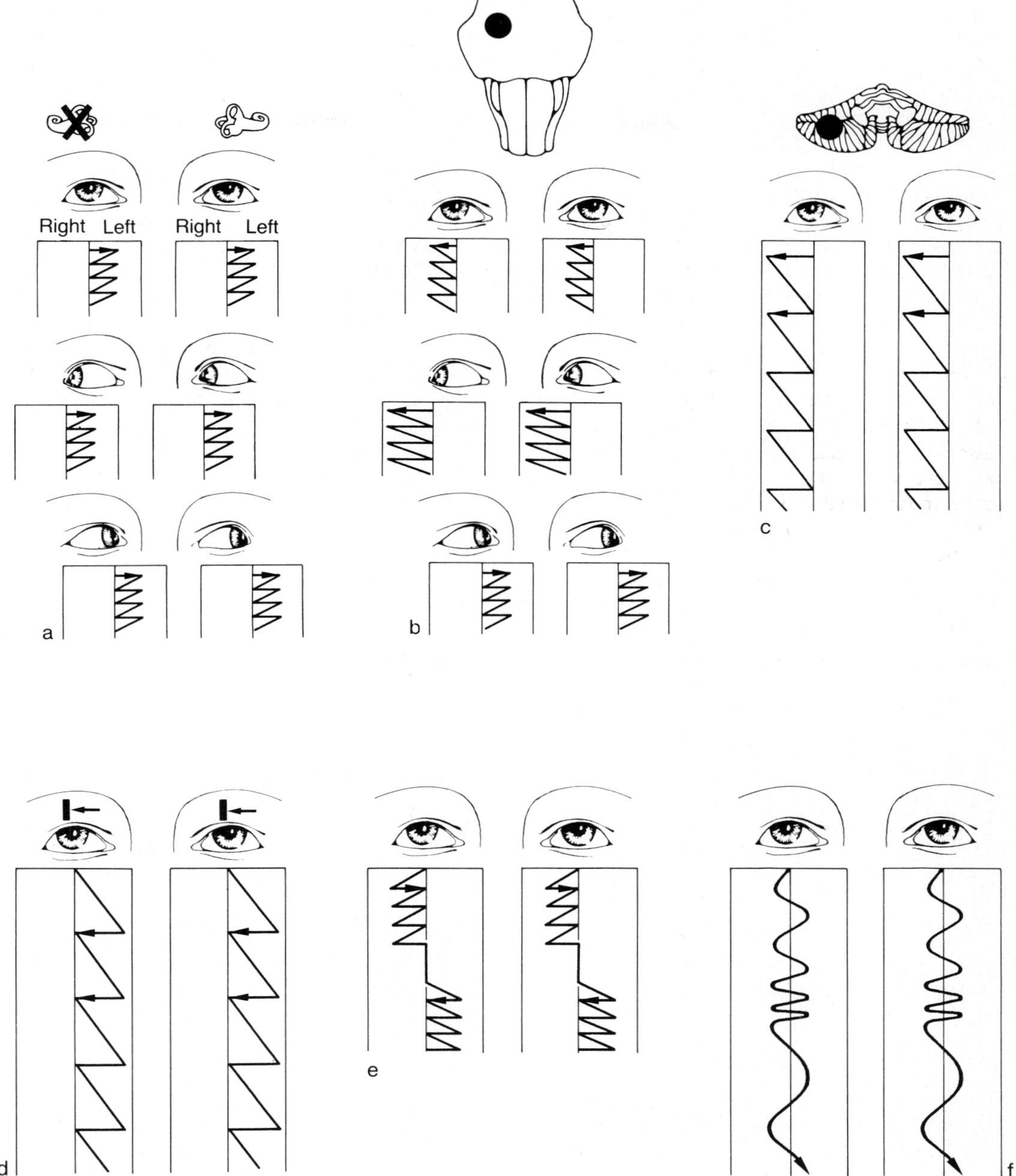

Fig. 24a–q   Type of nystagmus according to site of lesion. **a** Vestibular cochlear nerve; **b** brain stem lesion; **c** cerebellar lesions; **d** gaze paretic nystagmus; **e** optokinetic nystagmus; **f** with early visual disturbances; (continued)

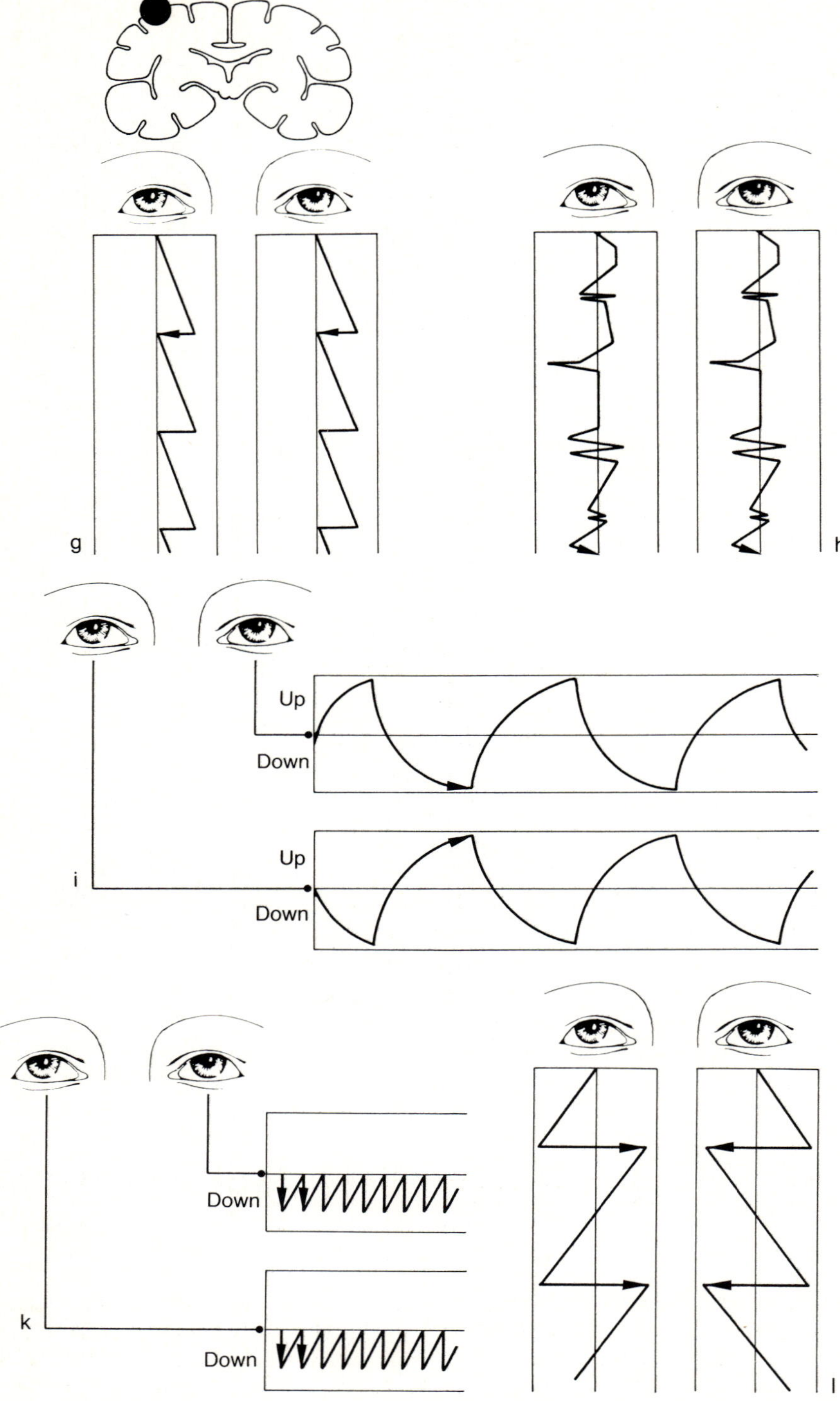

Fig. 24 (cont) **g** cortical nystagmus; **h** voluntary nystagmus; **i** see-saw nystagmus; **k** down-beating nystagmus; **l** convergent nystagmus

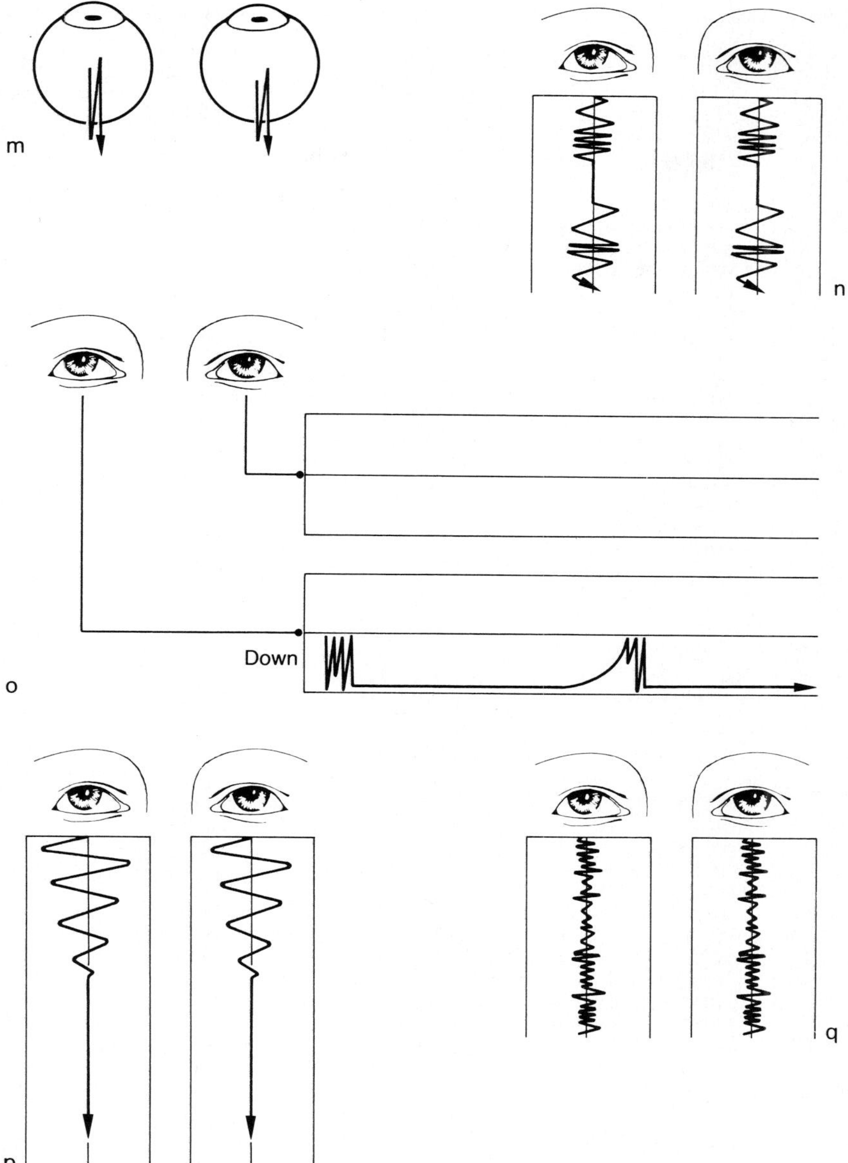

Fig. **24** (cont) **m** nystagmus retractorius; **n** opsoclonus; **o** ocular bobbing; **p** ocular dysmetria; **q** ocular flutter. (See Table 15 for characteristics and localization of lesions **a–q**)

- manifestations and increasing deafness, and positive recruitment)
- Lermoyez syndrome (similar to Meniere's disease, but with diminished hearing prior to attacks and improvement in hearing during the attacks of dizziness)
- vestibular neuronitis (isolated, rarely recurring attacks of rotatory vertigo lasting hours to days with no tinnitus or hearing loss). The attacks may abate for days but can be elicited again by changes in position. Each attack is followed for weeks by

Table 15 Characteristics of various types of nystagmus and nystagmus-like eye movements according to site of lesion[a,b]

	Characteristics	Localization	Cause and examples
Vestibular Peripheral vestibular apparatus	Nystagmus is directional; away from lesion (in all directions of gaze; nystagmus always in same direction, i.e., to side opposite lesion, most marked horizontally; occasionally, spontaneous nystagmus disappears within several weeks; influenced by eye closure (increasing) and changes in position of head	Peripheral vestibular apparatus	See 2.7.1
Vestibular cochlear nerve (a)		Vestibular cochlear nerve	See 2.7.1
Brain stem lesions (b)	Usually toward lesion, increases with gaze toward the side of lesion. Occasionally, rotatory nystagmus, dissociated nystagmus, or gaze nystagmus in all directions of gaze	Vestibular nuclei and their central connections	See 2.7.1
Cerebellum (c)	Coarse nystagmus; toward side of lesion; increases with gaze toward lesion; decreases with eye closure; head movement has no influence		
Ocular Gaze (eye muscle)-paretic nystagmus (d)	Mostly slow, coarse beating; rapid component in direction of impaired gaze; associated with supranuclear lesions, with nuclear or peripheral eye muscle paralysis; occurs only in affected eye – monocular nystagmus	Supranuclear or in other parts of oculomotor system	See 2.8.1
Optokinetic nystagmus (e)	Normal; rapid component; reposes eyes into neutral position; frequency dependent on rapidity of movement in visual field	When impaired, optomotor fibers from area 18	After trauma; with infarctions and tumors
With early visual loss (f)	Pendular nystagmus, changing in frequency; occasionally slow, conjugate movement of both eyes around neutral position with unilateral amblyopia; rarely unilateral, occasionally also vertical	?	Visual impairment severe; congenital or acquired within first 2 years of life
Latent (congenital) (without visual impairment)	As above; disappears with voluntary eye closure. Increased by fixation in congenital nystagmus, always accompanied by strabismus, visible with unilateral eye occlusion	?	No significant visual loss
Cortical nystagmus (g)	Slow deviation of eyes away from irritating lesions, then rapid correction to midline; later, predominance of normal frontal eye centers and conjugate deviation toward side of lesion	With irritation of frontal eye centers in areas 6 and 8 of second frontal convolution	Ischemia; tumors as irritative focuses; trauma

(continued)

Table 15   (continued)

	Characteristics	Localization	Cause and examples
Voluntary nystagmus (h)	Rapid, fine, short duration, conjugate pendular nystagmus; inconstant, often accompanied by fluttering of lids; no spontaneous nystagmus; mostly horizontal, rarely vertical		
See-saw nystagmus (i)	Alternate up and down movements of each eye in opposite direction with associated rotatory movements	Upper brain stem or diencephalon	Tumor, multiple sclerosis, vascular cause, or syringobulbia
Abnormal eye movements confused with nystagmus Down-beat nystagmus (k)	Vertical nystagmus with rapid downward component	Lesions caudal to medulla oblongata. B_{12} deficiency	As above; diphenylhydantoin intoxication; drugs
Convergent nystagmus (l)	Slow abduction followed by rapid adduction of eyes	(Rostral) mesencephalon	As above
Nystagmus retractorius (m)	Sudden backward movement of both eyes into orbits; usually associated with other disturbances of eye movements	Midbrain	Rare; tumor, multiple sclerosis, vascular cause
Nystagmus with lid retraction	Vertical nystagmus with rapid upwards component synchronous upper lid retraction	Pons or aqueduct	Often vascular
Nonocular nystagmus	With intranuclear ophthalmoplegia As ictal phenomenon in epilepsy	Medial longitudinal fasciculus	Very rare as part of seizure
Opsoclonus (myoclonus, dancing eyes) (n)	Spontaneous group movements, with rapidly changing, nonrhythmic conjugate eye movements; random side-to-side movements of eyes	Brain stem and cerebellum	Paraneoplastic, with neuroblastoma; multiple sclerosis; encephalitis
Ocular bobbing (o)	Rapid, nonrhythmic downward movement of eyes, which remain there for several seconds before slow elevation to midposition; unilateral, although other side often exhibits extraocular muscle weakness and usually oculomotor paresis (may be accompanied by synchronous palatal movements)	Pons; compression due to cerebellar bleeding (lesion of central tegmental tracts)	Tumor, ischemia, bleeding
Ocular dysmetria[c] (p)	Overshooting of eye movements on fixation; compensatory correction	Cerebellar	Multiple sclerosis
Ocular flutter (ocular myoclonus) (q)	Rapid, irregular to-and-fro movement around fixation point	With opsoclonus and ocular dysmetria	

[a] See also Table 14.
[b] (a) to (q) refer to Figure 24.
[c] For ocular apraxia see 2.8.1.

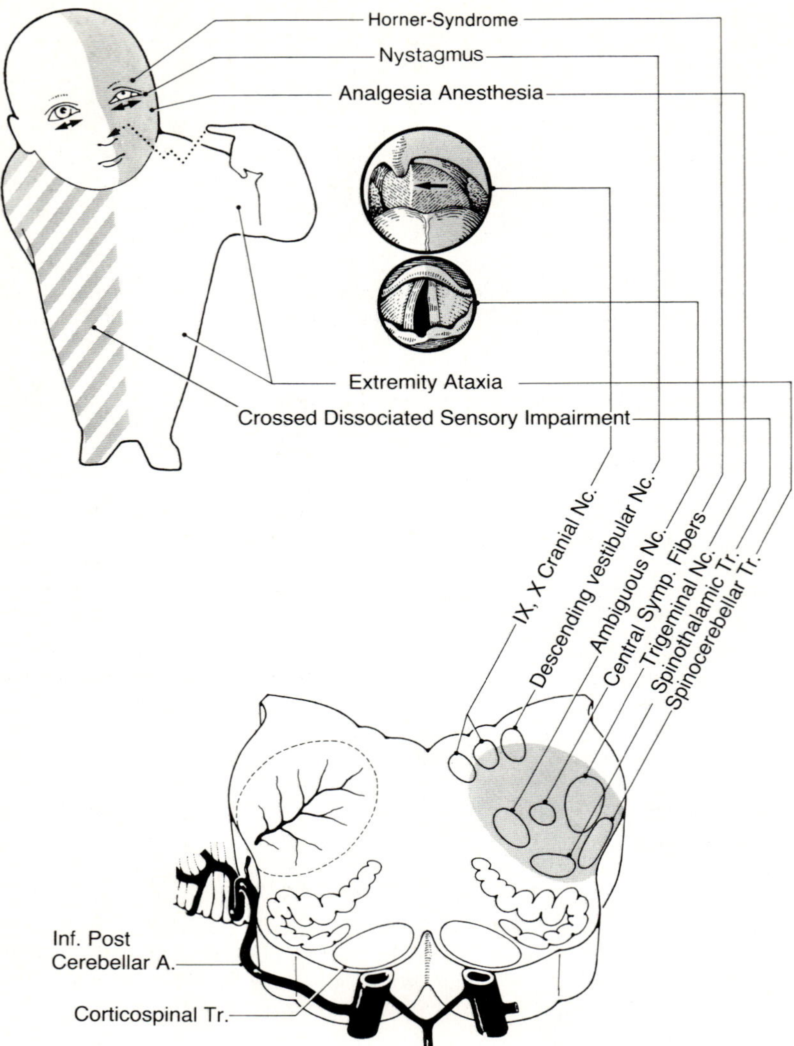

Fig. 25   Localization of lesion, anatomic basis and symptoms of a left Wallenberg syndrome (lateral medullary infarction)

instability during rapid movement. Similar symptoms occur in epidemic vertigo and vertigo after tick bites

- benign paroxysmal positional vertigo (vertigo triggered by certain head positions, with rotatory vertigo provoked by rapid recumbency from the sitting position with head rotated 30 degrees to one side)
- direct trauma or infection (otitis media) of the semicircular canals with (surgically approachable) perilymphatic fistula

- toxic or pharmaceutical damage, resulting especially from alcohol, streptomycin, quinine, barbiturate, diphenylhydantoin, tranquilizers, and antihistamines
- vascular apoplectic insults to the labyrinth, usually acute, unilateral, and associated with loss of hearing (risk factors)
- infections, such as herpes zoster (manifested by pain, vesicles, noises in the ear, paresis of other cranial nerves, particularly the facial nerve) or mumps. Lesions of the

vestibular apparatus with infectious causes are often bilateral, associated with swelling of the parotid glands and their surroundings and with antibodies
- irritation of the semicircular canals by water penetration during diving in subjects with perforated ear drums
- Cogan syndrome (interstitial keratitis, tinnitus, nystagmus, and progressive deafness)
– Lesions of the vestibular cochlear nerve:
- fracture of the skull (results in impairment of hearing and tinnitus; indicated in history)
- tumors, particularly acoustic tumors (tinnitus is often present, a slowly progressive decrease in hearing occurs, later other cranial nerves are involved, and negative recruitment is noted)
- chronic basal meningitis (distinguished by impairment of multiple cranial nerves, appropriate CSF findings)
- meningeal carcinomatosis (*see* 2.9.2)
– Lesions of the central vestibular apparatus (nuclei and their connection). Such lesions do not involve hearing and are distinguished by acute symptoms, often lasting longer than those produced by peripheral lesions, special nystagmus features (Table 15) and eventually other brain stem symptoms:
- vascular causes associated with brain stem infarction, such as the Wallenberg syndrome (occurs mostly in elderly patients, with clear sensorium, acute rotatory dizziness with vomiting, hoarseness, nystagmus, homolateral Horner's syndrome, deficient trigeminal system function, palatal weakness, asymmetry of faucial pillars, ataxia of extremities, and contralateral dissociated sensory loss of the extremities) (Fig. 25). Vascular insufficiency may be transient in patients with basilar migraine
- tumors, for example, brain stem gliomas (marked by slowly progressive symptoms and involvement of other brain stem structures; soon accompanied by an increase in cranial pressure due to obstruction of the aqueduct)
- multiple sclerosis (*see* 2.13.2.5.1; also test auditory evoked potentials)

2.7.2 Dizziness and Unsteadiness with Disorders of Afferents Arising in the Periphery

With such lesions, symptoms do not appear suddenly, and there is neither rotatory vertigo nor nystagmus. Unsteadiness is never present during complete rest, as while sitting. It does, however, increase during twilight or with eye closure, and also with rapid head movement (in situations, therefore, in which input of other afferents important for equilibrium is removed).

Common causes are

– Diffuse lesions of peripheral nerves or spinal roots
- polyneuropathies (*see* 1.3.5)
- polyradiculitis (*see* 1.3.1)
– Posterior column lesions (particularly in cases with disturbances of joint position sense and of movement of skin folds on trunk, with massive ataxia, without motor deficits or distal sensory loss, and with unimpaired reflexes):
- tabes dorsalis (marked by pupillary abnormalities, impaired pain sensation, serologic findings)
- subacute combined degeneration with vitamin B_{12} deficits (resulting in massive disturbances of joint position sense with ataxia and eventual pyramidal signs) or malignant disease (manifested in general or local signs of tumors)
- degenerative diseases, such as spinocerebellar atrophy, Friedreich's ataxia, and others, mostly familial, very slowly progressive, and accompanied by evidence of other system degeneration

2.7.3 Dizziness and Unsteadiness with Lesions of the Cerebellum and the Extrapyramidal Control and Regulatory Systems

With these disorders, there are no acute disturbances and, notably, no rotatory vertigo. The abnormalities are apparent only during movement. Movements are therefore limited in range, and coordination is impaired, causing disharmony and unsteadiness.

– Cerebellar disturbances. There is hypotonia, ataxia, dysmetria, wide-based gait, and instability of the trunk when sitting. General cere-

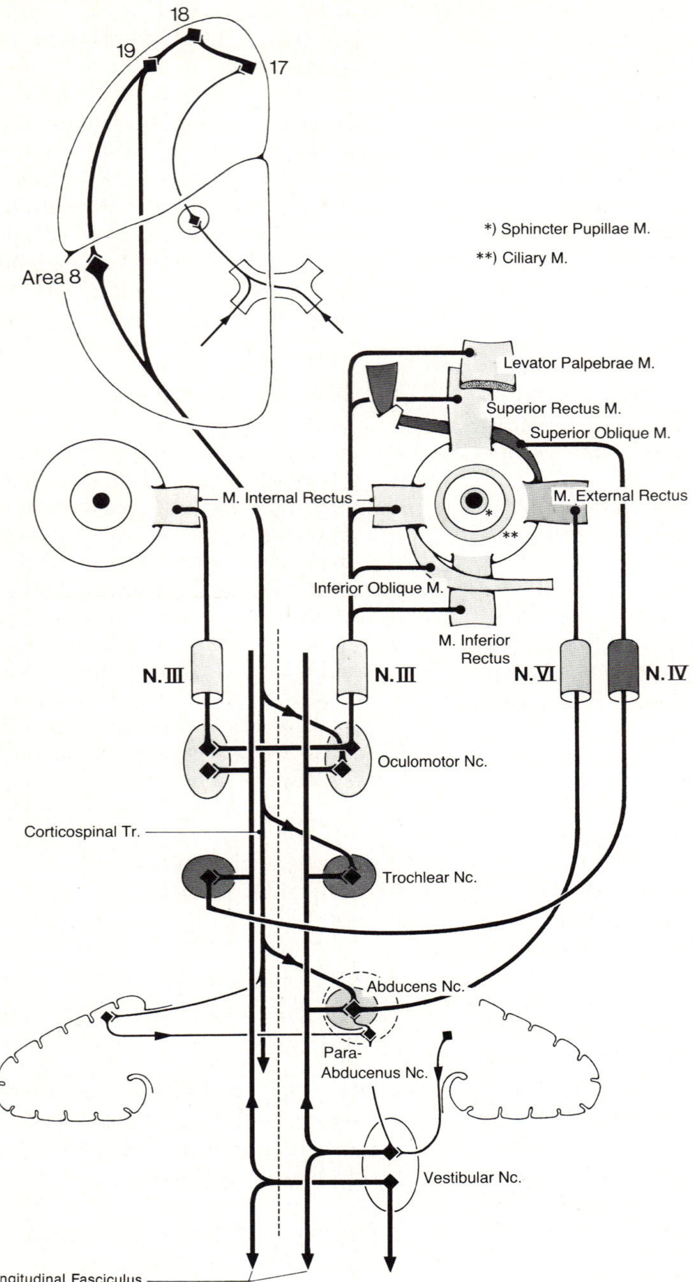

Fig. **26**   The anatomic background of ocular motility

bellar symptoms, their localizing value, and causes of cerebellar disease are given in 1.1.4
— Extrapyramidal disorders. Such syndromes are marked by unsteadiness resulting from disturbances of automatic movements, an increase in tone (as in Parkinson's syndrome), or interference by involuntary movements with normal movement (as in chorea, athetosis, or torsion dystonia) (*see* 1.1.3.1)

2.7.4 Other Causes of Vertigo and Unsteadiness

- The Barré-Lieou syndrome with cervical spondylosis, also known as the syndrome of the upper body quarter (symptoms include poorly defined unsteadiness, neck pain, burning facial sensations, tinnitus, disturbances of swallowing, and often brachialgias)
- autonomic dizziness (marked by palpitation, sweating, orthostatic difficulty, fearfulness)
- Tetany (*see* 2.3.2)
- Focal epileptic attacks with lesions of the posterolateral temporal lobe cortex near the sylvian fissure. The patient experiences a rotatory sensation, occasionally attack-like in character, which might later on generalize to a complex epileptic attack)
- Temporal lobe epilepsy (*see* 2.3.3). At the beginning of attacks the patient often describes dizziness.

2.8 Disturbances of Ocular Motility, Ptosis, and Pupillary Abnormalities

The anatomic substrate of ocular motility is summarized in Figure 26. There are four main components:

- The six extraocular muscles whose innervation and function are detailed in Table 16 and Figure 27
- The three cranial nerves concerned with ocular motility and their nuclei (Fig. 26), comprising the peripheral motor neuron of the extraocular muscles. A lesion affecting these structures always causes a deviation of the eyes and practically always double vision
- The supranuclear visual centers and their connections with each other and with both oculomotor nuclei:
  - in area 8 the frontal convolution gives rise to impulses for voluntary eye movement, particularly of conjugate gaze (and head movement) toward the opposite side. The impulses pass through the corticonuclear tract of the internal capsule and the medial parts of the pyramids and then, after synapsing, through intermediate neurons in the reticular formation of the rostral midbrain (with area representation for upward and downward gaze and for rotatory eye movement). Lastly the impulses pass through the medial longitudinal fasciculus to the oculomotor nuclei
  - in the occipital 'visual center' of area 19 arise the fibers that are triggered by visual afferent impulses related to visual reflex eye movement. The impulses reach this area along fibers that travel, paralleling the visual radiation, to the cortical area related to vertical eye movement and via the medial longitudinal fasciculus to the pontine field of the opposite side, which is related to horizontal eye movement. There are, however, also subcortical connections via association fibers from the occipital to the frontal eye fields through which at least some of the impulses for reflex eye movements are also conducted
  - the pontine field for horizontal eye movement (the pontine eye center; nucleus paraabducens) receives and transmits impulses from both cortical centers mentioned above and distributes them mainly through the medial longitudinal fasciculus to the nuclei concerned with coordinated movement of the eyes
- Integrated into the above-mentioned circuitry are impulses, related to reflex eye movements, received:
  - in areas 18 and 19, arriving from the visual system via the cortical eye centers in area 17 and their connections
  - in the oculomotor nuclei, but also in areas concerned with eye movement in the rostral midbrain, arriving from the vestibular system via the medial longitudinal fasciculus (but probably also after synapsing in the cerebellum)
  - in pontine eye centers, arriving from proprioceptors in the extremities and trunk but also particularly from the neck via ascending fibers of the medial longitudinal fasciculus

These structures enable coordinate (conjugate) movements of the eye and ensure that the reflex activity and movements of the eyeballs maintain the image on the fovea of the retina even when the object or the observer is moving in space.

Lesions of the above-named structures have varying effects upon eye motility, enabling the site

Table 16 Functions of oculomotor nerves and external ocular muscles; position of paretic eye; and double image

Nerve	Muscle	Main function	Subsiary function	Position of paretic eye (deviation from primary position)	Double image	
					Direction of gaze and maximum separation	Position and type
Oculo-motor	Internal rectus	Adduction of eye	None	Temporal	Nasal	Side by side, crossed
	Superior rectus	Elevation, action increasing in abducting eye; no function if eye adducted	Adducts eye and rotates vertical meridian inward; action improving when eye adducted; elevates upper lid	Down and temporal	Temporal and superior; greatest oblique separation: nasal and superior	Oblique
	Inferior rectus	Depresses eye, action improving with abducted eye; no action when eye adducted	Adduction of eye and rotation of vertical meridian outward, this activity increasing when eye adducted; depresses lower lid	Superior and temporal	Temporal and down; greatest oblique separation: nasal and superior	Oblique
	Inferior oblique	Elevation of eye, action increasing with adducted eye; no activity when eye adducted	Abducts eye and rotates vertical meridian outward, this activity increasing when eye abducted	Down and nasal	Nasal and superior; greatest oblique separation: temporal and superior	Oblique
Trochlear	Superior oblique	Depresses eye, action increasing with adducted eye; no activity when eye abducted	Abducts the eye and rotates vertical meridian outward, this activity increasing when eye abducted	Superior and nasal	Nasal and down; greatest oblique separation: temporal and down	Oblique
Abducens	Lateral rectus	Abducts eye	None	Nasal	Temporal	Images side by side, uncrossed

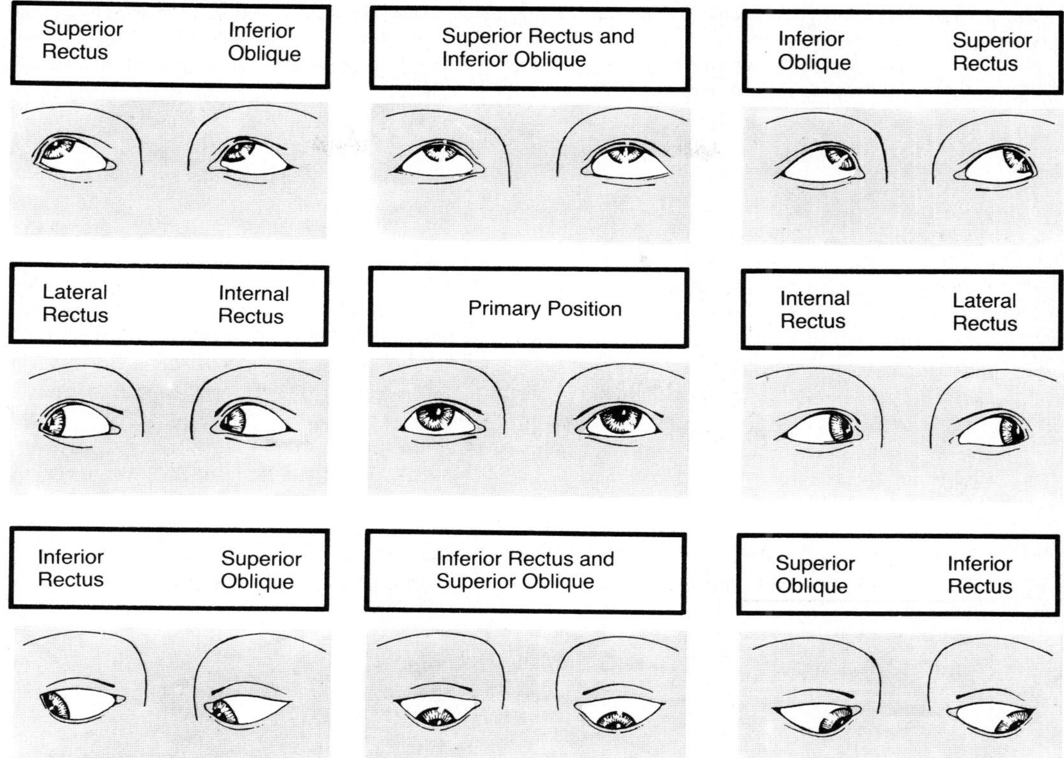

Fig. 27   The function of individual eye muscles. The scheme of Hering gives the direction in which the function of the muscle is predominantly involved. To move the eye to each position, other eye muscles are also activated (M. Mumenthaler: Neurology, 7th ed. Thieme, Stuttgart 1982)

of the lesion to be determined. For purposes of differential diagnosis, disturbances of eye movement can be divided into those with and those without double vision.

2.8.1 Disturbances of Ocular Motility with Double Vision

The presence of double vision in a patient with sufficient visual acuity implies that ocular muscles or ocular motor nerves or their nuclei are involved. A deviation of the eye from the neutral position, a squint, is always present and can be demonstrated either on confrontation or by instruments. Such a paralytic strabismus can result from the following three lesions, given with their characteristics:

– Muscular lesions or mechanical orbital disturbances resulting in disordered visual motility.

These do not show the normal characteristic of double vision found with lesions of extraocular muscle innervation (*see* below). They can be slowly progressive (oculomotor dystrophy), rapidly progressive (ocular myositis), or sudden and intermittent (Brown syndrome), or they can show varying intensity and varying localization (myasthenia gravis). The causes of these symptoms and signs are

- ocular muscle dystrophy (progressive over years, always showing marked ptosis, eventually involving neck and shoulder muscles)
- acute ocular myositis, also called pseudotumor of the orbit (rapidly progressive within days, usually bilateral, marked by periorbital edema, proptosis, pain)
- Kearns-Sayre syndrome (which includes pigmentary degeneration of the retina, heart block, ataxia, deafness, and small stature)

- orbital tumors (unilateral, resulting in slowly) progressive proptosis and eventually pupillary and optic nerve involvement)
- hyperthyroidism manifested by exophthalmos, which may be unilateral; positive Graefe sign; other signs of hyperthyroidism (*see* 2.13.1.1)
- Brown syndrome, which is mechanical impediment of the tendons of the superior oblique muscle in the trochlea (distinguished by sudden onset, transience, recurring symptoms, inability to move the eye up and inward with resulting double vision)
- myasthenia gravis (involving the eye muscles with varying localization and intensity, usually with ptosis evident, increasing during the course of the day, and usually affecting other facial muscles and swallowing)

The typical aspects of myasthenia gravis are shown in Figure 28.

– Lesions of oculomotor nerves. Depending on the nerve affected, such lesions cause paralyses that can be easily defined. They are, in part, described in Table 16 and are more fully defined below. The clinical aspects and the position of the double images of right-sided oculomoor paresis are shown in Figure 29. With such paralysis, mild exophthalmos may also be present, resulting from the hypotonia of the rectus muscles and the preserved tone of the oblique muscles, which tend to push the globe outward. The appearance of the pupil with oculomotor paralysis is described in 2.8.4.1. For differential diagnosis of the ptosis with oculomotor paralysis, *see* 2.8.3. The appearance of a patient with paralysis of the oculomotor nerve is shown in Figure 30. The clinical aspects and position of the double image with (right-sided) trochlear nerve paralysis are shown in Figure 31, with the manifestations of abducens paralysis (right) in Figure 32.

The following etiologic considerations apply to lesions of one or more oculomotor nerves:

- trauma (evident from history; can sometimes result in bilateral orbital hematomas or, in extreme cases, rupture of the oculomotor nerve)
- compression by tumor, particularly parasellar tumors producing slowly progressive paresis, often associated with involvement of the optic nerve and of the first division of the trigeminal nerve
- other space-occupying lesions such as supraclinoid or infraclinoid aneurysms of the carotid artery (indicated above all, in slowly progressive involvement of the oculomotor nerve and eventually leading to pain, impairment of sensation in the first division of the trigeminal nerve, and occasionally to calcification visible in the aneurysm in a plain film of the skull; later acute subarachnoid bleeding may set in)
- arteriovenous fistula in the cavernous sinus (the result of several [minor] traumas. Eventually leads to pulsatile exophthalmos, pulse-synchronous bruits that are always audible, and by engorgements of conjunctival veins and of the fundus). With compression of the oculomotor nerve, mydriasis is an early symptom, often appearing before paralysis of ocular motility
- generalized increase in intracranial pressure, usually involving the abducens nerve first, and eventually the oculomotor nerve (marked by general evidence of increased intracranial pressure but occasionally no localizing symptoms)
- after lumbar puncture (resulting in paralysis of the abducens nerve but with spontaneous recovery)
- the Tolosa-Hunt syndrome and the paratrigeminal syndrome of Raeder (very painful conditions showing external ophthalmoplegia and sometimes involvement of the first division of the trigeminal nerve; spontaneous regression within days or weeks; steroid treatment effective; recurrences rare)
- infectious diseases such as diphtheria and botulism intoxication (marked by paralysis of swallowing and accommodation difficulties), and parainfectious and other diseases (also with spontaneous recovery)
- nonspecific febrile illnesses (can result in paralysis of the abducens, particularly in children)
- meningitis (including signs such as fever, meningismus, generalized symptoms, affection of other cranial nerves; may be bilateral)
- neoplastic and leukemic meningeal infiltration (*see* 2.9.2)
- in sarcoid isolated cranial nerves most frequently the facial nerve
- as side effect of various drugs e.g. internuclear or total external ophthalmoplegia

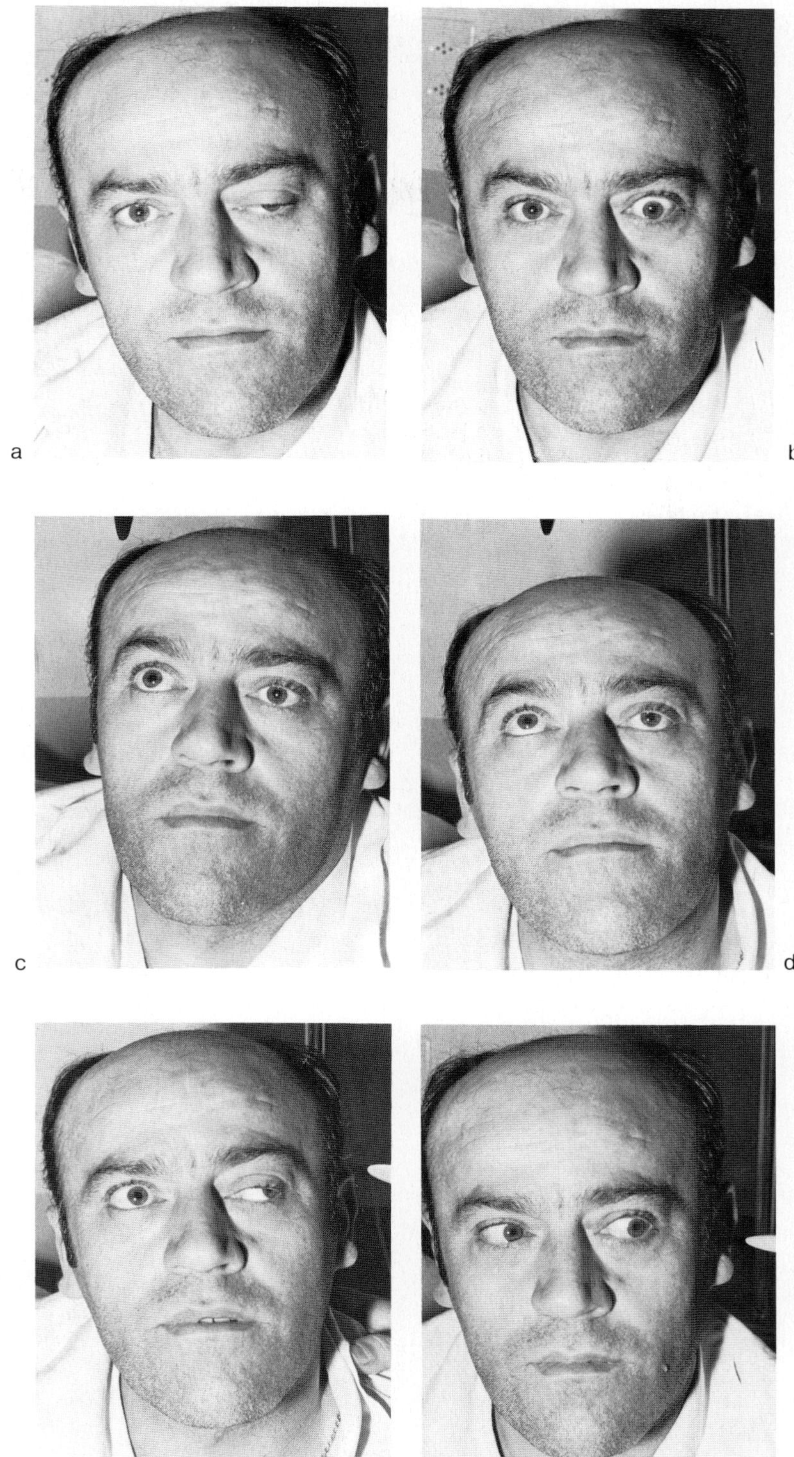

Fig. **28a–f** Disturbed ocular motility with myasthenia gravis. (M. Mumenthaler and J. Lutschg: Schweiz. Arch. Neurol. Neurochir. Psychiatr. 118 [1976] 23–56). Various eye positions before (**a, c,** and **e**) and after (**b, d,** and **f**) injection of 10 mg edrophonium chloride (Tensilon)

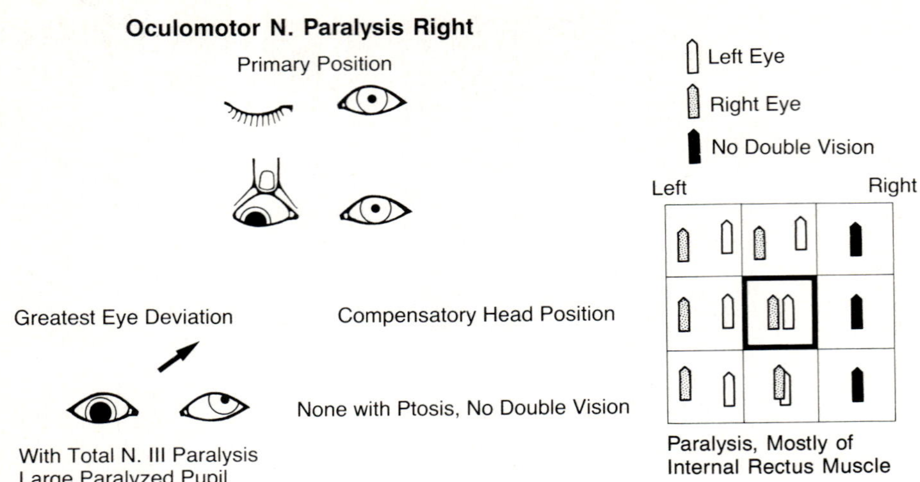

Fig. 29   Position of eyes and of double images with oculomotor paralysis on the right

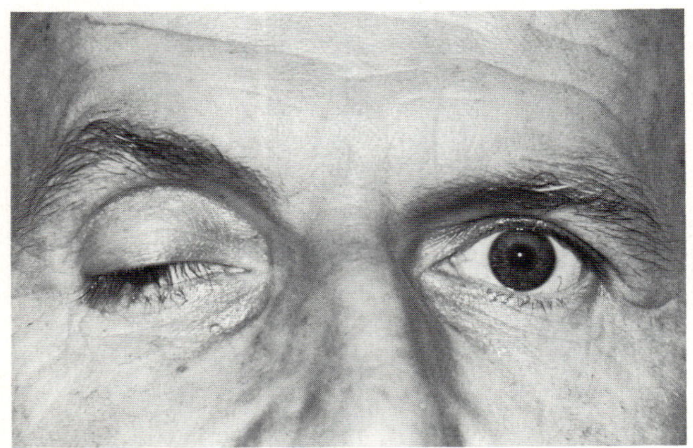

a

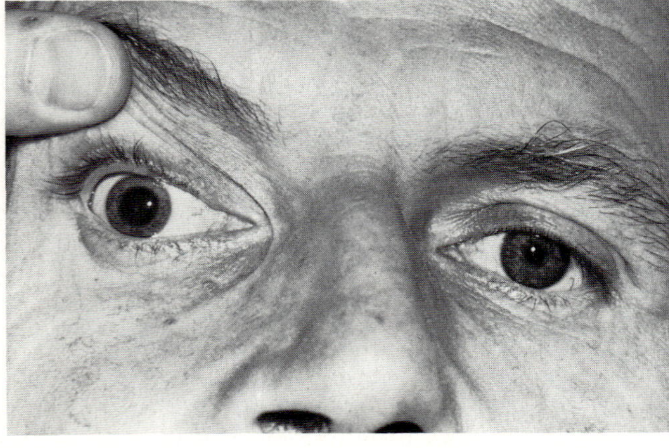

b

Fig. 30 a and b   Patient with total right-sided oculomotor paralysis resulting from a carotid aneurysm. **a** Ptosis with lateral deviation of the right eye. The patient attempts to overcome the deficit due to paralysis of the levator palpebrae by contracting the frontalis muscle. **b** On passive elevation of the upper eyelid, the large nonreactive pupil can be seen

Trochlear N. Paralysis N. IV

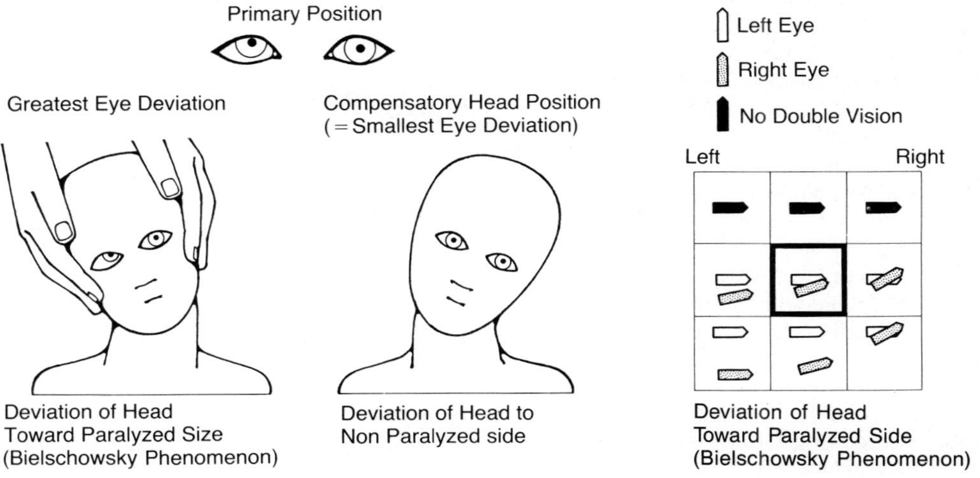

Fig. 31　Position of the head, of the eyes, and of the double images with paralysis of the right trochlear nerve

Paralysis of Abducens + N. VI

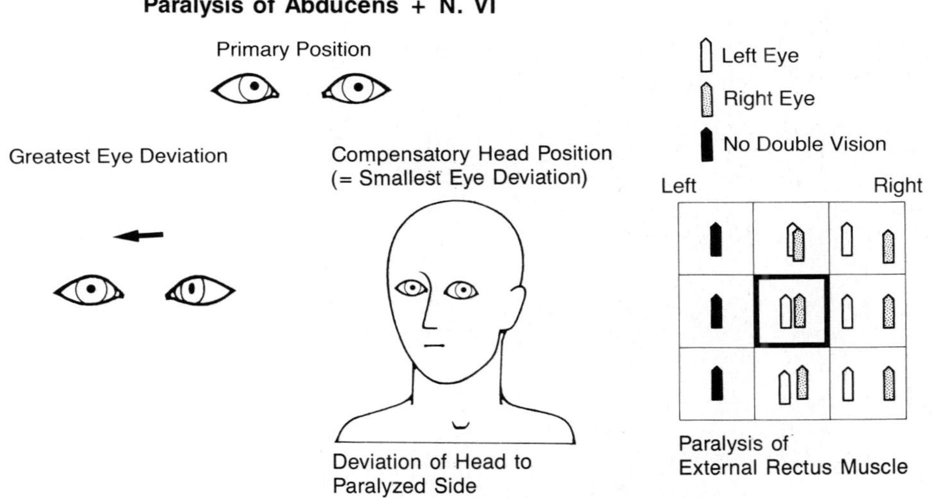

Fig. 32　Position of the head, of the eyes, and of the double images with paralysis of the right abducens nerve

due to tricyclic antidepressants or phenytoin. Abnormal saccades or nystagmus resulting from taking numerous other drugs

- cranial polyradiculitis as part of a spinal polyradiculitis of the Guillain-Barré type (predominantly motor paralysis with areflexia, always involving the facial nerves when extraocular muscles are affected; *see* 1.3.1)
- isolated polyradiculitis, as in Fisher syndrome (often showing only external bilateral ophthalmoplegia; also marked by ataxia, areflexia, eventual facial paralysis, and, in the CSF, dissociated albuminocytologic findings)

- diabetes mellitus (occasional complication of even light diabetes with involvement of the oculomotor or abducens nerves, sparing of pupil; a very painful condition that ends in spontaneous recovery within 3 months)
- ophthalmoplegic migraine (a rare complication of migraine; check for a history of migraine, but always search for other causes)
- multiple sclerosis (*see* 2.13.2.5.1). Lesions of oculomotor nerves are often the first symptoms, usually associated with disturbances of ocular motility
- isolated paralysis of the abducens nerve (most often found in children) or oculomotor paralysis, cryptogenic and totally reversible (these two conditions comprise about half of the cases of isolated paresis of extraocular muscle nerves)

Table 17 shows the various syndromes in which paralysis of extraocular muscles is present sometimes in combination with paralysis of other cranial nerves.

- Lesions of oculomotor nuclei have as a principal consequence a 'peripheral' paralysis that results in double vision. Because of the prox-

Table 17   Syndromes of localizing value in combinations of extraocular muscle nerve paresis and other cranial nerve involvement

Syndrome	Characteristics	Localization	Common cause
Orbital apex	Paralysis of III, IV, and VI nn, first division of trigeminal and optic nn (unilateral visual field defect)	Apex of orbit	Tumor
Superior orbital fissure	Paralysis of III, occasionally also of IV and VI nn; eventually paralysis of first division of V n	Varying extent of involvement of superior orbital fissure	Tumor, fracture
Cavernous sinus	Paralysis of III, IV, and VI nn, and first division of V n	Adjacent to sphenoid within the cavernous sinus	Septic thrombosis, tumor, arteriovenous fistula
Gradenigo	Paralysis of VI n, associated with pain; paresis of first division of V n; eventually impairment of hearing	Petrous temporal apex	Osteitis after suppurative otitis
Clivus	Paralysis of III n; occasionally only mydriasis	Clivus region	Increased intracranial pressure e.g. after trauma or bleeding
Cerebellopontine angle	Impaired hearing, eventually tinnitus; impaired balance; later paresis of V and VII nn; cerebellar symptoms and contralateral pyramidal signs	Angle between pons and cerebellum, often adjacent to pyramids	Tumor
Siebenmann	Paralysis of IX, X, and XI nn, with hoarseness, palatal palsy, and paralysis of soft palate and sternocleidomastoid m	Jugular foramen	Trauma, thrombosis of jugular vein, tumor
Garcin	Unilateral, multiple, caudal cranial nerve involvement	Base of skull, either intracranially or extracranially	Tumor, osteomyelitis of base of skull

imity of the oculomotor nuclei to other structures of the brain stem, lesions of these nuclei are associated not only with paralysis of extraocular muscles but also with other symptoms and signs that distinguish them from lesions of the nerves proper:

- such lesions are almost always associated with other central nervous system symptoms
- with nuclear oculomotor paralysis the various muscles supplied by the oculomotor nerve rarely exhibit the same degree of weakness. Ptosis usually appears only after paralysis of extraocular muscles ('the curtain falls last'). The internal ocular muscles (located farthest cranially) often are spared
- internuclear ophthalmoplegia (*see* 2.8.2, Table 18, and Fig. 26), though not associated with double vision, characteristically results in strabismus in certain directions of gaze

- The most common causes of nuclear disturbances of ocular motility are
  - vascular insults to the brain stem (sudden in onset, accompanied by other brain stem symptoms, predominantly crossed symptoms and dizziness [*see* also 1.1.3]). The brain stem syndromes that typically include nuclear disturbances of ocular motility are given in Table 18
  - tumors, particularly brain stem gliomas and metastasis (*see* 2.7.1)
  - trauma with hematoma in the brain stem (evident in history and in severe initial dysfunction)
  - syringobulbia (nonprogressive for long periods, eventually slowly progressive; marked by symptoms of long-tract involvement and eventually by dissociated sensory loss in the face)

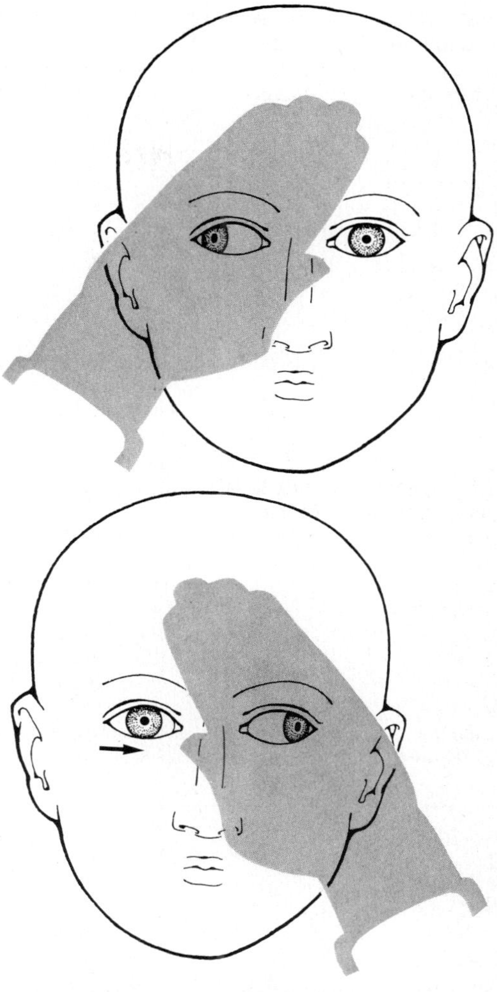

Fig. **33 Cover test:** With divergent alternating concomitant strabismus, the covered eye (nonfixing eye) deviates outward. With fixation there is restoration of the eye to normal position with outward deviation of the other eye

2.8.2 Disturbances of Ocular Motility without Double Vision

If ocular motility is disturbed without double vision, the disturbance is assumed to be supranuclear in origin. In clinical examination, gaze palsy is found on conjugate ocular gaze, that is, both eyes show an identical deficit in ocular motility, and the globes remain parallel in the preserved direction of gaze. If, however, there is a skewed deviation of the eyes without double vision, one of two other disturbances is present.

- So-called concomitant strabismus, which has the following characteristics:
  - present since childhood
  - often associated with marked reduction in visual acuity (amblyopia)
  - on examination of ocular motility in both eyes, a squint is noted, that is, one eye does not participate in certain directions of movement

Table 18 Brain stem syndromes, including those with disturbances of ocular motility of nuclear origin and pupillary abnormalities

Syndrome	Localization	Homolateral symptoms	Contralateral symptoms	Remarks
Chiray-Foix-Nicolesco (upper rubral)	Midbrain, red nucleus	No oculomotor paresis	Hemiataxia, hyperkinesia, intention tremor, hemiparesis (often without Babinski sign); eventually sensory disturbance	
Benedikt (upper rubral)	Midbrain, red nucleus	Oculomotor paresis; eventually gaze palsy toward side of lesion	Eventually hemiataxia, intention tremor, hemiparesis (often without Babinski sign)	Ataxic gait
Claude (lower rubral)	Midbrain, red nucleus	Oculomotor paralysis	Hemiataxia or hemiasynergia, hemiparesis	No hyperkinesia
Weber	Lower midbrain	Oculomotor paralysis	Motor hemiparesis	
Perinaud	Quadrigeminal plate region	Impairment of upward gaze (rostral quadrigeminal plate) and downward gaze (caudal quadrigeminal plate), impairment of convergence, and often absence of light reflex		
Nothnagel	Quadrigeminal plate	Oculomotor paralysis	Hemiataxia	
Raymond-Cestan	Upper dorsal pons	Gaze palsy toward side of lesion	Impaired sensibility (sometimes involving trigeminal area), occasionally hemiparesis	
Gasperini	Distal pons	Paralysis of facial, abducens, trigeminal, and auditory nn	Sensory impairment	Occasionally nystagmus
Millard-Gubler	Distal pons	Facial weakness (peripheral)	Motor hemiparesis	
Brissaud	Distal pons	Facial spasm	Motor hemiparesis	
Foville	Distal pons	Abducens and occasional facial weakness	Motor hemiparesis	
Babinski-Nageotte	Dorsolateral part of pontobulbar border zone	Cerebellar ataxia, Horner syndrome	Motor, hemiparesis, sensory disturbances	Nystagmus, lateropulsion (supply territory of posterior inferior cerebellar artery)
Wallenberg	Dorsolateral medulla oblongata	Horner syndrome; paralysis of vocal cord, soft palate, posterior wall of pharynx; impairment of trigeminal function; hemiataxia	Dissociated sensory loss	
Cestan-Chenais	Lateral medulla oblongata	Horner syndrome; paralysis of vocal cord; paresis of soft palate and posterior wall of pharynx; hemiataxia	Motor hemiparesis, hemihypesthesia	

(continued)

Table 18   (continued)

Syndrome	Localization	Homolateral symptoms	Contralateral symptoms	Remarks
Avellis	Lateral medulla oblongata	Paralysis of soft palate, posterior wall of pharynx vocal cord	Motor hemiparesis, heminypesthesia	
Schmidt	Lateral medulla oblongata	Paralysis of soft palate, posterior wall of pharynx, vocal cord, sternocleido mastoid and upper trapezius mm, tongue	Motor hemiparesis, hemihypesthesia	
Tapia	Lateral medulla oblongata	Paralysis of soft palate, posterior wall of pharynx, vocal cord, tongue	Motor hemiparesis, hemihypesthesia	
Vernet	Lateral medulla oblongata	Paralysis of soft palate, posterior wall of pharynx, sternocleidomastoid m; loss of taste on posterior third of tongue; hemihypesthesia of pharynx	Motor hemiparesis	
Jackson	Lower medulla oblongata	Paralysis of tongue	Motor hemiparesis	
Internuclear ophthalmoplegia	Medial longitudinal fasciculus	With lateral gaze, contralateral eye does not cross midline; with accommodation to near, convergence possible bilaterally; nystagmus in caudal lesions, occasionally also paralysis of external rectus; rostral lesions, also impairment of convergence without nystagmus		

After M. Mumenthaler: Neurology, 9th ed. Thieme, Stuttgart 1990.

- on separate examination of the ocular motility of each eye while the other eye is occluded, each eye has full motility
- the nonfixing eye (covered by the examiner) drifts to one side (concomitant divergent or convergent strabismus). This phenomenon may alternate in both eyes (concomitant alternate strabismus; for example, divergent) and can be recognized with the cover test (Fig. 33). Such strabismus is due to a congenital or early acquired disturbance of ocular muscle equilibrium, is generally associated with marked amblyopia of one eye, and has no specific neurologic significance

- Internuclear ophthalmoplegia produces a disturbance of ocular axes without double vision. A lesion of the medial longitudinal fasciculus between the pontine gaze center and the nucleus of the oculomotor nerve (Fig. 26) interrupts impulses for lateral gaze passing from the pontine center and the homolateral abducens nucleus to the rostrally situated nucleus of the third nerve, which controls the internal rectus of the opposite eye

- the abducting eye freely moves laterally
- the other adducting eye does not move across the midline
- however, convergence is preserved in both eyes because of impulses passing to both eyes from the rostrally situated center for convergence (Perlia's nucleus), enabling the previously paretic eye now to move inward together with the unaffected eye
- complete internuclear ophthalmoplegia is rare, but there are many patients with partial internuclear ophthalmoplegia manifested by slowed saccades of the adducting eye only

The cause of internuclear ophthalmoplegia is usually a brain stem vascular lesion; occasionally it is multiple sclerosis or tumor. Only rarely does disturbed ocular motility with deviation of axes without double vision result from other causes — for example, as part of giant cell arteritis syndrome (*see* 2.5.1.2).

Disturbances of ocular motility without deviation of ocular axes are known as conjugate paralyses. They are always caused by lesions of the supranuclear centers of gaze either in the brain stem or cortex. Gaze-paretic nystagmus (Table 15) is often associated with such disturbances. Differentiation from advanced ocular muscle dystrophies (slowly progressive disease often associated with ptosis and also disturbances of pharyngeal muscles) with complete paralysis of all ocular motility with parallel axes of the eyes is occasionally difficult. Among conjugate paralyses, inability to gaze voluntarily to the side can be due to

— Lesions of the pontine visual center ('nucleus paraabducens') in the caudal part of the pons. With a lesion in this site, there is inability to look toward the affected side.

  Causes: vascular (common in elderly patients, sudden in onset, always associated with other disturbances of function), tumors (*see* 2.7.1), multiple sclerosis (see 2.13.2.5.1), intoxications (for example, with carbamazepine)

— Lesions of the frontal, cortical gaze center in area 8. With excitation, there is deviation of the eye and head toward the opposite side, sometimes culminating in an epileptic aversive seizure. The damage to this region results in gaze and head deviation toward the side of the lesion because of the predominance of activity of the opposite area 8 (conjugate deviation); the patient looks toward the damage. Several days after appearance of the lesion, the patient will be capable of gazing straight ahead but still have trouble looking toward the opposite side. With time, even this function is restored. But gaze-paretic nystagmus (Table 15) persists with the rapid component of the nystagmus toward the opposite side. The pursuit movements of the eyes are preserved.

  Causes of lesions of the frontal gaze center include vascular insults (*see* 2.3.1.2), tumors

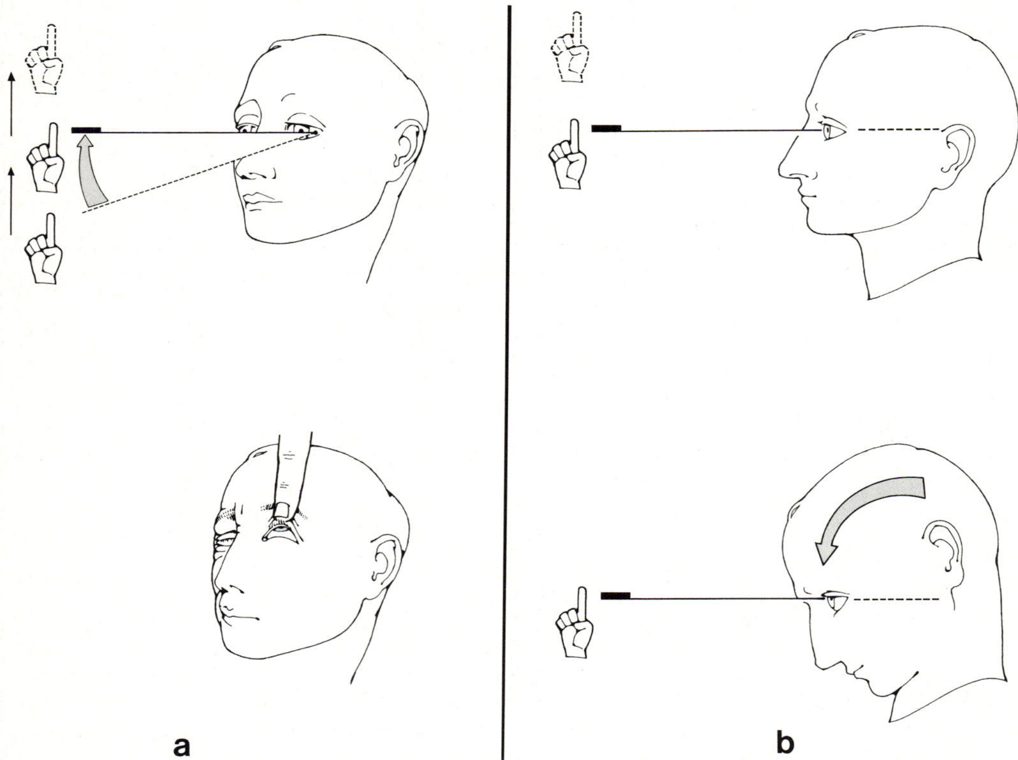

a

b

Fig. **34a and b** Differentiation of supranuclear gaze palsy from paralysis of the elevators of the eye. **a** While voluntary upward gaze is not possible on forceful closure of the eye, the Bell phenomenon is demonstrated. **b** Voluntary upward gaze is not possible, but on passive downward movement of the head with the eyes fixed on an object, there is a relative upward movement of the eye within the orbit (doll's eye phenomenon) (often associated with irritative symptoms and sometimes frontal psychic disturbances [*see* 2.1]); atrophic processes (in elderly patients, associated with dementia and other cortical, in part neuropsychologic, dysfunction); trauma (evident from history and sometimes from external injuries, fractures of the skull, subjective signs of cerebral concussion, bloody CSF, and occasionally other neurologic dysfunction)

Inability to gaze upward as well as disturbed downward gaze (called Perinaud syndrome when associated with disturbed convergence) points to a lesion in the tectal area of the rostral midbrain. It is to be noted, however, that many persons, particularly elderly, severely ill, or stuporous patients have trouble looking upward. True paralysis of upward gaze can be recognized (and distinguished from peripheral paralysis of the extraocular muscles) by the following findings:

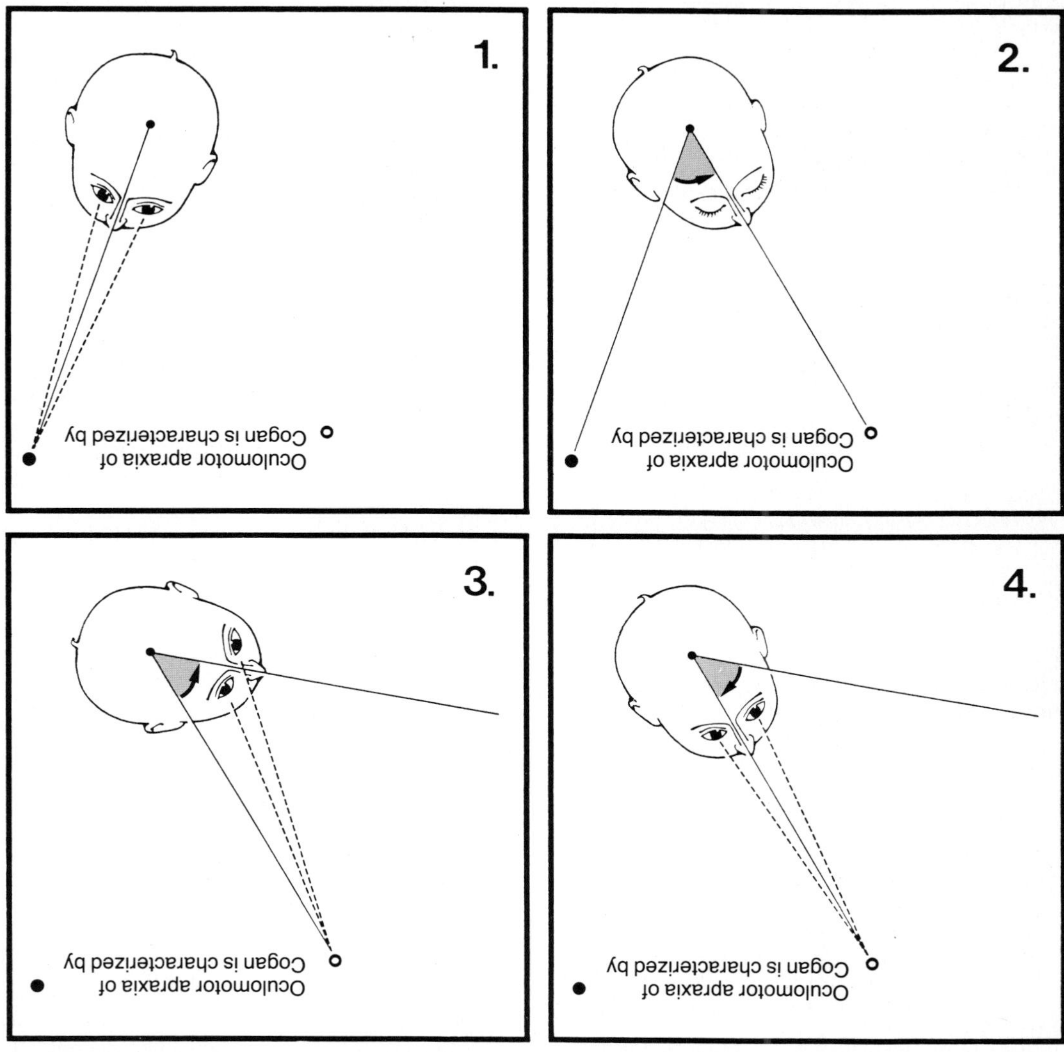

Fig. 35 Cogan's oculomotor apraxia. The patient, when attempting **1**, to fix on an object to the left, **2**, turns the head leftward with eyes closed, **3**, rotates the head beyond the target and fixes on the object, and **4**, then turns the head back into the direction of gaze

- The Bell phenomenon may be present: the patient attempts forceful closure of the eyes while the examiner passively elevates the upper lids; reflex-induced upward rotation of the eye becomes visible (Fig. 34a)
- The doll's eye phenomenon is present: when the patient fixes on an object in front of the eye while the examiner bends the patient's head forward, the vision remains fixed on the object so that upward rotation of the eyes is induced (Fig. 34b)

Causes of progressive vertical ophthalmoplegia may be

- A brain stem tumor (a common cause, manifested by other disturbances of ocular motility, paralysis of convergence, other neurologic dysfunction, mesencephalic signs, headaches, signs of increased intracranial pressure, and, with pinealomas, precocious puberty also)
- Noncommunicating hydrocephalus (marked by signs of increased intracranial pressure and in children, increased head circumference)
- Progressive supranuclear palsy, Steele-Richardson-Olszewski syndrome (seen in elderly patients and associated with akinetic Parkinson's syndrome, dementia, and eventually total external ophthalmoplegia)
- Whipple's disease (with uveitis, dementia, gastrointestinal disturbances)
- Wilson's disease (*see* 2.14.1.7)
- Huntington's chorea (*see* 2.14.1.8)
- Progressive multifocal leukoencephalopathy in association with malignant disease

Other disturbances of gaze (which manifest themselves partly as reading difficulty) must also be mentioned briefly:

- Ocular dysmetria, in which the eyes overshoot and eventually oscillate on a fixing object. This disorder is found in diseases of the cerebellum (Table 15)
- Congenital ocular apraxia or Cogan syndrome. The patient must move the head beyond the fixing target for the eyes to finally reach the target. When the eyes have fixed, the head can now be moved back into the proper direction (Fig. 35). This process leads to bizarre movements of the head, which must be distinguished from a tic, and also to difficulty in reading and writing, which must be distinguished from congenital alexia

- Forceful deviations of the eyes to one side or, more commonly, upward are known as oculogyric crisis. Most often seen in association with postencephalitic Parkinson syndrome, it is sometimes an early symptom of this disorder (which is also suggested by a history of febrile illness and other extrapyramidal symptoms both of which permit its differentiation from hysterical dysfunction)

2.8.3 Ptosis, Paralysis of Upper Lids, and Horner Syndrome

Ptosis is the abnormal lowering of the upper lid, narrowing the opening of the eye. It can be unilateral or bilateral.

As is evident from the relevant anatomic substrate shown in Figure 36, ptosis can occur

- With involvement of the striated lid elevator muscle (the levator palpebrae superioris)
- With a lesion of the nerve supplying this muscle (the oculomotor nerve or its nucleus)
- With apraxia of eye opening as a manifestation of supranuclear paresis, as in Parkinson's syndrome or in attacks as a manifestation of localized cataplexy in patients with the narcolepsy-cataplexy syndrome
- With impaired sympathetic innervation of the smooth muscle fibers of the superior tarsal muscle
- As apparent ptosis due to retraction of the eye, or exophthalmos of the opposite side

2.8.3.1 Affection of the Striated Lid Elevator Muscles

The ptosis under these circumstances is mostly bilateral or (with myasthenia gravis) inconstant, shifting occasionally from side to side. Possible causes are

- Congenital ptosis (muscular or neurogenic?), usually unilateral, present from birth, and nonprogressive, occasionally associated with weakness of extraocular muscles. Bilateral disturbances are often familial, and the head is typically tilted backward
- Progressive ocular muscular dystrophy (very slowly progressive over the years, bilateral, with involvement of other muscles and eventually also involvement of neck muscles and muscles of deglutition (*see* 2.8.1)

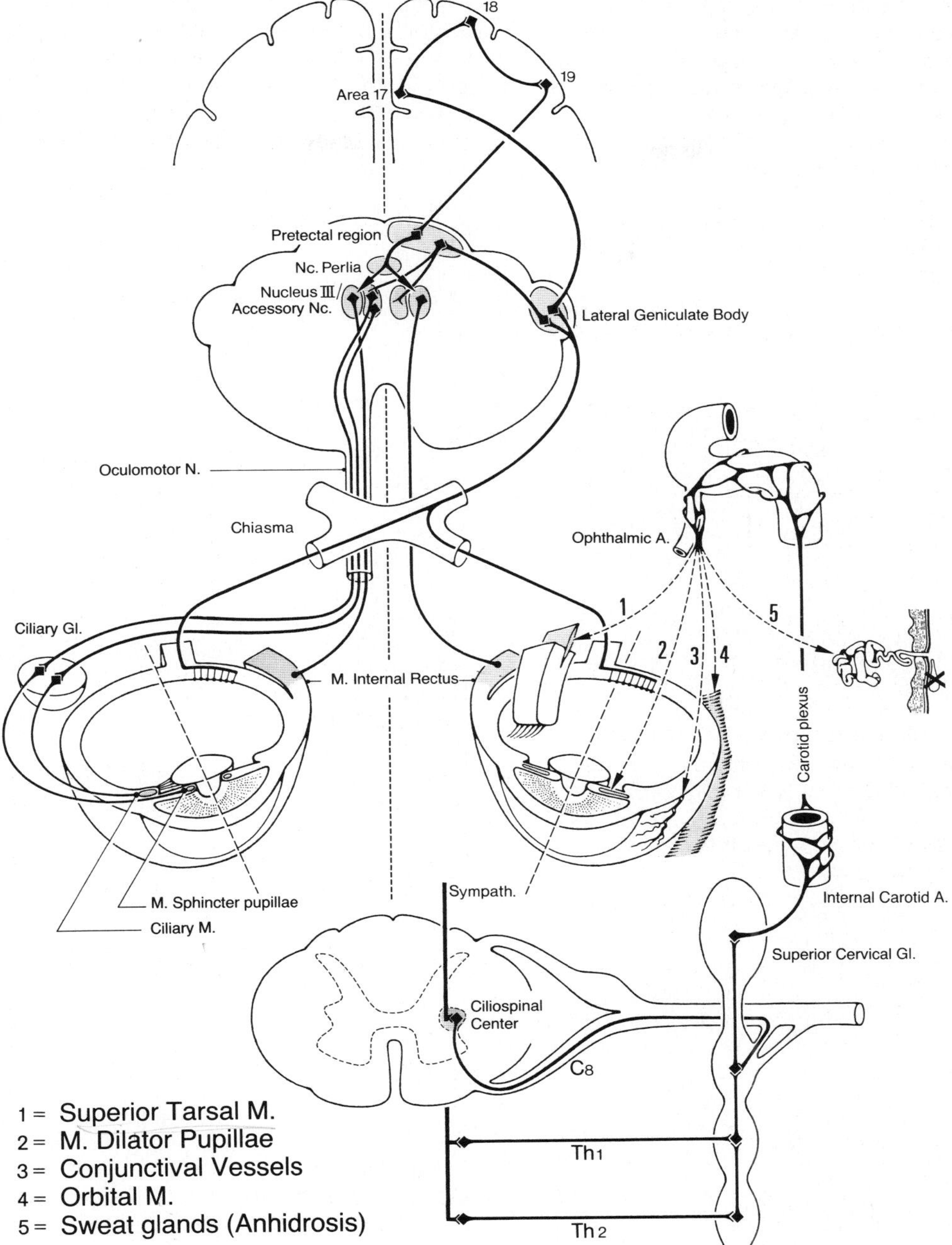

Fig. 36   Anatomic basis of ptosis, Horner syndrome, and pupillary innervation

— Myotonic dystrophy of Steinert (*see* 2.9.2)
— Myasthenia gravis (results in changeable dysfunction during the day, increasing toward the evening, disappearing while the patient is rested, and generally involving extraocular muscles to differing degrees; ptosis increases markedly after several forceful eye-opening attempts against resistance)

- In patients with polyradiculitis there may initially be unilateral or bilateral ptosis without impairment of ocular motility and facial weakness. These patients must be differentiated from those with myasthenia gravis
- In hyperthyroidism there may occasionally be ptosis rather than the usual lid retraction

2.8.3.2 Lesions of the Oculomotor Nerve and Oculomotor Nuclei

Ptosis is often an early symptom of oculomotor nerve disturbances (often associated with mydriasis), because the fibers for the levator palpebrae and parasympathetic fibers to the constrictor of the pupil are peripherally situated in the oculomotor nerve. Under these circumstances the difference in palpebral fissure size is accentuated with upward gaze (in Horner syndrome, however, upward gaze decreases the difference in palpebral fissure size). With lesions of the oculomotor nuclear region, ptosis often appears after paresis of extraocular muscles ('the curtain falls last'). In every case, however, it is eventually accompanied by other signs of dysfunction of other cranial nerves (*see* causes in 2.8.1).

2.8.3.3 Lesions of the Sympathetic Innervation of the Eye and Horner Syndrome

Such lesions can cause ptosis alone, without other signs of Horner syndrome

- Isolated denervation of the superior tarsal muscle may result from chronic infection of the conjunctival sac. Mostly however such denervation is without obvious cause and gives rise to ptosis. An important diagnostic test is the conjunctival instillation of one drop of 10% phenylephrin
- The pseudo-Horner syndrome may also belong in this section. Ipsilateral to the ptosis is also miosis. However, this miotic pupil (unlike the pupil in the true Horner syndrome) dilates with the instillation of 10% cocaine drops.

This form of ptosis (paralysis of the smooth superior tarsal muscle), together with more or less marked miosis (paralysis of the dilator pupillae), with less impressive hyperemia of the conjunctiva (vasomotor paralysis), with exophthalmos (paralysis of the smooth orbital muscle [Muller muscle]) that usually is even less discernible, and, often, with impaired sweating of the upper body quarter, constitutes the Horner syndrome. The difference in palpebral fissure size decreases with upward gaze in the Horner syndrome (because of activation of the intact and powerful striated levator palpebrae superioris muscle). A Horner syndrome can result from:

- Lesions of the central sympathetic homolateral pathways passing among the hypothalamus, the dorsolateral medulla oblongata, and the lateral columns of the spinal cord. The following always result in Horner syndrome as well as other central nervous system dysfunction:
  - vascular insults, particularly in the brain stem, such as Wallenberg syndrome (*see* 2.7.1 and Table 18)
  - tumors
  - syringomyelia
  - progressive hemifacial atrophy (*see* 2.9.4)
- Lesions of the paravertebral sympathetic chain and its radicular afferents. If single components of the paravertebral sympathetic chain are affected there are no functional disturbances of the nervous system. However, with lesions of the stellate ganglia, the Horner syndrome occurs in association with anhidrosis of the face. The Horner syndrome does not occur when the lesion involves the (ventral) roots of C8 to T2 (where, however, dysfunction of a radicular nature is found). With paravertebral sympathetic chain lesions immediately caudal to the stellate ganglion, the result is isolated anhidrosis of the face without Horner syndrome. Possible causes are
  - impingement by tumor upon the paravertebral sympathetic chain (often associated with a distal brachial plexus dysfunction)
  - root or chain damage due to trauma (root avulsion with lower brachial plexus paralysis as a radicular syndrome C8–T1; prevertebral hematoma)
  - cluster headache, which is commonly associated with Horner syndrome (*see* 2.17.1)

2.8.4 Abnormalities of the Pupils and of Pupillary Reactions

The anatomic basis of pupillary motility is depicted in Figure 36. Abnormalities of the pupils can manifest themselves as

- Abnormalities in form or size or as pupils of different dimensions
- Anomalies in pupillary reactivity to light or convergence or both

2.8.4.1 Abnormalities of the Pupil at Rest

Bilateral large pupils (mydriasis) occur

- As a harmless peculiarity in vegetative labile sympathotonic individuals
- In wearers of contact lenses
- With midbrain lesions
- As a result of impaired reaction to light (often with deep coma)
- With the topical or internal use of mydriatic drugs (also with the secret application of atropine preparations) (Fig. 37)

Bilateral abnormally small pupils (miosis) occur

- As harmless peculiarities
- As a normal reaction to intensive light in the examination room
- With lesions of the pons, occurring along with other neurologic symptoms and often associated with impaired consciousness
- With drugs administered locally (pilocarpine in glaucoma patients) or internally (morphine derivatives)
- In syphilis (*see* 2.8.4.2; Fig. 37)

A difference in size of the two pupils at rest (anisocoria) indicates either a unilateral pathologically large or abnormally small pupil.

- Unilateral abnormally large pupil occurs
  - with oculomotor paralysis (accompanied by ptosis and often by associated paralysis of extraocular muscles; *see* 2.8.1)
  - with Adie syndrome, commonly unilateral or unilaterally prominent (absence of light reflex with preservation of convergent reaction and with tonic dilatation, often absence of muscle tendon reflexes; mostly found in women; occasionally familial) (Fig. 37)
  - unilateral application of mydriatic drugs
  - ciliary ganglionitis (Fig. 37)
  - unilateral affection of the anterior components of the eye (often accompanied by marked blood vessel dilatation, deformity of the pupil [see below], and synechiae)
  - 'Iron mydriasis' without other symptoms and caused by an iron splinter in the anteri-

or compartment of the eye (particular attention before MRI)
  - unilateral mydriasis with migraine (but often also miosis with Horner syndrome, particularly in cluster headache, *see* 2.17.1)
- Unilateral abnormally small pupil occurs with
  - Horner syndrome (*see* 2.8.3.3)
  - unilateral application of miotic drugs
  - certain unilateral local affections of the anterior chamber of the eye
  - syphilis – rarely may be unilateral (*see* 2.8.4.2 and Fig. 37)
- Harmless central anisocoria. Difference in pupil size is rarely greater than 1 mm and is more marked in poor light; the size of the smaller pupil often changes

Abnormal forms of one or both pupils (oval or otherwise deformed) occur.

- With congenital ectopic pupils, in which the distortions are mostly upward and outward and are often associated with dislocated lenses and other ocular anomalies
- With partial absence of the iris with acquired synechia and with partial iridic atrophy (for example, in tabes dorsalis)

Among other abnormalities is hippus of the pupils (spontaneous, partially rhythmic contractions that can appear in normal individuals but also may appear with incipient cataracts, multiple sclerosis, meningitis, and contralateral vascular insults or after recovery from oculomotor paralysis).

2.8.4.2 Abnormal Pupillary Reactions

The normal pupil reacts directly and uniformly around its circumference to light and on convergence. The anatomic substrate is diagrammed in Figure 36.

The most common abnormalities in pupillary reaction are illustrated in Figure 37.

Causes of the abnormalities shown in Figure 37 are

- Associated damage to the optic nerve (*see* 2.5.1)
- Associated damage to the oculomotor apparatus (*see* 2.8.1)

Other causes are:

- Adie syndrome (*see* 2.8.4.1)
- Acute ciliary ganglionitis, in which a large pupil, nonreactive to light or convergence, sud-

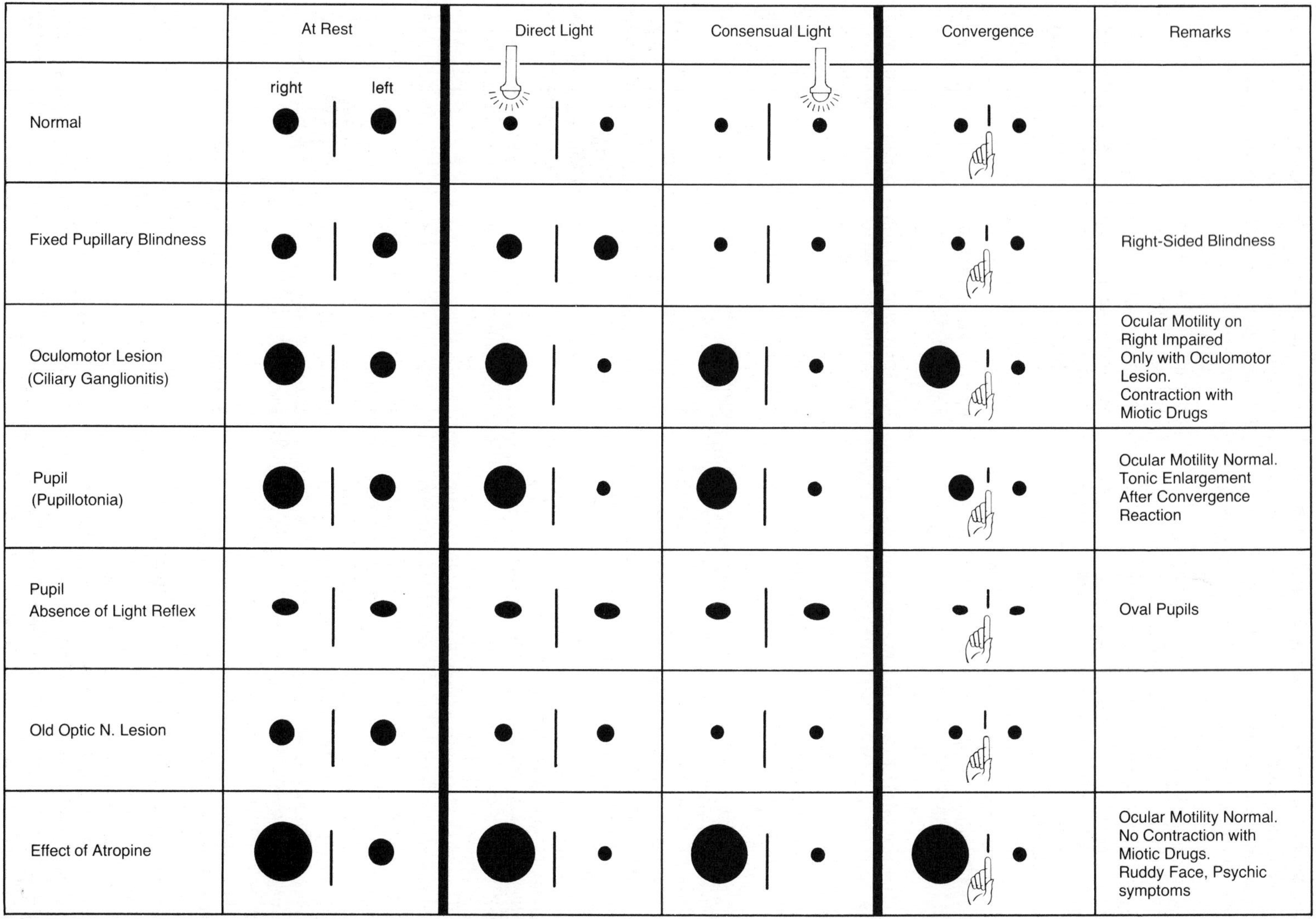

	At Rest	Direct Light	Consensual Light	Convergence	Remarks
Normal					
Fixed Pupillary Blindness					Right-Sided Blindness
Oculomotor Lesion (Ciliary Ganglionitis)					Ocular Motility on Right Impaired Only with Oculomotor Lesion. Contraction with Miotic Drugs
Pupil (Pupillotonia)					Ocular Motility Normal. Tonic Enlargement After Convergence Reaction
Pupil Absence of Light Reflex					Oval Pupils
Old Optic N. Lesion					
Effect of Atropine					Ocular Motility Normal. No Contraction with Miotic Drugs. Ruddy Face, Psychic symptoms

Fig. 37   Disturbances of pupillary reaction (the right pupil is abnormal) (M. Mumenthaler: Neurology, 9th ed. Thieme, Stuttgart 1990)

denly appears several days after an infection or trauma; initially there is also impaired accommodation, but ocular motility remains normal
— Pandysautonomia (*see* 2.20). Special mention should be made of the reflex pupillary paralysis with absence of light reaction but preserved convergence reaction (Fig. 37). This abnormality has been described in a variety of affections (neurosyphilis, Adie syndrome (*see* 2.8.4.1), diabetes mellitus, pinealoma, abnormal regeneration after paralysis of the oculomotor nerve, encephalitis, multiple sclerosis, ophthalmic zoster, trauma to the eye; myotonic dystrophy, amyloidosis, pandysautonomia, familial dysautonomia [Riley-Day syndrome], Fisher syndrome, and Type I HMSN [Charcot-Marie-Tooth disease]).

2.9 Paralysis and Other Abnormalities of Facial Muscles and of the Face

The facial muscles, including the platysma, are supplied by the facial nerve. The facial nucleus lies in the caudal part of the pons. Associated in part with the facial nerve are efferent pathways for the salivary glands, the lacrimal glands, and the glands of the nasal mucosa, and afferent sensory taste fibers from the anterior third of the tongue. In its course through the petrous temporal bone, the facial nerve passes close to the middle ear. The cortical pontine fibers to the facial nerve's motor nucleus reach its cranial portion, which contains the motor neuron for the frontal muscles and includes fibers from the opposite and homolateral precentral gyrus. These relationships are depicted in Figure 38. The mandibular branch of the facial nerve runs along the mandible, a terminal branch of the mandibular division penetrating from below, around the border of the mandible, to the perioral muscles. Certain clinical details complement these anatomic relations: During reinnervation following complete interruption of axons (even when there is no macroscopic disturbance of continuity of the nerve), regeneration is misdirected in all branches of the facial nerve. This leads to the innervation of muscles by ganglion cells to which they were not connected originally. The result is pathologic synergy in facial movement and a "mass innervation." In attempting to show the teeth on the previously paretic side the patient

may simultaneously close the eye because of pathologic innervation of the orbicularis oris. Other abnormal simultaneous movements may also appear (Fig. 39).

The general clinical aspects of facial paralysis are the following:

— With peripheral facial paralysis, the muscles of the face, including the forehead and periorbital muscles, are equally involved. With marked paralysis there is incomplete closure of the eye, leaving the sclera partially visible. The reflex upward movements of the eyes during Bell's phenomenon are clearly evident (Fig. 40). Other symptoms are also depicted in Figure 38 (there is also a disturbance of taste in the anterior two thirds of the tongue, impaired lacrimation, and saliva secretion, occasionally hyperacusis)
— With central paralysis the branch to the frontalis muscle is less affected than in peripheral paralysis (although a degree of paresis is almost always to be found). When the eye is closed the sclera is always completely covered (Fig. 41). (The same is true, of course, in incomplete peripheral facial palsy.) Other hemisyndromes and symptoms are commonly present, for example, deviation of the tongue toward the paralyzed side, homolateral paralysis of extremities, and reflex disturbances

Incomplete central and peripheral paralysis can usually be recognized by a few remaining deficits:

— Closure of the eye on the paralyzed side is somewhat less forceful, with the eyelashes remaining more prominent (the so-called *signe des ciles*); (*see* Fig. 47)
— With the fingertips lightly applied to the upper lids, the examiner perceives the vibration of the forcefully contracting muscle on the unaffected side only
— The contraction of the platysma as the patient shows the teeth is less prominent or totally absent on the affected side

2.9.1 Unilateral Facial Paralysis

The most marked paralysis of the face occurs with peripheral facial nerve lesions.

— Causes of acute paralysis are
  ● unknown. So-called cryptogenic or idiopathic rheumatic or *e frigore* paralysis is accompanied by retroauricular pain; often

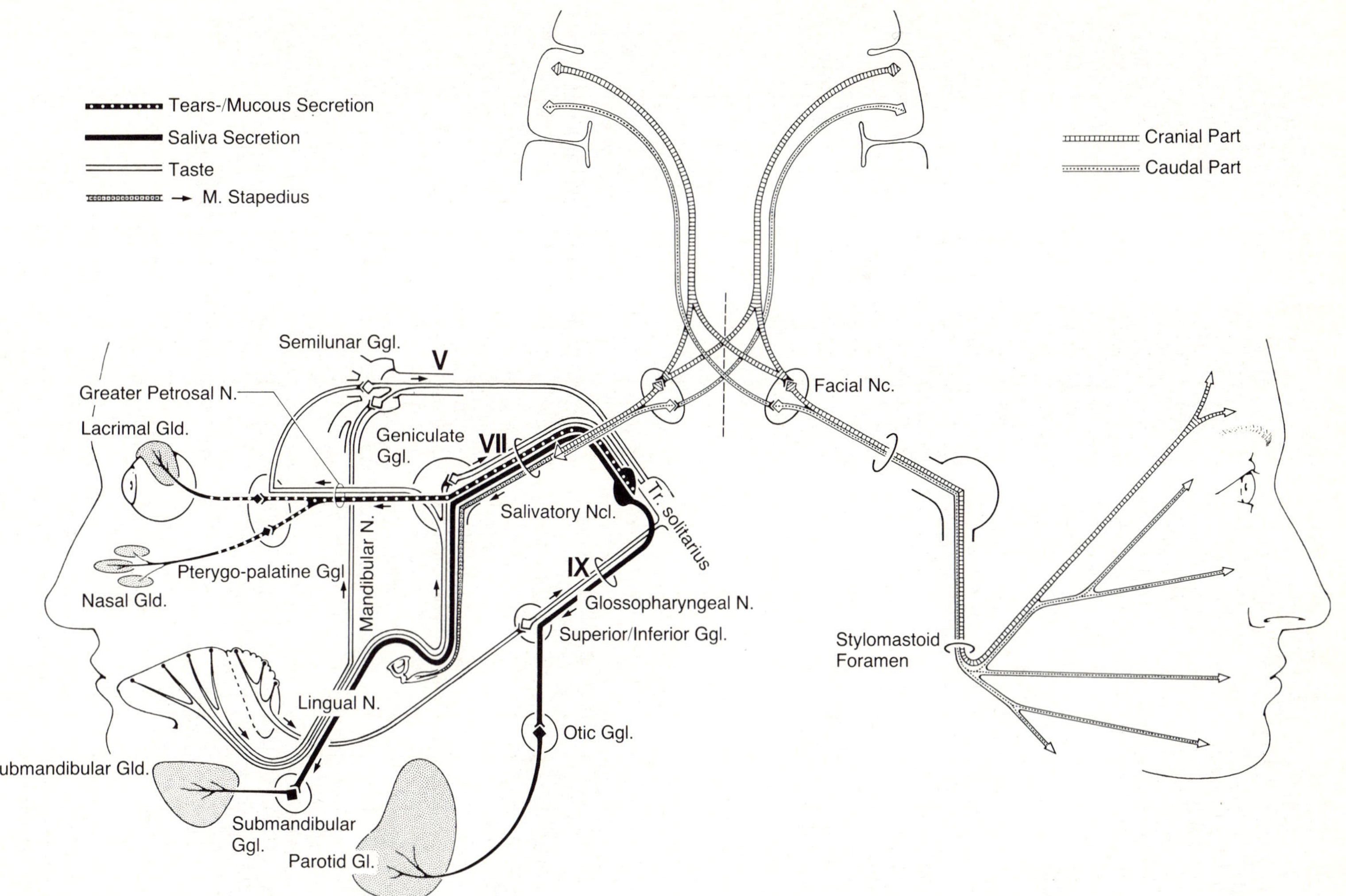

Fig. **38**   Anatomy of the facial nerve (After M. Mumenthaler: Neurology, 9th ed., Georg Thieme Verlag, Stuttgart 1990)

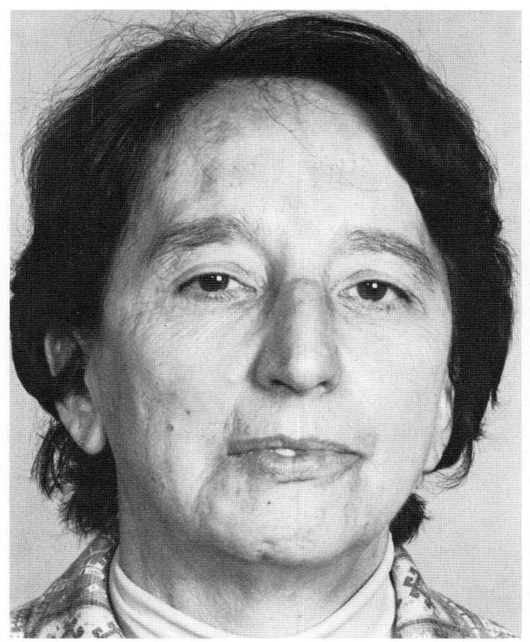
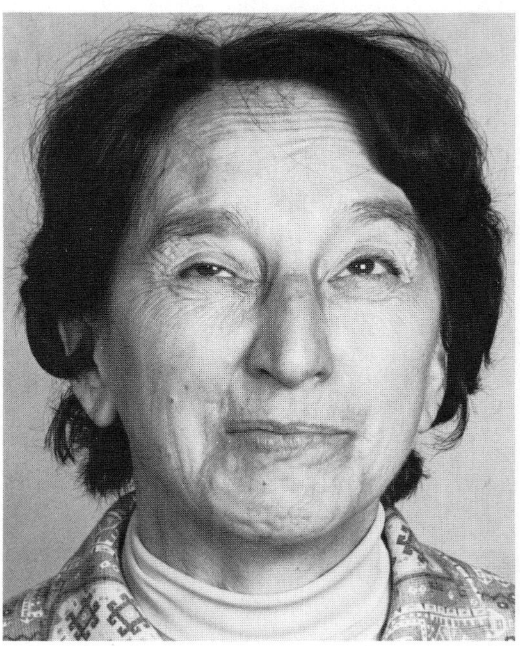

Fig. **39a and b**   A 58-year-old patient five years after idiopathic right peripheral facial paralysis. **a** No significant abnormality at rest. **b** Attempt to wrinkle forehead leads to pathologic activation of the orbicularis oculi and orbicularis oris muscles on the right

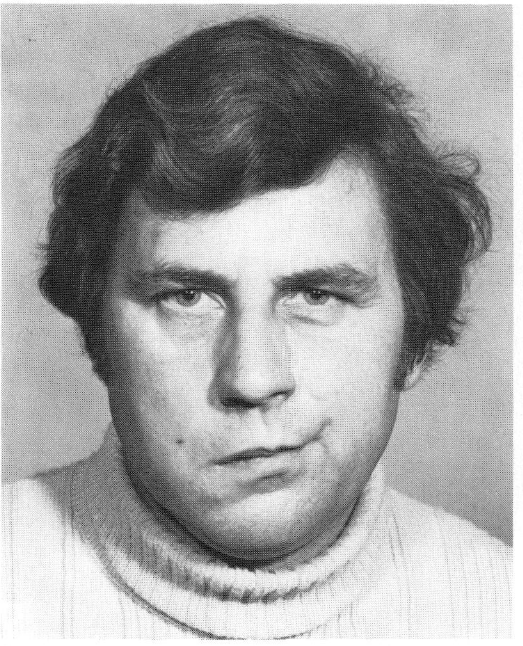
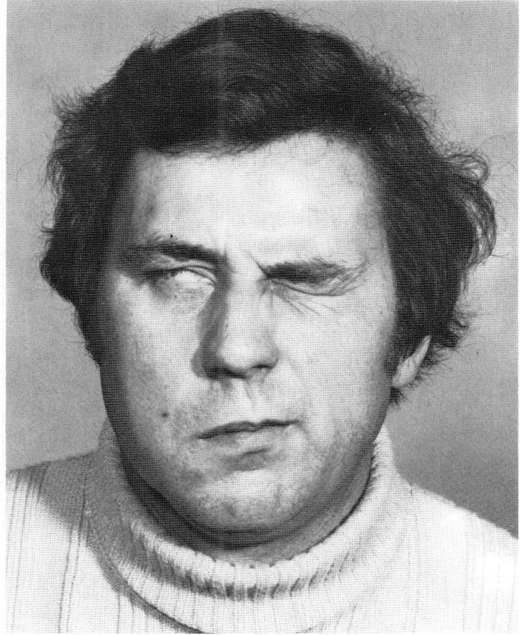

Fig. **40a+b**   A 44-year-old patient with typical idiopathic complete peripheral facial paralysis on the right. **a** At rest there is flaccid paralysis with the corner of the mouth and the cheek lower on the right side. **b** An attempt to close eyes is unsuccessful on the paralyzed side. Part of the eye remains visible. Bell's phenomenon is clearly evident on the right the onset occurs overnight, accompanied by disturbances of taste and occasionally disturbance of tear secretion (Fig. 40)

- infection with associated signs as above. Postinfectious facial paralysis is particularly common after otic zoster or herpes zoster over the neck (vesicular painful eruption)
- Melkersson-Rosenthal syndrome (resulting in recurring episodes of facial swelling with geographic tongue)
- Heerfordt syndrome (resulting in bilateral facial paralysis associated with sarcoidosis with swelling of the parotid glands and visual symptoms)
- head trauma with basal fracture and especially fracture of the pyramid. (With a fracture across the pyramid, the statoacusticus is involved immediately; with a longitudinal fracture the statoacusticus may not be involved for up to 14 days. Such a fracture may be otoscopically visible.)
- otitis and middle ear tumors such as glomus tumor (*see* 2.6) (Paralysis following such disorders is always associated with hearing loss and otoscopic and radiologic findings.)
- basal meningitis, carcinomatous or leukemic meningeal infiltration (other cranial nerves are always involved as well; the paralysis is often bilateral and its onset rapid, although rarely a matter of hours)
- mechanical lesions of the mandibular branch of the facial nerve due to pressure or trauma (usually affecting peribuccal musculature on one side only)
- congenital facial paralysis with Möbius syndrome (always accompanied by impairment of ocular motility, and in particular by difficulty in abduction, sometimes apparent bilaterally)
- congenital aplasia of the depressor anguli oris visible from birth, particularly on crying (Fig. 42)

– Causes of slowly progressive unilateral peripheral facial paralysis are:

- slowly progressive compression of the facial nerve by tumors, particularly in the cerebellopontine angle (paralysis occurs in combination with involvement of other cranial nerves, particularly the statoacusticus and eventually by central nervous system dysfunction)

'Peripheral' facial paralysis can occur with lesions of the motor nucleus of the facial nerve in the caudal part of the pontine tegmentum. Frequent causes are:

– Vascular brain stem insults such as Millard-Gubler syndrome (in which facial paralysis occurs with contralateral hemiparesis), Foville syndrome (facial paralysis in combination with homolateral paralysis of the abducens nerve and contralateral hemiparesis)
– Brain stem tumors (*see* 2.7.1)
– Poliomyelitis (here, with the acute appearance of facial paralysis always associated with paralysis and atrophy of other nuclear muscles)

Unilateral central paralysis of the face results from lesions of the contralateral central motor neurons, either in the region of the precentral gyrus or its efferent pathways (for symptoms, *see* 2.9). Isolated facial paresis occasionally accompanied by pseudobulbar signs is often seen in lacunar infarcts of the internal capsule and/or corona radiata. Common causes are:

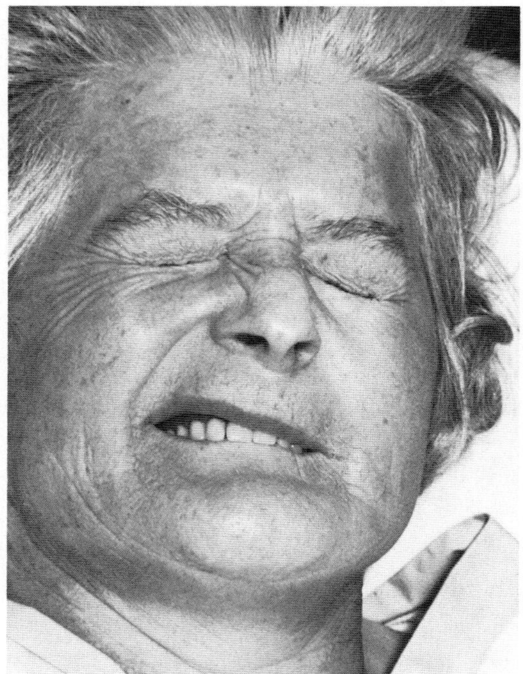

Fig. **41** **a** 62-year-old patient with left-sided hemiparesis (resulting from thrombosis of the right internal carotid artery). Unlike the patient in Figure 40, this patient can close the eyes on the paralyzed side. Nevertheless, the eyelashes remain visible (*signe des ciles*)

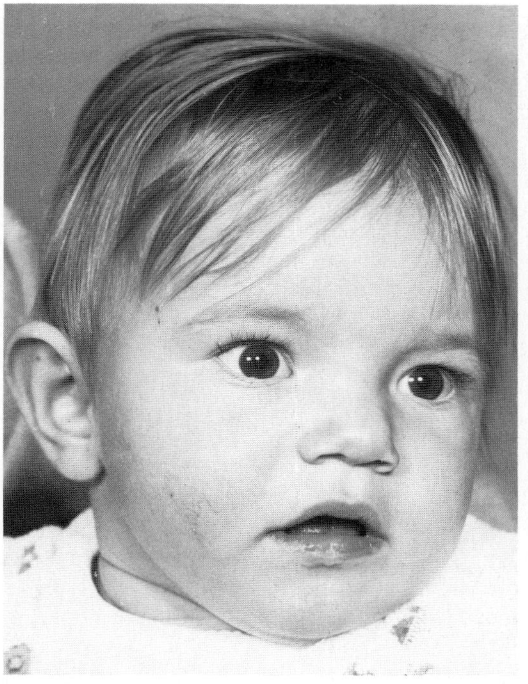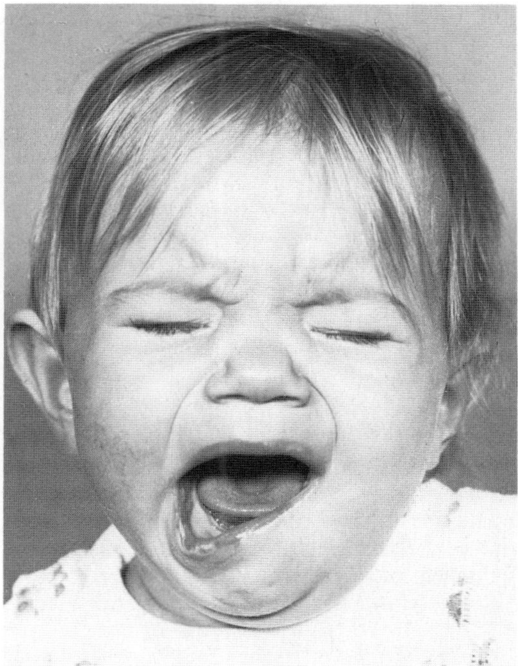

Fig. **42 a and b** Congenital aplasia of the left depressor anguli oris in a one-year-old girl. **a** At rest the face appears to be that of a normal child. Occasionally the lower lip on the affected side may be smaller. **b** While the baby is crying the lower lip on the left side is not displaced downward as it is in the healthy right side. (Courtesy of the Section of Neurology of the Pediatric Clinic, Zurich University. Chief physician, Prof. W. Isler)

— Vascular insults (*see* 2.3.1.2)
— Trauma (evident in history, sudden onset, other cortical dysfunction, psychologic deficits)
— Tumor (resulting in slowly progressive paralysis, usually accompanied by weakness of the hand and later by evidence of increased intracranial pressure and seizures)

2.9.2 Bilateral Paresis or Weakness of Facial Muscles

Causes of facial nerve lesions resulting in bilateral peripheral facial paralysis are

— Cranial polyradiculitis occurring in a setting of ascending Landry-Guillain-Barré syndrome (*see* 1.3.1)
— Cranial tetanus (local injury, trismus)
— Basal meningitis (resulting in meningismus, fever, involvement of other cranial nerves)

— Meningeal carcinomatosis (indicated by pain, rapid progress, involvement of several cranial nerves, rapid appearance of abducens paralysis, increased CSF cell count with pathologic cells, low CSF sugar)

Bilateral nuclear paralysis of the facial muscles occurs

— In rare cases of poliomyelitis (*see* above)
— As congenital paralysis with Möbius syndrome (*see* 2.9.1)

Bilateral weakness of facial muscles is also found with some myopathies, particularly with myotonic dystrophy of Steinert (a very slowly progressive bilateral syndrome with ptosis, "tired" facial expression, bilateral atrophy of temporal muscles, frontal baldness, distal muscle atrophy of the extremities, percussion myotonia of the tongue and thenar eminence; also apparent after forceful clenching of the fist).

Bilateral stiffness of the facial muscles and paucity of facial movement occur

- With Parkinson's syndrome (*see* 2.15.1.3)
- With depression (evident from mood, history, behavior)
- As one manifestation of pseudobulbar palsy with bilateral lesions of the corticobulbar fibers (*see* 2.11.2)
- As an isolated dysfunction of voluntary motor activity, with preservation of automatic motor activity, of mouth and swallowing muscles due to bilateral softening in the anterior part of the operculum, the so-called Foix-Chavany-Marie syndrome. In young patients this may be due to multiple sclerosis and may be reversible.

2.9.3 Involuntary Facial Movement

Typically this consists of hemifacial spasms (synchronous contractions of all muscles innervated by the facial nerve on one side and also contraction of the platysma) [Fig. 43]. The cause is largely unknown, although occasionally it results from vascular compression of the facial nerve root.

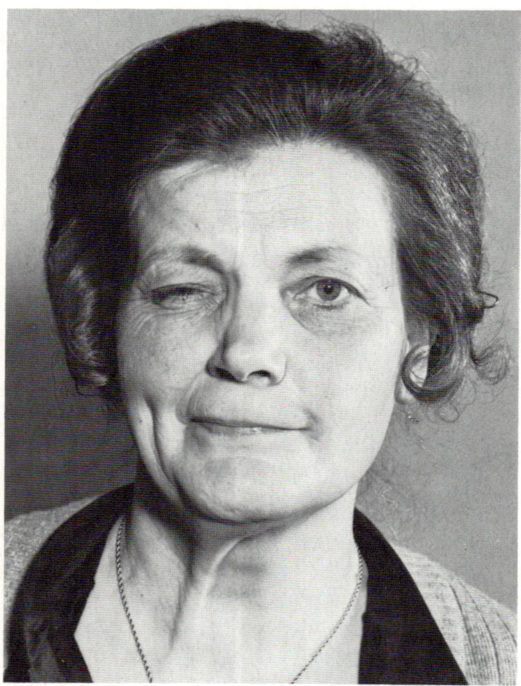

Fig. 43 A 47-year-old patient with right-sided hemifacial spasm. All muscles, including the platysma, innervated by the facial nerve, contract simultaneously, involuntarily, and repeatedly

Such movements occur in rare cases after facial nerve paralysis or benign processes in the cerebellar pontine angle and with brain stem glioma or vascular insults (*see* 1.1.3.3) as a manifestation of the Brissaud syndrome (homolateral peripheral facial palsy with contralateral hemiparesis).

Hemispasm of masticatory muscles is rare. This causes episodic trismus lasting several minutes. The etiology may be similar to that of hemifacial spasm.

Facial myokymia (continuous worm-like contraction of the muscles of the face) occurs with multiple sclerosis (without facial palsy), occasionally occurs as a manifestation of brain stem tumors (with facial weakness), and can be observed with polyradiculitis.

Impressive abnormal movements of the face can occur with chorea (in which other muscle groups also have involuntary movements [*see* 1.1.3.1 and 2.14.1.8]) or facial buccolingual dystonia (*see* 1.1.3.1 and 2.14.11), particularly in elderly individuals after treatment with phenothiazine derivatives.

Blepharospasm (bilateral, irregular spasm of the eyelids, increasing with stress and excitement) can be a manifestation of incipient organic extrapyramidal disorder, but is sometimes difficult to distinguish from a tic.

2.9.4 Other Abnormalities of the Face Important in Neurologic Differential Diagnosis

Progressive hemifacial atrophy, often beginning with scleroderma in a facial scar, affects mostly skin and muscles, but also skeletal structures and brain on one side. It is sometimes combined with a Horner syndrome, with difficulty in ocular motility, and with contralateral focal epileptic attacks, and is slowly progressive. It can be confused with asymmetry of the facial muscles resulting from a unilateral chronic mandibular dislocation.

2.10 Disturbances of Swallowing

The anatomic substrate of the swallowing act consists of

- The striated muscles of the tongue, palate, and pharynx as well as the smooth muscles of the esophagus

– The glossopharyngeal, vagus, and hypoglossal nerves
– The motor nuclei of these nerves
– The sensory afferents from the mouth and pharynx, which pass through the trigeminal, glossopharyngeal, and vagus nerves
– The supranuclear innervations of the mouth and pharynx, which arise in the precentral gyrus and pass through the corticobulbar tracts

The clinical symptomatology consists primarily of disturbance of swallowing, that is, dysphagia. This may be manifested by difficulty in initiating the swallowing act or by frequent coughing and regurgitation up through the back of the nose. The clinical manifestations of the dysphagia and of accompanying dysfunctions, particularly dysarthria (*see* 2.11), may hint at the anatomic site of the lesion. The following lesion sites may account for dysphagia:

– The pharyngeal muscles, in very rare cases, are the location of the disease causing dysphagia.

  ● with very slowly progressive ocular-pharyngeal muscle dystrophy apart from the extraocular muscle involvement. There are also ocular-pharyngeal forms in which the muscles of deglutition and the neck muscles are affected
  ● with myasthenia gravis there are sometimes varying difficulties in swallowing that may be a marked initial symptom of the disease (of varying intensity but increasing during the course of a meal, almost always accompanied by extraocular muscle weakness)
  ● with myotonic dystrophy of Steinert (*see* 1.4 and 2.9.2), difficulties in swallowing are known but rare

– A lesion of the peripheral caudal cranial nerves IX, X, and XII, if unilateral, gives rise to only slight disturbances of swallowing that are soon compensated. When the lesions affect the glossopharyngeal and vagus there may be some swallowing difficulty. There is always a sensory disturbance in the pharynx, with dysfunction of the soft palate and impairment of pharyngeal reflexes. There is usually impairment of taste on the posterior third of the tongue, although this is difficult to demonstrate (Fig. 38). With unilateral lesions of the glossopharyngeal and hypoglossal nerves there is typically weakness of the soft palate on the ipsilateral side, and in gagging, movement of

the raphe toward the unaffected side on contraction. Causes for these lesions may be
  ● Isolated benign unilateral palatal palsy particularly in children predominantly in boys sometimes preceded by a viral illness with spontaneous recovery. Other cranial nerves may also be homolaterally involved on rare occasions
  ● Siebenmann syndrome with paralysis of the glossopharyngeal, vagus, and accessory nerves (Table 17), occurring, for example, with a fracture at the base of the skull, thrombosis of the jugular vein or glomus tumor
  ● Garcin syndrome (Table 17) with extracranial tumors at the base of the skull (examine for enlargement of glands at the mandibular angle)
  ● sarcoid may affect any cranial nerve either unilaterally or bilaterally
  ● Sjögren's syndrome, where there may be recurrences
  ● rarely multiple sclerosis, with lesions of the brain stem affecting the intramedullary parts of the cranial nerves

– Bilateral lesions of the caudal cranial nerves cause severe dysphagia (and dysarthria). Among their causes are:
  ● diphtheria resulting in paralysis of the palate (associated with nasal speech, paralysis of extraocular muscles)
  ● widespread tumors of the base of the skull
  ● cranial polyradiculitis (always associated with facial paralysis as well, and almost always occurring in conjunction with spinal nerve and root syndromes [*see* 1.3.1]), may be commonly also a partial manifestation of infection with *Borrelia burgdorferi* (Lyme disease) (in 50% known tick bite followed by chronic erythema migrans)
  ● chronic meningitis or carcinomatous meningitis (*see* 2.9.2)
  ● cryptogenic benign recurring cranial nerve paralyses (predominantly affecting nerves V, VII, VIII, and also XII)

– A lesion in the medulla oblongata affecting the motor nuclei of the nerves that supply the muscles of swallowing causes a permanent peripheral type of palsy of the corresponding muscles. Causes of unilateral lesions of this type are predominantly vascular disturbances of the brain stem, and the persistent severe swallowing difficulty, is often known as cricopharyngeal achalasia. This is the result of an increase in tone of the cricopharyngeal muscle which does not relax during the act of swallowing. This occurs, for example, in:

- Wallenberg syndrome (*see* 2.7.1)
- Cestan-Chenais syndrome (homolateral Horner syndrome, paralysis of the soft palate, paralysis of the pharynx and vocal chord with hemiataxia, contralateral hemiparesis, and hemihypesthesia)
- Avellis syndrome (homolateral swallowing and contralateral vocal chord paresis)
- Schmidt syndrome (homolateral swallowing paresis, but also contralateral involvement of trapezius and tongue)
- Tapia syndrome (homolateral paralysis of the soft palate and pharynx, vocal chord, tongue, contralateral motor and sensory hemiparesis)
- Vernet syndrome (homolateral paralysis of soft palate, pharynx, and sternocleidomastoid muscle; loss of taste in the posterior third of the tongue; contralateral motor hemiparesis)
- Jackson syndrome (homolateral paralysis of the tongue, contralateral motor hemiparesis)

Rarely lesions of the motor nuclei involved in swallowing are caused by syringobulbia or intramedullary tumors (for example, gliomas) with slow or rapid progression. Such lesions are soon accompanied by long-tract signs and obstructive hydrocephalus with increased intracranial pressure.

- Bilateral damage of cranial nerve nuclei leads to severe impairment of swallowing and dysarthria with atrophy of the involved muscles, particularly the tongue, which grows wrinkled and cannot be protruded beyond the teeth or moved from side to side. With chronic degenerative processes, fibrillation of the tongue can also be seen. Common causes are:
  - degenerative process such as true bulbar paralysis, mostly in association with amyotrophic lateral sclerosis (for effects on tongue and speech see above; other signs include involvement of muscles of the extremities as well as increasing atrophy and paralysis, fasciculations, and pyramidal signs), rarely in orthostatic hypotension of multiple system atrophy (Shy-Drager) (*see* 2.20.1.1)

- vascular accident with extensive softening of the medulla oblongata, leading to acute bulbar paralysis (acute in onset and bilateral, associated with distal cranial nerve paralyses, severe bilateral paralysis of the extremities, miosis)

- With lesions of the supranuclear structures, the predominant symptoms are due to damage of the corticobulbar fibers important in the act of swallowing. With such lesions facial reflexes are increased, and there is no muscle atrophy or fasciculations. Only bilateral lesions of this type cause disturbances of swallowing and speech, which are termed pseudobulbar paralysis. Causes of these symptoms are

- vascular lacunar state (*see* 2.15.1.1)
- degenerative affection (or perinatal trauma) of bilateral motor pathways. This is the cause, for example, of childhood pseudobulbar paralysis (from the earliest age, the patient experiences difficulty in drinking and feeding; food remains in the mouth for long periods and must be propelled backward with the fingers; among other signs are decreased movements of the tongue, increased periaural reflexes, disturbed development of speech, and even anarthria)
- amyotrophic lateral sclerosis. In adults the supranuclear part of the disease may be so prominent as to give rise to a clinical picture of pseudobulbar paralysis

Other non-neurologic diseases also causing disturbances of swallowing must be distinguished from the above. Dysphagia is found, for example, with scleroderma in iron deficiency anemia and with stenosing esophageal processes such as tumors or esophageal diverticula.

2.11 Speech and Language Disturbances

The anatomic structure involved in speech are schematically represented in Figure 44. It can be seen that the causes of speech and language disturbances may be variously localized and consequently may have distinguishing characteristics, which are summarized in Table 19 and discussed in topical order below.

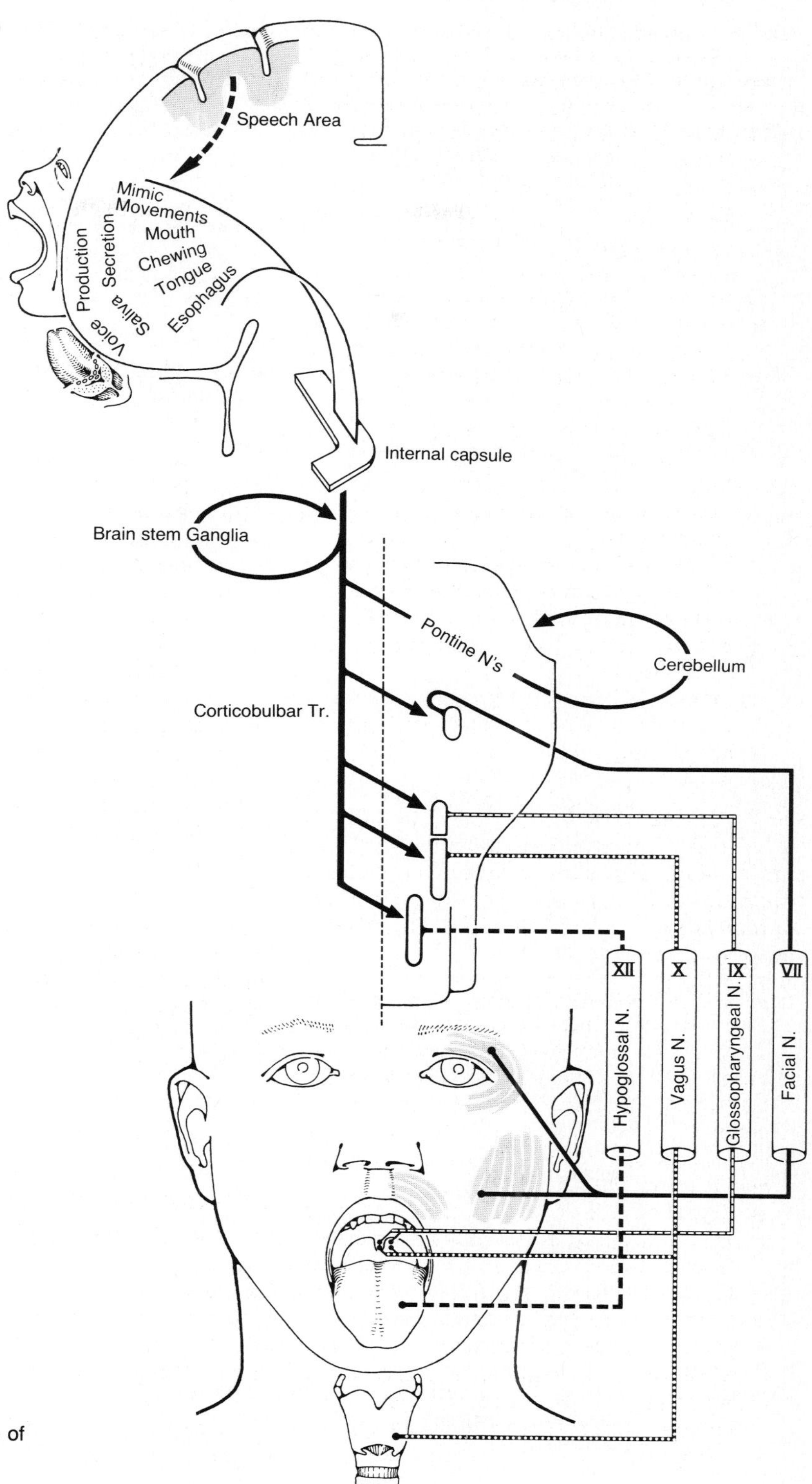

Fig. **44**   Anatomic basis of speech

Table 19 **Speech and language disturbances, characteristics, localization, and causes**

Disturbance	Characteristics	Localization	Causes
Aphasia	Disorder of language; use of overlong words and jargon, incorrect grammatical construction	Dominant hemisphere	Trauma, tumor, disordered blood flow, atrophic processes
Facial apraxia (buccofacial apraxia)	Disorder of mouth-tongue movements, usually associated with aphasic disturbances	Motor association area in vicinity of cortical mouth representation	As above
Echolalia	Uncontrollable repetition of words or sentences	Hemisphere, cortex, diffuse damage	Atrophic processes, also psychogenic in tics
Logoclonia	Uncontrollable repetition of syllables	As above	As above
Dysarthria	With correct speech planning, speech is unclearly articulated (with poor coordination of speech-forming tools)	Central (pseudobulbar) or peripheral (bulbar) motor neurons	Lesions of corticobulbar pathways with vascular brain stem processes, always bilateral; degenerative diseases; lesions of cranial nerve nuclei with degenerative atrophic processes, e.g., amyotrophic lateral sclerosis; true bulbar paralysis; syringobulbia; acute infarction of brain stem
Paroxysmal dysarthria	As above, but paroxysmal	Brain stem, particularly pons; occasionally cerebellar foci	Multiple sclerosis
Pseudobulbar and bulbar speech	As with dysarthria	As with dysarthria	As with dysathria
Iteration	Several involuntary repetitions of each sentence, associated with monotonous, soft, poorly modulated speech	Basal ganglia disorders of hypokinetic rigid type	Parkinson's syndrome, psychogenic depression
Palilalia	As above, but affecting phrases rather than sentences	As above	As above
Explosive speech	Inharmonic, irregular, loud, and explosive	Cerebellum	Variety of cerebellar disturbances (*see* 1.1.4)
Scanning speech	Halting, explosive, with exaggerated pauses between sentence parts	Cerebellum	Multiple sclerosis
Akinetic mutism	Absence of speech but consciousness appears preserved	Organic lesions of central gray or basal ganglia; psychogenic	Encephalitis, ischemia, anoxia, subarachnoid bleeding, depression, catatonia, hysteria

Table 19   (continued)

Disturbance	Characteristics	Localization	Causes
Open nasal speech	Escape of air through nose while speaking	Epipharynx	Paralysis of soft palate as with myasthenia, lesions of cranial nn IX and X, after diphtheria
Closed nasal speech	Abnormal closure of epi-pharynx against nasal passages		Space-occupying lesion in epi-pharynx
Dysphonia	Difficulty in speaking (i.e., in prosody) due to disorder of voice-producing organs, in-cluding larynx	Larynx	Paralysis of vocal cords
Spastic dysphonia	As above, with accompanying involuntary contractions of facial muscle		Psychogenic
Hoarseness	Form of dysphonia	Larynx	Unilateral paralysis of vocal cords, autonomic neuropathy (alcohol, vit B_1 deficiency)
Aphonia	Loss of voice	Larynx	Bilateral total paralysis of vocal cords, psychogenic factors

2.11.1 Cortical and Subcortical Lesions

With lesions in the cortical speech centers, aphasic disorders – disturbances in the scheme and organization of speech – can be expected. Facial apraxia (buccofacial apraxia) occurs with lesions of afferent fibers to the motor representation of the muscles for speech in the lower third of the precentral gyrus (*see* Fig. 1 and 2) and with lesions of the connections to the motor association cortex. Its characteristics are discussed in 2.1. The large majority of such patients also have aphasia (resulting from disturbed mouth movement while speaking, a condition known as parapraxia). Speech is markedly impaired in the Foix-Chavany-Marie-syndrome but spontaneous facial expression (e.g. smiling), is preserved (*see* 2.9.2). With diffuse cortical disturbances (for example, atrophic processes [*see* 1.1.2 and 2.1]) there is paucity of speech eventually with echolalia (meaningless repetition of words or sentences) and logoclonia (repetition of single syllables). The speech of the deaf mute, who has no control of his production of language, sounds like a foreign language learned with difficulty and spoken without harmony.

- causes of cortical language disturbances include trauma, tumors, vascular insults, and atrophic processes

2.11.2 Lesions of the Corticobulbar Pathways

Such lesions cause permanent and significant disturbances of language only when they are bilateral. Speech in such cases is poorly articulated and dysarthric. Perioral reflexes are increased, and swallowing is often also disturbed (for disturbances of swallowing with pseudobulbar paralysis [*see* 2.10]). There usually are signs of bilateral pyramidal lesions in the extremities, a short-paced step, and no fasciculations. The causes of lesions resulting in this disturbance of speech are similar to those causing pseudobulbar paralysis with disordered swallowing (*see* 2.10). In addition, paroxysmal dysarthrias that may last only a very few seconds occur after brain stem encephalitis and multiple sclerosis with lesions of the brain stem.

2.11.3 Lesions of Basal Ganglia and Cerebellum

These structures influence the smoothness, coordination, and harmony of voluntary and automatic motor acts and thus also influence speech. With hypokinetic rigid extrapyramidal syndromes, particularly Parkinson's syndrome (*see* 2.12.1 – 2), the speech is soft and monotonous, with little rhythmic and melodic modulation. Iteration and palilalias (several repetitions of sentences or parts thereof, involuntary iteration with tics only are present [*see* 2.11.8]). With lesions of the central gray matter and basal ganglia, the hypokinesia of the act of speaking can be so pronounced that akinetic mutism occurs (Parkinson's syndrome, brain stem encephalitis, anoxic damage, medication-induced basilar blood-flow disturbances, subarachnoid bleeding). With hyperkinetic extrapyramidal syndromes (*see* 2.14.1.8), involuntary movements of the mouth-tongue can interfere with the act of speaking. With disorders of the cerebellum, speech is harmonically disturbed, irregular, loud, and explosive. The speech disturbance in multiple sclerosis is due to foci in the cerebellum, and takes the form of staccato explosive speech with exaggerated pauses between parts of sentences and words, as in scanning speech.

2.11.4 Lesions of Cranial Nerves

Lesions of the nuclei of cranial nerves VII, IX, X, and XII cause peripheral paralysis of the muscle fibers corresponding to their innervation by these nerves, with atrophy of appropriate muscles and, in chronic processes, fasciculations. The resulting disturbance of speech is acoustically similar to that due to supranuclear lesions of the corticobulbar pathways: The speech is unclear and poorly articulated, sounding as though the patient has something in his mouth. This form of dysarthria is also designated bulbar speech. Appropriate disturbances of swallowing are always present as well (*see* 2.10). If central neurons are also affected (for example, in amyotrophic lateral sclerosis with bulbar involvement) then there is also exaggeration of perioral reflexes. Causes are the same as those described above for disturbances of swallowing (*see* 2.10).

2.11.5 Extracerebral Lesions of Distal Cranial Nerves

These lesions produce peripheral paralysis of distant nerves that innervate muscles involved in speech production. Sensation in the pharynx is often disturbed with such lesions.

Paralysis of the glossopharyngeal nerve causes recognizable disturbances of speech only if it is bilateral. The open nasal speech that results in accompanied by arreflexia of the pharynx, paralysis of swallowing, and ageusia of the posterior third of the tongue. Causes are

— Diphtheria (evident in history, involvement of extraocular muscles)
— Cranial polyradiculitis (*see* 1.3.1 and 2.8.1)
— Carcinomatous meningitis or extensive invasion of the base of the skull by tumor (*see* 2.9.2)
— Fractures involving the jugular foramen or thrombosis of the jugular vein (giving rise to Siebenmann syndrome with dysfunction of the glossopharyngeal, vagus, and accessory nerves [Table 17])

Paralysis of the vagus nerve, even if unilateral, causes dysfunction of the recurrent laryngeal nerve with paralysis of vocal cords, hoarseness, and soft speech. If the disorder is unilateral the speech becomes normal again after several weeks. Bilateral paralysis of the vagus causes aphonia. With bilateral lesions of the posterior branches of the recurrent laryngeal nerve, abductor paralysis occurs with the vocal cords assuming a cadaveric position, and there is danger of asphyxiation. Proximal lesions of the vagus cause symptoms similar to those of glossopharyngeal lesions, with additional parasympathetic disturbances manifested by tachycardia, dysfunction of the ocular cardiac reflexes, dysphonia, and dry mouth. Causes of vagus lesions are identical to those of glossopharyngeal paresis.

Involvement of the recurrent laryngeal nerve results in vocal cord paralysis. Tumor of the thyroid gland, thyroidectomy, mediastinal processes such as aortic aneurysm, tumor, inflammatory lung and esophageal diseases can all cause such involvement. Paralysis of the hypoglossal nerve, if unilateral, causes deviation of the tongue toward the paretic side, but no important speech disturbance. Bilateral hypoglossal paralysis causes total paralysis of the tongue with great difficulty in articulation, speech disorders, and pronounced difficulty in swallowing. Causes are predominantly tumors of the base of the skull and postoperative ("neck dissection").

2.11.6 Diseases of Muscles Involved in Speech

Among myopathies, only myasthenia gravis leads to significant speech disturbances. Abnormal fatigability of muscles resulting in progessively softer speech with a nasal quality occurs—symptoms that are temporarily relieved by silence. They are often associated with problems of swallowing and double vision.

2.11.7 Diseases of Sound-Producing Structures

With these disorders the sound and quality of words are impaired while word selection remains normal. A few examples are hoarseness with disease of the larynx, closed nasal quality of voice with hypertrophy of the tonsils or epipharyngeal tumors, open nasality of voice with cleft palate, impairment of speech after laryngectomy.

2.11.8 Functional Disorders of Speech

Most cases of stuttering are probably of psychogenic origin. Spastic dysphonias accompanied by irregular contractions of facial muscles during speech are of similar origin. The speech in Gilles de la Tourette syndrome—which is of organic nature—is characterized by explosive and involuntary loud words, often accompanied by cursing or swearing (coprolalia), and by logoclonia and iteration. Psychologic disorders that may result in disturbed speech include depression (soft monotonous voice), schizophrenia (for example, neologisms), hysterical neurosis (aphonia). All three disorders may lead to mutism.

2.12 Disorders of Muscle Tone

Muscle tone is the physiologic tension of muscles, whereas muscle tension is produced by voluntary or involuntary activation of the muscle nerves. The anatomic basis of muscle tone is identical to that of the central motor pathways (Figs. 1, 3, 6, and 45), but elements of spinal reflex arcs are also important. These parts are schematically represented in Figure 45. The assessment of normal tone requires experience, a relaxed patient, and the correct method of examination (involving non-rhythmic, passive movements, both slow and rapid, of various parts of the limbs). Many individuals (tense or uncooperative patients, medical personnel) are unable to relax, making a correct examination of tone impossible. The following abnormalities are found (Fig. 46).

- An increase in tone (hypertonia), manifested as
  - spasticity (Fig. 46a), which implies increased initial resistance to passive movement with rapidly decreasing resistance as the movement proceeds (clasp-knife phenomenon)
  - rigidity (Fig. 46b), that is, resistance to passive movement throughout the range of motion
  - a special intermittent form with more or less rhythmic and always perceptible increases in tone, the so-called cogwheel phenomenon (Fig. 46c)
- A decrease in tone (hypotonia) (Fig. 46d)

2.12.1 Increase in Muscle Tone

Spasticity is clinically regarded as an expression of a lesion in the pyramidal system. However, excision of the precentral gyrus or interruption of the corticospinal pathways in the peduncle causes flaccid paralysis or only transient paresis. Only when such excision is combined with dysfunction of the supplementary motor area on the medial surface of the hemisphere is the result spastic paralysis. In practice, however, supranuclear motor paralysis is always associated with dysfunction of wide cortical areas due to the convergence in the corona radiata, and the internal capsule, or in the lateral parts of the spinal cord of their efferent fibers. There is always involvement of numerous efferents arising in extrapyramidal structures and of afferent fibers as well. Such widespread dysfunction is very commonly associated with spastic paralysis.

Lesions causing spastic paralysis can be located in any part of the pyramidal system (which is interwoven with fibers coming from other areas related to motor activity). With a small lesion and slight damage, the spastic increased tone may be

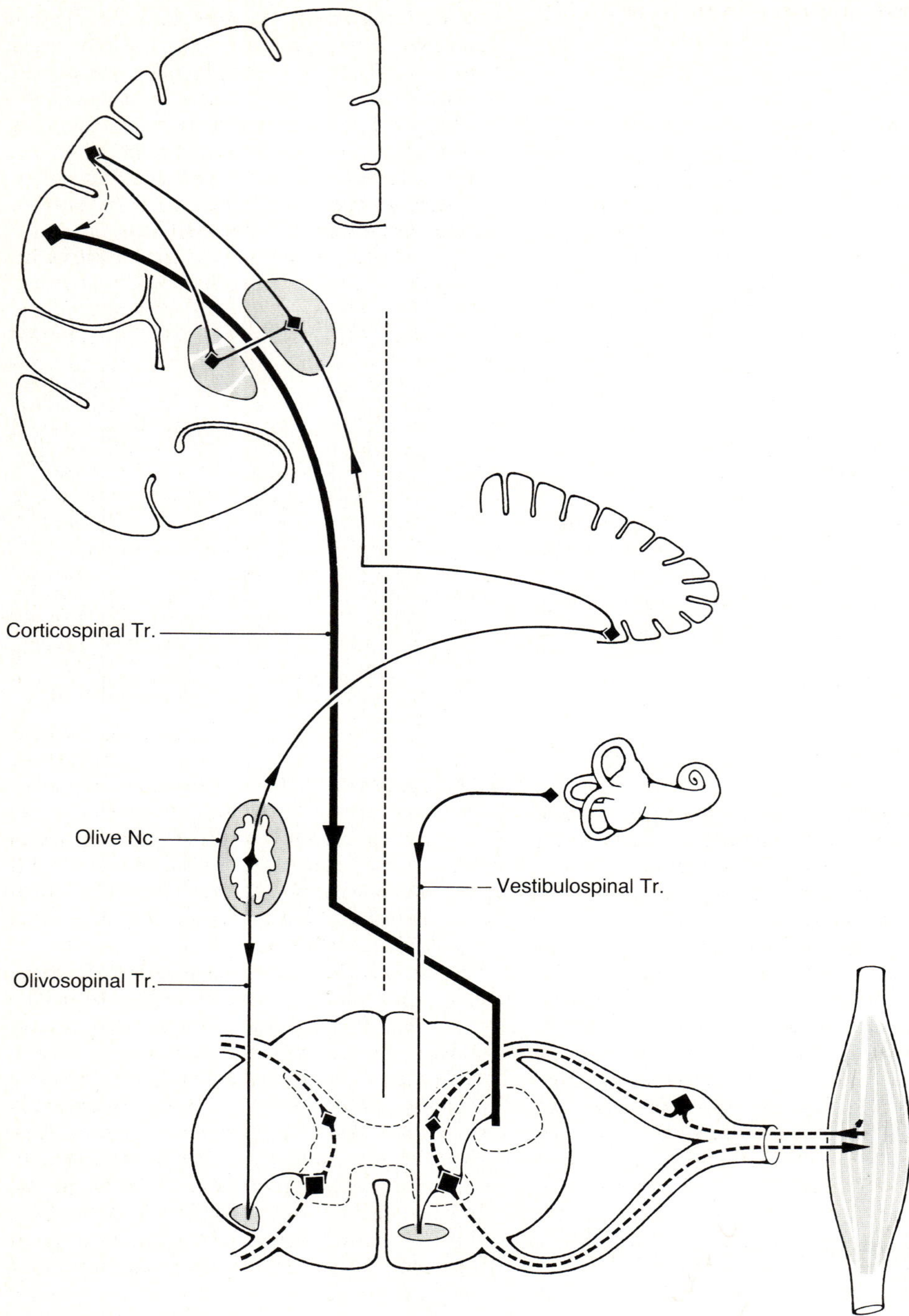

Fig. **45** Anatomic structures important in muscle tone

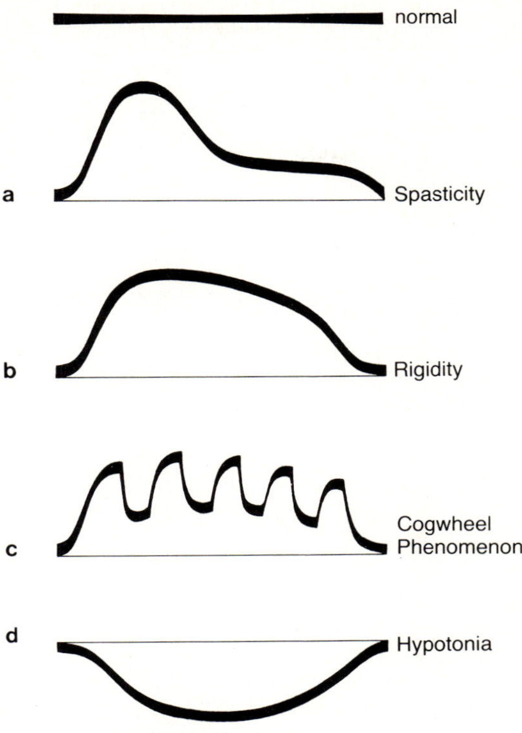

Fig. 46   Abnormalities of muscle tone

present throughout the range of passive motion, even increasing slightly toward the end of the movement. The clasp-knife phenomenon is evident only with marked spasticity (*see above*).

An isolated bilateral increase in tone of the legs is termed paraspasticity and is generally due to damage of the thoracolumbar spinal cord (the result of compression by space-occupying lesions or a narrow spinal canal, degenerative [familial] spastic spinal paralysis, multiple sclerosis, trauma, Little's disease with adductor spasticity, or affection of pyramidal fibers with metabolic disorders and intoxication as in hyperthyroidism and lathyrism). In rare cases, spastic paraplegia is due to a parasagittal cerebral process (pure motor as with bilateral ischemia in the supply territory of the anterior cerebral artery, meningiomas, corpus callosum lipomas, or a process impairing the function of both hemispheres such as bilateral subdural hematoma). Spastic tetraplegia points to a lesion in the cervical spinal cord or higher (resulting from compression of the cervical spinal cord – for example, by cervical spondylosis – anomalies of the cranial-cervical junction, chronic atlan-

toaxial dislocation, or multiple sclerosis). Spastic tetraplegia also occurs as a partial manifestation of amyotrophic lateral sclerosis with lesions of the pyramidal pathways and as a disturbance of movement of cerebral origin following birth trauma. A hemispastic disorder has the same significance as incipient motor hemiparesis (*see* 2.13.2.5).

Intermittent hemispasticity is a manifestation of tonic brain stem fits (*see* 2.3.1.1).

Decerebrate posture represents an extreme increase in spasticity of all antigravity muscles, resulting in extensor spasticity, extension of the body, inward rotation of arms and legs; it is often associated with opisthotonus. This is sometimes designated the appallic syndrome. It is caused by midbrain damage, particularly due to crowding in the tentorium, resulting from supratentorial processes such as temporal lobe tumor, brain hemorrhage with intraventricular extension, severe brain contusion, and brain stem hemorrhage, or due to encephalitis or anoxic or toxic conditions. The apallic syndrome may occur intermittently in so-called cerebellar fits, which can be triggered by external stimuli. With total interruption of the descending impulses in the spinal cord, most often by acute transection of the spinal cord, flexion spasticity is seen.

Rigidity (Fig. 46b) is a manifestation of damage in the extrapyramidal system. It is found in the various types of Parkinson's syndrome (together with akinesia, the cogwheel phenomenon, and often tremor) and may begin unilaterally. It also accompanies other degenerative diseases with Parkinson-like components, for example, olivopontocerebellar atrophy, orthostatic hypotension, Creutzfeldt-Jakob disease.

Other forms of increased muscle tone to be distinguished from those mentioned above include
– Neuromyotonia, although not completely identical to the syndrome of continued muscle fiber activity or the stiff-man syndrome, is manifested by painful, hard, contracted muscles, often associated with plastic spasms, slow painful movement, and fine muscle activity with worm-like contractions. Of diagnostic significance is the EMG, which shows continuous muscle action potentials. Most cases are idiopathic. Sometimes a syndrome of continued muscle fiber activity with myokymia has appeared after gold therapy. The Schwartz-Jampel syndrome (small stature, abnormal facial features, and stiff marionette-like gait, hypoplasia, and stiff muscles, particularly in the shoulder girdles) is a related disorder

- Tetanus, which can also be local in its effects (painful attacks of spasms and stiffness of muscles, rapid progression). A subacute injury is the antecedent
- Some types of myotonia (*see* 1.4), which include recurring episodes of muscle stiffness, particularly after activity (myotonia congenita [Thomsen disease]) or after exposure to cold (paramyotonia congenita [Eulenburg disease])
- Painful cramps of the calves (easily identified)

2.12.2 Decrease in Muscle Tone

A significant decrease in muscle tone (hypotonia) is usually associated with exaggerated extensibility of the joints and often with decreased reflexes or areflexia. Hypotonia (Fig. 46d) is found with the following lesions:

- Extensive brain stem damage, in which hypotonia occurs with deep coma and bulbar syndromes (mostly dilated nonreactive pupils, absence of vestibular ocular reflexes, and oculocephalic reflexes, disturbances of respiration, and abnormal vasomotor function). For causes of this clinical picture, see decerebrate rigidity (2.12.1)
- Lesions of the cerebellar hemisphere, in which hypotonia is seen homolateral to the lesion (occasionally bilateral), together with cerebellar symptoms. Causes and characteristics of these symptoms are listed in 1.1.4
- Cord transection. Specific lesions or disorders leading to hypotonia include
  - sudden disruption of descending pathways in the spinal cord (acute transverse syndrome) manifest as spinal shock (diaschisis) with areflexia and absence of pyramidal signs, with hypotonia lasting at the most 3 weeks after injury
  - extensive central medullary softening almost always due to vascular lesions (*see* 1.2.1.3), resulting in permanent hypotonia
  - hyperkinetic-hypotonic extrapyramidal diseases (*see* 2.14.1.8), together with abnormal movements
  - isolated white matter lesions of the cord, which usually cause single sensory disorders, particularly of deep sensibility-position sense and epicritic touch. In the cases of posterior column lesions (*see* 1.2.2) and extensive posterior root lesions (for ex-

ample, lues), these sensory losses often occur without associated motor weakness
  - muscle atrophies and motor paralysis without sensory disturbances
  - anterior horn cell disease, such as acute anterior poliomyelitis or chronic spinal muscular atrophy (*see* 1.2.3) if associated with faciculation
  - fairly advanced myopathies (for symptoms and etiology, *see* 1.4 and 2.13.1.1)
- In association with polyradiculitis (*see* 1.3.1) and polyneuropathies (*see* 1.3.5), in which hypotonia is associated with a combination of progressive motor and, above all, distal sensory deficits
- In infants, hypotonia can appear as the only symptom (the so-called floppy child syndrome):
  - in the early stages of a cerebral movement disorder (CP), upon which a spastic or dystonic disorder soon becomes superimposed
  - as an early symptom of neuromuscular disease, most often spinal muscular atrophy of Werdnig-Hoffmann (*see* 1.2.3)
  - as a manifestation of atonic astatic syndrome of Foerster or of amyotonia congenita of Oppenheim, both being diagnostic wastebaskets for etiologically poorly defined cases

The hypotonia predicted theoretically and verified experimentally with vestibular lesions is never found clinically. On the other hand, distinct hypotonia can be found with cerebellar lesions.

2.13 Weakness and Fatigue

Weakness is a complaint that often brings the patient to the neurologist, especially localized weakness, which is often interpreted as paralysis. The discussion below is confined to weakness as a dominant symptom.

Weakness can be a generalized manifestation of asthenia, a general affection with direct effects on the neuromuscular apparatus, or an affection primarily of the central or peripheral nervous system. There is also pure neurovegetative or psychogenic weakness. The differential diagnosis of weakness is best attempted by categorizing the disease according to the location and development of the weakness and its accompanying symptoms and findings.

2.13.1 Generalized, Poorly Localized Weakness

2.13.1.1 Generalized Weakness that is Gradual in Onset and Eventually Slowly Progressive

Patients complain of generalized listlessness and asthenia, and they may feel psychologically tired, easily fatigued and lack drive. Causes are:

- Generalized internal diseases without direct affection of neuromuscular function, such as chronic infection, tuberculosis, sepsis, Addison's disease, or malignant disease. (The weakness is usually associated with specific symptoms of the underlying disease; a general clinical and physical examination is important in diagnosing this cause)
- General diseases with known direct effects on the neuromuscular apparatus. The weakness with such diseases is often predominantly proximal, that is, particularly prominent in the girdle areas. In this category belong:
  - endocrinopathies, such as hypothyroidism (characterized by skin that is cold, pale, doughy, and dry; lack of drive, constipation; thick tongue; hoarseness; bradycardia; myoedema, slow ankle jerk relaxation; and so on; occasionally associated with other neurologic symptoms such as paresthesia, ataxia, carpal tunnel syndrome, and muscle cramps); hyperthyroidism (characterized by proximal muscle weakness with difficulty in rising from a squatting position; *signe du tabouret*; sweating; tachycardia, tremor; warm skin; heat intolerance; diarrhea and the like; and rarely by neurologic symptoms such as pyramidal signs); hypoparathyroidism (marked by muscle weakness and cramps, tetany, headache, fatigability, ataxia, nausea, epilepsy, occasionally hallucinations, and choreoathetotic symptoms); hyperparathyroidism (distinguished by true diffuse myopathy with muscle atrophy; depression; lability of mood, irritability, confusion, constipation); Cushing's disease as well as others
  - certain metabolic disorders such as glycogenoses (marked by heart and liver involvement), hypercalcemia (due to hyperparathyroidism or due to other causes) or diabetes mellitus
  - some intoxications and pharmaceuticals, which can result in slowly progressive generalized weakness. Chronic forms of alcoholic myopathy develop over weeks or months and are accompanied by atrophy of proximal muscles. With chloroquine medication, vacuolar myopathy has been observed; with cortisone particularly fluorohydrocortisone) and with long-term colchicine administration there is a reversible myopathy
  - malignant disease, which may be accompanied by polymyositis (*see below*) as well as by generalized weakness
  - collagen diseases, particularly lupus erythematosus and scleroderma, in which muscle symptoms can occur in association with polymyositis (*see below*)
  - sarcoidosis. Granulomas may clinically involve muscles, particularly the proximal muscles
- Many true myopathies, for example, the hereditary muscular dystrophies. (For more details, *see* 1.4)
  - some painful syndromes impair strength (*see* 2.17)
- Psychogenic weakness (*see* 2.13.3)

2.13.1.2 Acute and Rapidly Progressive Generalized Weakness

Here too the proximal muscles are most involved. Causes are

- Internal diseases, such as hypocalcemia of various causes, which can lead within several hours to widespread severe weakness (*see* 2.3.1.2.2)
- A number of substances interfere with neuromuscular transmission. These include curare, alkylphosphates (insecticides, nerve gas) and tetrodotoxin produced by the Pacific puffer fish
- Myopathies, particularly acute paroxysmal myoglobinuria (rhabdomyolysis) (characterized by pain and red urine); myasthenia gravis in its rarer generalized form and occasionally a symptomatic form due to penicillamine therapy. Drug-induced myasthenic syndrome has been described with the administration of beta blockers, carnitin, lithiumcarbonate, numerous antibiotics, chloroquine, lidocaine, phenytoin and other drugs. (With myasthenia gravis the weakness increases with effort, and

the patient is easily fatigued but improves with rest and in the morning); polymyositis (often associated with red violet patches in the skin and face, painful muscles, and weakness that is predominantly proximal); rarely trichinosis (painful generalized muscle weakness, eosinophilia.)

— A diffuse fasciitis with accompanying eosinophilia and high sedimentation rate (Shulman syndrome) is associated with scleroderma-like changes and edema. Occasionally this condition is accompanied by painful muscle weakness and this must then be distinguished from true polymyositis

— The eosinophilia-myalgia syndrome (painful diffuse muscle weakness and high eosinophilia) attributed to intake of tainted L-tryptophan as a dietary supplement

— Actual affections of the nervous system. Weakness that is more or less generalized clinically can result from infectious anterior horn ganglion cell involvement, such as poliomyelitis (weakness without sensory loss, accompanied by fever, areflexia, CSF findings), a variety of virus infections, and toxic causes, such as the toxic state following tetanus in the newborn. The polyradiculitis of Guillain-Barré is usually associated only with discrete paresthesia distally and some sensory changes (*see* 1.3.1). The rarer acute polyneuropathies (*see* 1.3.5), such as porphyria (abdominal symptoms, constipation, epileptic attacks, tachycardia, and light sensitivity of the urine) also result in weakness with little sensory change

— Psychogenic weakness (*see* 2.13.3) sometimes manifested as acute loss of tone (falling attacks [*see* 2.3.1.21])

2.13.1.3 Intermittent or Recurring Generalized Weakness

In this category the following diseases can be listed:

— Diseases of muscle, in particular myasthenia (*see above*) and muscle phosphorylase deficiency (McArdle), which produces hypokalemic paralyses that appear together with pain and weakness with generalized effort

— Diseases of the central nervous system; intermittent compression of the spinal cord by the odontoid process, resulting in intermittent tetraparesis; vertebrobasilar insufficiency (*see*

2.3.1.2.1), resulting in drop attacks. For further discussion, *see* 2.3.1.2.1

2.13.2 More or Less Localized Weakness

Most of the following disorders can appear in various muscle groups and lead to varying patterns of weakness. The discussion that follows, however, takes into account the tendency of certain diseases to show particular manifestations. Reference is made to affections discussed in other chapters.

2.13.2.1 Weakness Predominantly in the Head, Neck, and Facial Muscles

Causes of this disorder are

— A myasthenic syndrome, particularly with paralysis of extraocular muscles (resulting in ptosis and double vision [*see* 2.8.3 and 2.8.1]) and difficulty in swallowing (*see* 2.10)

— Myasthenia and certain muscle dystrophic processes, for example, myotonic dystrophy of Steinert (*see* 1.4 and Table 11), causing paralysis of muscles of mimicry. A lesion of the facial nerve can also cause such paralysis (for acute facial paralysis, *see* 2.9.1)

— Paralysis of muscles of mastication may be more or less isolated, particularly in myasthenia

— Soft palate myopathy ('hypertrophic branchial myopathy'), a rare syndrome with weakness and hypertrophy of the muscle of mastication

— A lesion of the motor part of the mandibular division of the trigeminal nerve causing unilateral paralysis of muscles of mastication, usually associated with sensory impairment in the trigeminal distribution. It also causes deviation of the jaw toward the paralyzed side as the mouth is opened

— Bilateral lesions of the accessory nerve causing paralysis of the sternocleidomastoid (as a consequence, for example, of bilateral basal skull tumor, neck dissection, fracture at the base of the skull with bilateral Siebenmann syndrome [Table 17]). A similar clinical picture can occur after poliomyelitis or with prolonged malnutrition resulting in symptoms sometimes seen in prisoners of war; myasthenic symptoms with ptosis and generalized fatigability, particularly of the neck muscles (the Japanese kubisagari, "one with a hanging head").

2.13.2.2 Weakness Particularly in the Shoulder, Arm, and Hand

More or less symmetric weakness confined to these areas is almost always due to neuromuscular affection. A progressive muscle dystrophy, for example, fascioscapulohumeral dystrophy (type I) or trunk girdle form (type II) causes predominantly proximal weakness (very slowly progressive with eventual involvement of other muscles, mostly familial in occurrence and accompanied by atrophy). With polymyositis, similar weakness occurs, but progression is more rapid. With myasthenia the distribution of weakness is often asymmetric, and the degree of weakness variable (*see* 1.4).

With pseudomyopathic spinal muscular atrophy, Kugelberg-Welander type or a Vulpian-Bernhardt type, there are fasciculations and, in early stages of the former type, similar involvement of pelvic girdle musculature. In poliomyelitis the proximal or distal muscles may be involved symmetrically or asymmetrically, sometimes resulting in acute arm weakness. A more or less symmetric weakness predominantly localized distally is found in dystrophia myotonica of Steinert or in the vary rare distal myopathy of Welander or the juvenile form of Biemond (a hereditary disorder, usually involving other muscles as well, progressing very slowly). In Charcot-Marie-Tooth disease (peroneal muscle atrophy), distal progressive atrophies and paresis of the hand usually follow involvement of the distal lower extremity (*see* 2.13.2.4.2). More marked weakness of the arms that is slowly progressive, distal or proximal and occasionally asymmetric, with atrophy and rarely also fasciculations, can be seen with intermedullary processes in the cervical spinal cord, for example, syringomyelia or tumors. These can lead to flaccid atrophic paralyses of the arms. With such processes, signs of involvement of long spinal tracts may be absent, but the (segmental) dissociated sensory loss is always found. Lesions of single peripheral nerves in the arm can, on occasion, be bilateral and cause difficulties in differential diagnosis. This is particularly so in cases of bilateral carpal tunnel syndrome (bilateral atrophy of the thenar eminence, usually with nocturnal pain and sensory disturbances); bilateral cervical ribs and other lesions of the brachial plexus (the dominant hand is usually more involved and always shows the first symptoms of the disorder); rare bilateral pressure palsies of the radial nerve or ulnar nerve, occurring after prolonged pressure resulting from inappropriate positioning during

coma or, under unusual circumstances, certain habitually assumed postures.

Unilateral weakness in certain areas of the upper limb can be the initial phase of muscle weakness that later is generalized (for example, spinal muscular atrophy, myasthenia, polymyositis, sarcoid with muscle involvement). Such weakness may, however, also remain localized, although muscles in other parts of the body may also be involved. With such a condition or with pure motor paralysis of acute onset, a likely cause is inflammatory involvement of the anterior horn cells, such as poliomyelitis or other virus infection. In children, persistent unilateral weakness occasionally appears after an attack of bronchial asthma. Localized proximal arm weakness (especially abduction and elevation) together with limb apraxia and weakness of the pelvic girdle muscles may be found in lesions of the contralateral premotor cortex (vascular tumor). Involvement of a single muscle most often results from an infection of a root, plexus, or peripheral nerve. With classic involvement of a single peripheral nerve there is weakness of the muscle supplied by the nerve, along with appropriate sensory loss or pain and paresthesia. Such symptoms or the presence of an appropriate injury make the diagnosis clear. Difficulty arises when there is no clear-cut external cause and pain and sensory impairment are absent. All or some of this confusion occurs, for example, in the shoulder-upper limb paresis after neuralgic shoulder amyotrophy (marked by pain that initially is acute and severe followed by shoulder weakness with winged scapula but without sensory impairment); in iatrogenic injury, as of the accessory nerve at the posterior border of the sternocleidomastoid muscle (dissection of glands in the lateral part of the neck followed by shoulder pain with paralysis of the trapezius muscle but without sensory impairment); after cryptogenic lesions (sometimes resulting from heavy lifting) of the long thoracic nerve (indicated by winged scapula) or of the musculocutaneous nerve (resulting in paralysis of the biceps muscles).

Localized paresis of the extensors of the forearm (together with weakness of the triceps) is found after sleep paralysis of the radial nerve and after clutch paralysis of the same nerve. This paresis can be recognized in careful examination as wristdrop and as sensory disturbance on the dorsum of the hand over the first interosseal space. With the supinator canal syndrome there is chronic damage to the perforating branch of the radial nerve alone (resulting in slowly progressive paralysis of dorsal extension of the fingers and hand without sensory impairment). Ischemic necrosis of deep forearm extensors is rarely a complication of forearm fracture or chronic pressure increase in the deep forearm compartment. It is followed (if untreated) by impairment of hand extension. With ischemic Volkmann contracture (usually after supracondylar fracture of the humerus with dislocation) there is fibrosis and shortening of the long hand and finger flexors. Initially there is also an ischemic lesion of the median nerve and of the ulnar nerve. Another disorder sometimes confused with neuromuscular affection is disruption of tendons, particularly of the extensor pollicis longus (drummer's paralysis) with isolated paresis of the dorsal extensor of the thumb. With strong ulnar deviation of the fingers at the metacarpophalangeal joints, the extensor tendon slips laterally, as the joint is flexed the tendon comes to rest below the point of rotation and, on purely mechanical grounds, is then unable to extend the joint.

The deep branch of the ulnar nerve, which is purely motor, is most often damaged by pressure in the hand or by a ganglion (paralysis of interossei). It must be differentiated from spinal muscular atrophy, which can begin asymmetrically (but muscles innervated by the median nerve are then also involved, and fasciculations are also present in clinically unaffected muscles).

2.13.2.3 Weakness Predominantly in Trunk Muscles

This is rare, found occasionally after poliomyelitis or as paralysis of hip flexors in disorders affecting the pelvic girdle muscles (*see below*) evident as weakness on sitting up. Unilateral diaphragmatic paresis may result from lesions of the 4th cervical root may be also the only manifestation of neuralgic amyotrophy of the shoulder and can occur after lesions to the phrenic nerve (e.g. due to cold after cardiac surgery).

2.13.2.4 Weakness Predominantly in Pelvic Girdle and Legs

The same circumstances as those mentioned in weakness of the upper extremities (*see* 2.13.2.2) are usually operative. However, lesions of the spinal cord and motor systems in the brain can result in lower extremity weakness while the upper limbs remain intact.

2.13.2.4.1 Symmetric, Global, or Predominantly Proximal Weakness of the Legs

This pattern of weakness is known as paraparesis (with total paralysis: paraplegia). Causes for this clinical picture are

— A cortical atrophic process, predominantly confined to the precentral gyrus, causing unilateral or bilateral motor loss, ranging from (para)paresis to tetraparesis, which is slowly progressive over years. The brain atrophy can be recognized with computed tomography. Unilateral paralysis is designated Mills paralysis (*see* 2.13.2.5.2)

— Lesions of the spinal cord above the sacral and below the cervical cord, particularly intraspinal space-occupying lesions. Signs include girdle pain, eventually bilateral impairment of radicular function, spastic paraparesis with pyramidal signs, bladder dysfunction, and sensory loss, occasionally well circumscribed at first; later a sensory level becomes apparent. Such lesions are evident on lumbar puncture and myelography. The foremost causes are tumors, which may progress over months to years (in the case of meningioma or neurinomas) or (in the case of metastasis) may cause paraplegia within days or weeks. On a plain film of the spine, particular attention should be paid to widening of the interpeduncular distance or deformity of the dorsal contour of vertebral bodies, destruction of peduncles, or enlargement of the spinal foramina. Another cause, epidural hematoma, can occur even without antecedent trauma, for example, during anticoagulant therapy, and lead to rapidly progressive painful paraparesis. Chronic, sometimes cystic, spinal arachnoiditis can cause slow loss of function.

A slowly progressive transverse syndrome of the spinal cord can give rise to the same signs as intramedullary lesions. Transverse myelitis may rarely be a manifestation of multiple sclerosis. This is usually of poor prognostic significance and, if the onset is acute, causes particularly severe paralysis accompanied by back pain. Myelopathy with paraparesis in combination with periphlebitis and retinal hemorrhages can be seen with Eales disease and with Vogt-Koyanagi-Harada syndrome. Spastic paraparesis can be found in myelopathy due to cervical spondylosis or, rarely, to calcification of the posterior longitudinal ligament in the cervical region. The paralysis is accompanied by paresthesia often, by glove-like sensory disturbances particularly prominent for temperature and pain in the upper limbs, and by ataxia; roentgenograms show a sagittal diameter in the cervical canal of less than 13 mm and in the thoracic canal of 9.5 mm or less.

Vascular causes of paraplegia (*see* 1.2.1.3) include spastic spinal paralysis (predominantly spasticity with less weakness without sensory disturbances), a familial disease; paraplegia also occurs, for example, with adrenoleukodystrophy, with ectodermal dysplasia of the Bloch-Sulzberger (incontinentia pigmenti) type, with hyperglycinemia, with Sjögren-Larsson syndrome, and in hyperthyroidism.

— Spinal muscular atrophies, particularly the progressive pseudomyopathic type of Kugelberg-Welander (*see* 2.13.2.2) or the rarer initially symmetric form of amyotrophic lateral sclerosis (resulting in pure motor paralysis with fasciculations and abnormally increased reflexes or pyramidal signs)
— Myopathies, in which the affection initially is often found exclusively or predominantly in the pelvic girdle and upper thighs. These include the pelvic girdle type of progressive muscular dystrophy (type II), Duchenne dystrophy (type III), a variety of other childhood manifestations of myopathies, (dermato)myositis, and so on. A similar localization of muscle weakness occurs rarely in myasthenia. Involvement of the same muscles in other diseases (*see* 2.13.1.1) is often most marked in the pelvic girdle (as in hyperthyroidism, Cushing's disease, and hyperparathyroidism, and also in a setting of uremia).

2.13.2.4.2 Mostly Symmetric, Predominantly Distal Weakness of Lower Extremities

Causes of this type of weakness are

— A lesion of the medial aspect of the hemisphere involving the precentral gyri, causing spastic, predominantly distal, paraparesis. The etiology is similar to that described with paraspasticity (*see* 2.12.1.1)
— A spinal cord lesion. Such processes cause predominantly distal spastic paraparesis only when they affect the cord bilaterally from the

periphery, thus involving the corticospinal tract and, in particular, its superficial fibers, which pass to the lower extremities. An intermedullary process (tumor or syrinx) in the region of the lower lumbar and upper sacral cord can affect the anterior horn cells of the muscles of the lower leg (resulting in slowly progressive paralysis, always associated with sensory loss, and often with disturbances of micturition). Spinal muscular atrophy rarely involves distal leg muscles first, and if it does, this is usually not symmetric. The occasional patient with amyotrophic lateral sclerosis is an exception

— Lesions of the conus and cauda equina causing bilateral distal paralysis of the leg (always associated with severe sensory loss and disturbances of micturition [For further details, *see* 1.3.1 and Table 4].)
— Peroneal neural muscle atrophy of Charcot-Marie-Tooth and its variants show exquisite bilateral, symmetric, distal lower leg atrophy with paralysis or paresis of the feet (a familial disorder, very slowly progressive, marked by high arched feet, absence of ankle jerks, well-developed thigh muscles ['storklegs', 'inverted champagne flask']. Hand muscles later become involved occasionally vibration sense may be disturbed distally in lower extremities; in some forms and nerve conduction velocities are greatly diminished.) A similar clinical picture can be seen with pure motor, usually familial, scapuloperoneal syndromes (although these syndromes also involve the shoulder girdle)
— Myopathies (the above-named syndrome may initially be myopathic in some). In rare cases, myopathies cause symmetric distal or predominantly distal weakness; among the variants are myotonic dystrophy of Steinert (*see* 1.4, 2.9.2, and Table 11) and hereditary distal myopathy of Welander (and of Biemond) (*see* 2.13.2). Such syndromes result in a pure motor deficit and frequently involve the upper limbs
— Polyneuropathies. The weakness, both at the onset and later in the disease, is more marked distally (and always accompanied by paresthesia, subjective disturbances of sensation, footdrop with high stepping gait, and absence of ankle jerks (*see* 1.3.5)
— Bilateral mechanical symmetric peroneal pressure palsy (found in thin individuals after a period of unconsciousness, and in other susceptible individuals at particular risk). This af-

flection results in bilateral exclusive involvement of the muscles of the anterior tibial compartment, peroneal muscle paralysis (without impairment of the calf muscles and with preservation of ankle jerks), and sensory loss on the dorsum of the foot and laterally on the lower limb

2.13.2.4.3 Unilateral Motor Weakness in Circumscribed Areas of the Legs

Such localized motor deficits are frequently the initial phase of an affection that later becomes generalized. This is particularly true, for example, in spinal muscular atrophy; amyotrophic lateral sclerosis, which frequently begins unilaterally with distal or proximal weakness; and polymyositis and myasthenia.

The causing localized motor deficit, most often lies in dysfunction of roots, plexuses, or peripheral nerves. The resulting motor deficits are usually accompanied by pain and sensory disturbances. With typical topographic distribution of deficits, and particularly when a classic history accompanies the signs, diagnosis is usually straightforward. Difficulties usually arise when clinical examination does not reveal the typical causes of local dysfunction, and when the distribution of motor deficits is atypical or not accompanied by sensory dysfunction.

Unilateral weakness of hip flexors and thigh muscles, resulting from lesions of the lumbar plexus, occurs with retroperitoneal hematomas and with diabetes mellitus, which is usually accompanied by severe pain (*see* 2.17.5). A similar situation may be found with superior subperiosteal hematomas of the upper ilium after trauma (electric cars at fairs are a common cause). A rare form of lumbar sacral plexus lesion after X-ray therapy or with certain retroperitoneal tumors also produces weakness, occasionally without pain (but with appropriate sensory loss). Femoral nerve lesions leading to paralysis of the quadriceps muscle (marked by inability to ascend steps and by absence of knee jerks) are accompanied by sensory loss on the thigh and medial part of the lower limb. (Such lesions may occur, for example, after surgical intervention.) Repeated intramuscular injections in a newborn can effect contracture of the quadriceps muscle (without paralysis). In adults, injection can result in paresis of the gluteus medius and gluteus minimus (Duchenne limp or Trendelenburg limp), often without pain.

In the lower leg, acute paralysis of dorsiflexors of foot and toes occurs as a result of ischemia of the anterior tibial artery (due to excessive activity or painful, primarily ischemic, swelling of the anterior tibial compartment). Such a syndrome is marked initially by absence of the dorsalis pedis artery pulse, frequently accompanied by transient ischemic participation of the perforating branch of the peroneal nerve, and later by contracture of muscles in the anterior compartment, resulting in a claw-like position of the big toe (which prevents footdrop). Achilles tendon rupture (a very painful condition) causes incomplete plantar flexion paresis (because the posterior tibial and peroneal muscles act together as foot flexors).

2.13.2.5 Hemiparesis

Most causes of this symptom have already been dealt with in discussions of other dysfunctions (*see* references to other sections below). With apparent hemiparesis, it is important to be sure that only one hemibody is symptomatic (occasionally, early tetraspasticity may be present even though the patient refers only to the more markedly affected side). For the diagnosis and causes of cerebrally induced hemisymptoms (*see* 1.1.1). (For 'sudden' paralysis with brain tumors, *see below*)

A lesion of the brain stem can induce acute hemiparesis (for example, with an ischemic brain stem insult). Such weakness is, however, accompanied by crossed sensory impairment on the face or extremities of the contralateral side (*see* 1.1.3). Similar considerations apply in the case of a high cervical spinal cord lesion (resulting from trauma, ischemia, or bleeding, as with angiomas). Here, too, crossed symptoms (dissociated sensory disturbances) are present on the contralateral side (*see* 1.2.1.2).

2.13.2.5.1 Subacute or Slow-Onset Hemiparesis

Here too the most common cause is a cerebral site for the lesion (*see above*). The appearance of discrete motor hemiparesis is depicted in Figure 47. Causes for this type of weakness are the following:

− Vascular processes, such as stroke, in evolution. Most often a stepwise progression is present. (This cause may be suggested by the age of the patient, stepwise progression, risk fac-

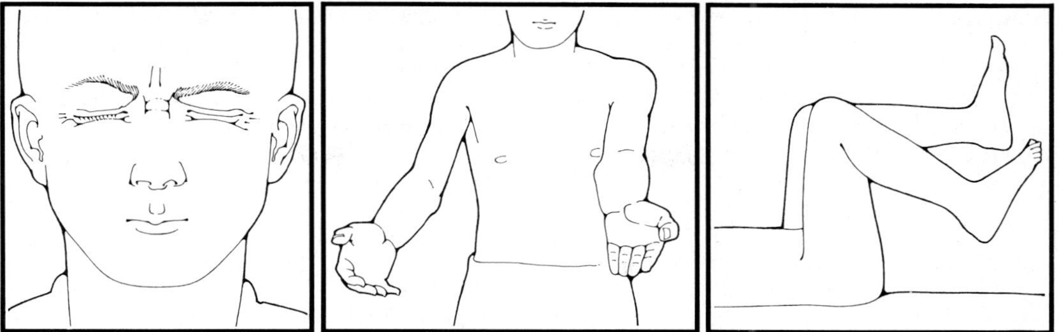

Fig. **47**   The discrete signs of central hemiparesis on the right side. The diagram on the left shows incomplete closure of the right eye, with the lashes remaining visible (*signe des ciles*) (compare with Fig. 41). With positioning of the arms (middle diagram) there is a drift of the right arm, flexion of the elbow and fingers, and pronation of the forearm. With positioning of the legs (right diagram), there is a drift of the right lower limb

tors, stenotic murmurs over arteries, and previous vascular episodes)

— Intracranial space-occupying lesions such as tumors (mostly progressive over weeks or months; usually accompanied by epileptic attacks, and in meningiomas by a history of epilepsy over years; eventually resulting in increased intracranial pressure, headache, and progressive psychic alterations), chronic subdural hematoma (mostly traumatic, sometimes suggested by light trauma in the history; always accompanied by headache, changing psychic alterations, relatively discrete neurologic symptoms, and usually pathologic CSF; abscesses (suggested by the presence of a source of infection, evidence of inflammation such as increased sedimentation rate, rapid progression). Through bleeding into the tumor mass, brain tumors can suddenly become symptomatic, giving rise to a hemisyndrome not unlike a stroke. This is particularly true of metastasis. With the sudden onset of symptoms one should also think of tumor emboli in blood vessels

— Localized unilateral cortical atrophy of the precentral region. The loss of function can be slowly progressive, sometimes taking years to develop into motor hemiparesis (Mills paralysis), and can be seen on CT. Pure motor hemiplegia may result from ischemic lesions in the internal capsule, corona radiata or basis pontis

— Multiple sclerosis. Hemiparesis can appear rapidly, over 1 to 2 days, and be very severe (common in younger patients, no early stepwise progression with other localization as in stroke, and quick recovery, accompanied by visual symptoms such as retrobulbar neuritis and transient double vision, precipitateness of micturition; frequently by optic nerve head pallor, pathologic visual evoked potentials, nystagmus, and pyramidal signs; and by CSF findings of increased plasma cells and IgG). The rare form of demyelinization that causes concentric sclerosis of Balo can produce a hemisyndrome

— Encephalitis. In rare cases, acute hemorrhagic herpes encephalitis, in particular, can cause a rapidly progressive hemisyndrome (with severe cerebral dysfunction, epileptic attacks, and pathologic CSF soon leading to a comatose state)

— Brain stem processes. Such processes, in rare cases, are associated with progressive hemisyndromes; the association of spinal cord processes with imposing hemisyndromes is even rarer. The presence of crossed symptoms is proof of such localization. In both sites the most common causes of symptoms are space-occupying lesions (tumor, aneurysm, spinal spondylosis, epidural hematoma, and abscess). (For Brown-Séquard syndrome *see* 1.2.1.2)

2.13.2.5.2 Sudden or Very Rapidly Progressive Hemiparesis

The most common sign of a central lesion as cause of this clinical symptom is the involvement of the face or visual fields.

Causes are

– A vascular process (the most common cause)
  ● a stroke with cerebral ischemia (*see* 2.3.1.2)
  ● an embolus (stemming from myocardial infarction, atrial fibrillation with mitral disease, mitral valve prolapse, ulcerated plaque in extracranial blood vessels)
  ● with complicated migraine and with hypoglycemia in diabetes mellitus (both mostly in juveniles with frequent recurrences and recovery)
  ● cerebral hemorrhage in a setting of hypertension or arteriovenous malformation (arteriovenous angioma or saccular aneurysm); with putaminal hemorrhage it may give rise to pure motor hemiplegia
  ● with cerebral venous thrombosis (occurring in the puerperium, or other risk factors such as Behçet's disease, cancer, cachexia, or thrombotic diathesis; marked by headache, epileptic attacks, disturbances of consciousness, xanthochromic CSF)
– In rare instances a tumor or tumor metastasis, usually associated with bleeding (suggested by a history of headache, epileptic attacks, and manifestations of primary tumor)
– Head trauma (indicated in the history). An accidental fall, with brain contusion, resulting from loss of consciousness due to an earlier cerebral event must be distinguished from a fall that causes the cerebral lesion

It is important to think of a lesion in the cervical cord when the sensorium is clear but there is associated sensory impairment without cranial nerve involvement (*see* Brown-Séquard syndrome [Table 4]). Such lesions may result from cord ischemia or contusion.

Without actual paralysis but a lack of use of the extremities on one side, the so-called motor neglect results as a rule from lesions of the right hemisphere, mostly parietal but also frontal and thalamic locations (vascular or tumor).

2.13.3 Nonorganic Weakness

A feeling of generalized weakness is found in a setting of depression and also in neurosis as a symptom of a neurasthenic syndrome (sleeplessness, irritability, easy fatigability, fear, body sensations, and hypochondria, often with an exhibitionist quality).

True hysterical (unconscious) mechanisms are rarely the cause of diffuse global weakness, but they frequently result in localized weakness. The following circumstances suggest a psychogenic mechanism of the weakness:

– Localization of weakness in a circumscribed area, not corresponding to any particular peripheral nerve supply territory or root
– Absence of sensory disturbances or their presence in a pattern (often circular) differing from known dermatomal distribution or affecting a whole limb or sharply limited to the exact midline and with total analgesia and anesthesia
– Absence of objective deficits, particularly and most importantly absence of atrophies (inactivity over long periods can lead to muscle atrophy), and of reflex abnormality or of pathologic reflexes
– Inappropriate strength in certain situations. For example, apparent total flaccid paralysis of dorsiflexion of the foot but absence of steppage gait; total flaccid paralysis of an arm, but lack of centrifugal, upward swing of the arm with rapid active or passive rotation of the body; apparent total absence of extension of hand and fingers, but reflex activation of extensor muscles on making a fist (note that this reflex is also preserved with organic central weakness. In this setting, however, other objective signs [reflexes and tone] and central spastic paralysis make differentiation possible)

The peculiarities of psychogenic weakness are also seen to a large extent in the case of sensory psychogenic deficits (*see* 2.16.4), and they are noted in unconscious hysterical paralyses and also in (conscious) simulated paralysis (malingering).

2.14 Involuntary Movement and Abnormal Movement Disorders

The anatomic substrate of motor activity is summarized in 1.1.1 and in Figure 1. Figure 3 shows the influence of the basal ganglia on movement and on the harmony of movement; Figure 6 shows the influence of the cerebellum. Pathophysiologically abnormal movements (uncontrollable movement) occur with epileptic discharges in cases of pathologic irritability of the cortex, and with lesions of the basal ganglia. The site and extent of such lesions, which may be functional (biochemical) or anatomic, determine the characteristics of the abnormal movement. Disturbances of the speed and purposefulness of movement, such as the hypokinesia in Parkinson's syndrome (*see* 1.1.3.1) and in cerebellar lesions (*see* 1.1.4), are also due to disturbances of basal ganglia.

The clinical aspects of abnormal movement and disturbed sequence of movement are summarized in Table 20. Descriptions of clinical pictures and most important causes of abnormal movement follow.

2.14.1 Abnormal Spontaneously Occurring Motor Phenomena

These are active motions, independent of movements voluntarily initiated by the individual, appearing uncontrollably and during rest. They are analyzed and described according to their site, extent, frequency, regularity, progress, and the degree to which they are provoked by external circumstances.

2.14.1.1 Epileptic Attacks

Epileptic attacks are mentioned here for the sake of completeness and to distinguish them from nonepileptic involuntary movements. Epileptic attacks are described in 2.3.1 as attack-like disturbances. They are the manifestation of a lesion in a part of the cortex or of the centrencephalic structures with primary projections to the cortex. Differentiation from other movement disorders is rarely difficult because of the sudden onset of the involuntary movements, their clonic, powerful twitching character, and the often-associated disturbances of consciousness. Forms of epilepsy without loss of consciousness, however, and particularly with short-lived motor phenomena, may in individual cases be difficult to distinguish from other forms of abnormal movement.

Such forms of epilepsy include

- Jacksonian motor epilepsy (*see* 2.3.1.1) (initially localized; extends to a whole limb or a whole region of the body ("march of convulsion") in clonic rhythmic attacks, repeated but irregular in occurrence, usually lasting for minutes)
- Epilepsia partialis continua of Koževnikov (*see* 2.3.1.1) (localized attacks, always recurring in the same areas of the body, with irregular, short, sudden clonic twitches, and lasting hours or even days)
- Oral and other automatisms of types of absence epilepsy (*see* 2.3.3) and, in particular, temporal lobe epilepsy (*see* 2.3.3)

2.14.1.2 Spasms and Cramps

Spasms are irregularly occurring, usually repetitive contractions of muscles and muscle groups. They are heterogeneous in characteristics and cause.

- Hemifacial spasms result when all the muscles of mimicry contract on one side of the face (*see* 2.9.3)
- In blepharospasm there are bilateral, irregularly occurring periorbital muscle contractions that may lead to prolonged and continued disturbance of eye closure or opening. The cause may be psychogenic (tic) even when there are no other clinical signs of psychic abnormalities in the patient. Blepharospasm can also be an early symptom of a complex extrapyramidal disorder or a manifestation of an isolated dystonic syndrome
- Occasionally there is spastic, clonic, repetitive, and rhythmic contraction of the muscles of eye closure, blepharoclonus
- Rhythmic upper lid retraction with upward beating vertical nystagmus is found mostly in pontine lesions (*see* 2.7.1 and Table 15)
- For other dystonic movement disorders of facial muscles (*see* 2.14.1.11). (For psychogenic tic *see* 2.14.1.12; for oculogyric crisis *see* 2.8.2.2)
- Among spasms affecting other body parts generalized spasm e.g. in hyperthyroidism have been observed, or spasms resulting in paw-like positions of the hand, and carpopedal spasms of the feet, occurring with tetany (*see* 2.3.2). Very painful cramps of hip flexors and abdominal muscles with rapidly appearing contractures can occur with Addison's disease
- True infectious tetanus may be localized and manifest by repeated painful local spasms (which later become generalized, progressively increasing in intensity and duration)

Cramps are very painful involuntary contractions of muscles that lead to transient contracture with fixed position. They appear predominantly in the calves, particularly at night. The cause is usually unknown (*see also* 2.17.5). (For writer's cramp *see* 2.14.1.11)

Table 20 **Involuntary and disturbed movement: characteristics, localization, and causes**

Movement	Characteristics	Localization	Causes	Remarks
Epileptic attacks	Sudden in onset, occurring at irregular intervals, with clonic, powerful twitches, often with disturbance of consciousness	Cortex	Brain damage resulting from anatomic alteration or toxic causes	Jacksonian epilepsy, other focal epilepsies, and epilepsia partialis continua of Koževnikov not accompanied by loss of consciousness
Spasms	Occurs at irregular intervals with variable frequency and extent; contractions of muscles or muscle groups, occasionally painful			
Hemifacial spasm	Synchronous contraction of all muscles innervated by the facial nerve	Facial nerve root or facial nerve nucleus	Mechanical lesions	
Blepharospasm	Bilateral periorbital muscle contractions, irregular in occurrence and often long lasting	Sometimes basal ganglia disease	Extrapyramidal disease; occasionally psychogenic	Compare with tic
Cramps	Long-lasting tonic contractions of single muscle or muscle groups, resulting in fixed joint position; often painful, particularly in calves	Muscular	Varied	*See* writers' cramp
Fasciculations	Irregular short contractions of single muscle bundles without movements of joint; visible with naked eye	Peripheral motor neurons	Predominantly chronic lesions of anterior horn cells, rarely peripheral nerve roots; occasionally benign	Provoked by percussion or injection of cholinesterase inhibitors
Myokymias	Contraction waves always in random fascicles of single muscle or muscle groups, without significant movement; visible as waves	?	?	Rare
Myorhythmias	Rhythmic twitches in same muscle group causing movement	Central structures		Contraction frequency of 1−3/sec
Palatal nystagmus		Central segmental tracts or olive	Vascular, degenerative	

(continued)

Table 20   (continued)

Movement	Characteristics	Localization	Causes	Remarks
Myoclonias	Nonrhythmic, rapid extensive, occasionally powerful twitches of single or several muscles with marked movement	Cortex, cerebellum	Hereditary, anoxic, or metabolic	For action myoclonus, see below
Tremor	Rhythmic, individually extensive motions that are constant in frequency, particularly prevalent under certain conditions, more or less constant in localization, usually with little movement manifest	Central nervous system	Hereditary, toxic, or degenerative	
Chorea	Relatively rapid, nonrhythmic, irregular movements of varying localization and short duration, more marked distally, leading to short-lived, extreme position of joints	Basal ganglia	Vascular, degenerative, occasionally hereditary metabolic disturbances, sometimes infectious	Occasionally unilateral, i.e. hemichorea
Athetosis	Like chorea, but slower, with exaggerated and longlasting extreme position of joints	Basal ganglia	Neonatal, jaundice, other perinatal damage	Hemiathetosis or double athetosis
Ballismus	Irregular, rapid, widely distributed flinging movements of several joints	Subthalamic nucleus	Like chorea	
Torsion dystonia	Irregular, slow movement that overcomes resistance of antagonists, often with rotatory components; involves large number of muscle groups in various body parts, leading to bizarre postures	Basal ganglia	Neonatal jaundice particularly	For localized forms, see below
Localized dystonia	As above, but localized to few muscles	Basal ganglia		
Torticollis	Slow movement of head with rotation, occasionally forced retraction (retrocollis), irregular in occurrence	Basal ganglia	Occasionally after neck trauma; organic	Can progress to generalized dystonia
Writers' cramp	Occurs only during writing, with dystonic position of fingers	Basal ganglia	Organic in origin	Remains localized
Facial buccolingual dystonia	Irregular writing movements confined to mouth and tongue muscles	Basal ganglia	Particularly after drugs; may be senile, degenerative	

(continued)

Table 20   (continued)

Movement	Characteristics	Localization	Causes	Remarks
Tic and tic-like movements	Irregular movement, confined to certain body parts, rapid, but not lightning-like	Psychogenic	Nonorganic	
Tic disease	Rapid, psychogenic tic with forced activity and coprolalia	?	Organic, occasionally hereditary; seen in rare cases after neuroleptic withdrawal	To be differentiated from organic spasms and dystonia
Spasmus nutans	Irregular flexion and flexed position of the head; nystagmus, more marked in one eye	?	Psychogenic? a result of prolonged stay in darkness? Similar symptoms with tumors of third ventricle and chiasm	Appears in first year of life; disappears at about 2 years
Ataxia	Deviation from intended line of movement with any voluntary motion and present throughout its range	Lesions of sensory afferents, cerebellum or motor efferents	Multiple	
Intention tremor	A tremor that increases as a movement near its target. Extensive deviation from the intended line of movement	Dentate nucleus and its efferents	Particularly common in multiple sclerosis	See Fig. 49
Action myoclonus	Powerful, lightning-like, extensive movements, suddenly appearing at the beginning of active movement	Cerebellum	Anoxia, degenerative, acute uremia	

2.14.1.3 Fasciculations

Not really movements but spontaneous, uncontrollable, irregular, short contractions of single muscle fiber bundles; fasciculations are visible with the naked eye, if there is not too much subcutaneous fat (as there is in newborns and small children). They are rendered more prominent by percussion and by injection of cholinesterase inhibitors (edrophonium chloride).

Fasciculations may be benign, particularly those that are localized in the orbicularis oculi or in the calf. Generalized, benign, spontaneous fasciculations that disappear after months are in rare cases the aftereffects of a variety of infections, including poliomyelitis or myelitis. Localized fasciculations (without muscle weakness, muscle atrophy, or reflex abnormalities may occur with chronic infection [sinusitis]). Occasionally they may be accompanied by pain and cramps.

Widespread or generalized fasciculations commonly are manifestations of chronic denervation. They are most often due to chronic progressive disappearance and death of anterior horn cells (with accompanying motor weakness, electromyographic changes due to disorders of motor units, and eventually other signs of motor system affection such as pyramidal signs), etiologically most often in chronic spinal muscle atrophy (*see* 1.2.3).

Fasciculations are found in rare cases in which there are (chronic) lesions of spinal roots or of a peripheral nerve. With peripheral nerve lesions the fasciculations are restricted to the muscles innervated by the nerve structures and are associated with paresis, sometimes with reflex abnormalities, and always with sensory disturbances. They can also appear occasionally in hyperthyroidism and in hexosaminidase deficiency in which their association with muscle atrophy and weakness mimics amyotrophic lateral sclerosis. Rarely they are a manifestation of chronic polyradiculitis. Because of the atrophy and pareses in this disorder spinal muscular atrophy must be considered. Recovery from polyradiculitis is, however, common.

2.14.1.4 Myokymias

Waves of contraction that repeatedly affect new fibers and pass over muscles or muscle groups are called myokymias. They do not produce significant movement, but are visible as continuous waves sweeping along the skin. They may be a symptom of continuous muscle fiber activity (*see* 2.12.1). In the face they appear as facial myokymia (*see* 2.9.3).

2.14.1.5 Myorhythmias

These are rhythmic twitches occurring with a frequency of 1 to 3 per second, repeatedly affecting the same muscle group with definitive, but not pronounced, movements. They are caused by organic disturbances of central structures that are only rarely more definitively localizable. Myorhythmias of short duration are found as harmless abnormalities, for example, in the region of the orbicularis oculi or platysma. Around the mouth they can cause rhythmic protrusion of the tongue (to be distinguished from faciobuccolingual dystonia *see* 2.14.1.11). Hiccough is myorhythmia of the diaphragm (occurring with encephalitis and other organic diseases of the brain, in toxic-metabolic coma, with cervical or mediastinal tumors and in pleuro-pulmonary or cardiac localized processes, and with local involvement of the diaphragm after abdominal or thoracic surgical procedures; most often, however, cryptogenic and benign).

Palatal nystagmus, occasionally occurring in synchrony with a rhythmic movement of the eyes, is always the manifestation of a lesion in the central tegmental tract or the dentate nuclei (mostly of vascular origin). (For myorhythmia and myoclonia of the eyes and particular forms of nystagmus *see* Table 15)

2.14.1.6 Myoclonias

Myoclonias are nonrhythmic, rapid, widespread twitches of single or several muscles, often with marked movement effects that result in injury of the limbs and falls (for action myoclonus *see* 2.14.2.3). Etiologically this may be a partial symptom of several forms of epilepsy: myoclonic astatic petit mal (which occurs in children in the first year of life and is marked by falls, disturbances of consciousness that commonly are very brief, typical EEG, and eventually clonic fits *see* 2.3.1.2.1); myoclonic epilepsy (occurs during childhood, with short bursts of marked twitches singly or in salvos, affecting in particular the upper extremity, and usually occurring in the morning without loss of consciousness; often combined with grand mal epilepsy); myoclonus epilepsy (familial, asymmetric, often involving only parts of muscle without great movement effects; provoked by sensory stimuli and active movement; associated with grand mal epilepsy and progressive dementia). Possibly the myoclonials of uremia and dialysis encephalopathy are also manifestations of epileptic disorders. Myoclonic encephalopathy has been observed with silver-salt intoxication and with bismuth poisoning. Myoclonus can be seen in lipidoses, spino-cerebellar degeneration, alcohol and drug withdrawal, encephalitis lethargica, subacute sclerosing panencephalitis, Jakob-Creutzfeldt disease and after anoxia.

Common harmless cryptogenic myoclonias are found during early sleep phases (marked movement of legs with simultaneous awakening known as sleep jerks).

Rare disorders are paramyoclonus multiplex (an affection lasting for years, with spontaneous irregular twitches, particularly of the shoulder muscles); fibrillary myoclonus multiplex or fibrillary chorea of Morvan (irregular, affecting various muscle groups or parts of muscle together with pain and autonomic disturbances, disturbances of sleep, and psychic alteration; sometimes a sign of mercury intoxication); and infantile polymyoclonia (irregular myoclonia, dancing eyes, ataxia, irritability, stepwise, prolonged disorder). Myoclonus occurs in the very rare early infantile glycine encephalopathy. Rarely local myoclonus of single muscle groups may occur after trauma to the brachial plexus.

2.14.1.7 Tremor

Fine, ordinarily invisible twitching of about 10 Hz can be recognized with special instrumentation in normal individuals. This spontaneous tremor is rhythmic with a fairly constant frequency in each individual. It usually remains well localized. It can become coarser and therefore more noticeable, most often in specific circumstances: for example, at rest — rest tremor — or with particular positions of the limbs — position tremor. The basis for this is a harmless (hereditary) 'vegetative' abnormality, a metabolic disturbance, or a disorder of the central nervous system.

The signs and symptoms of essential 'autonomic' tremor are identical to those of autosomal dominantly inherited familial tremor and senile tremor. In all three forms there is a mostly symmetric fine to midfrequency beating, a position tremor with a frequency identical to that of the invisible physiologic tremor — between 8 and 13 Hz; in older patients it is somewhat slower. In other cases the tremor may have from the beginning a frequency of 4 to 6 Hz. It affects, as a rule, the hands, and, occasionally, the head, increasing with anxiety and with attempts to hold an object firmly. It is improved with alcohol intake; in children who later develop familial tremor, there may be short-lasting attacks of shivering. The probability that a patient with essential tremor will develop Parkinson's disease later on is 25 times higher than the average.

The tremor of Parkinson's disease can initially appear as an isolated symptom. It is a rest tremor with a frequency of 4 to 6 Hz and is often, at least at the beginning, unilateral. It decreases or disappears altogether with movement, particularly intentional (for example, with the finger/nose test). Exceptions, however, in the form of a position tremor are also found. Initially the tremor is often rapid, but with increasing disability it becomes coarser, the so-called pill rolling or coin counting

tremor. On examination, rigidity and cogwheeling should be searched for.

Toxic forms of tremors are more or less symmetric, often somewhat faster and slightly more irregular than the essential tremor, occur usually as position tremors, and are most marked with hands outstretched and fingers separated. Such tremors occur also with hyperthyroidism, mercury intoxication, with some drug intoxications, for example, sodium valproate, after intake of a variety of other drugs, and particularly with chronic alcoholism.

In delirium (tremens) the tremor is often more marked in the lower limbs, and accompanies psychic dysfunction, agitated confusion, hallucinations, signs of alcoholic polyneuropathy, or epileptic attacks. Tremor can also occur in chronic polyneuropathy and in chronic recurring polyradiculopathy. In infants, attacks of tremor, together with epileptic fits, can be the manifestation of hypomagnesemia.

With lesions of the red nucleus and the brachium conjunctivum there is often a coarse positional tremor together with ataxia (*see* 2.14.2.1). The tremor is accompanied by marked one-sided flexion and extension movements, in particular of the fingers of one hand. This is sometimes termed a flapping tremor and is often accompanied by irregular extension and flexion movements of the extended arms. It is seen in diseases of the liver and in hepatolenticular degeneration (Wilson's disease).

The hysterical tremor seen in rare cases is irregular, often very coarse, and mostly confined to one extremity. If the examiner grasps the involved extremity firmly, the tremor often appears in another part of the body. If the attention of the patient is distracted from the tremulous part of the body, this psychogenic tremor decreases; organic tremors usually intensify.

2.14.1.8 Chorea and Athetosis

The involuntary movements of chorea are irregular, variously localized but more marked distally, short lived, rapid, and irregular in sequence. They are accompanied by very brief but exaggerated positions of the limbs; when they affect only one half of the body, they are designated hemichorea. The movements of athetosis are also irregular with varying localization but more marked distally, occurring in a time lapse tempo and resulting in exaggerated final position of the limbs, in particular the exaggerated extension and even subluxation (bayonet finger) of the joints (Fig. 48). Athetosis can also be confined to one half of the body; it is then known as hemiathetosis. Bilateral athetosis is sometimes designated double athetosis.

Commonly there are mixed clinical pictures. For example, choreoathetosis combines the signs of chorea and athetosis. Ballistic and dystonic movements can also occur concurrently (*see below*). All of these abnormal movements can disappear during sleep. They usually become exaggerated with excitement or with intentional movement. Pathophysiologically these abnormalities are usually caused by lesions in the region of the caudate or putamen, the outer part of the globus pallidus, and the subthalamic nucleus.

Common forms of chorea are

- Chorea minor or rheumatic chorea, also known as Sydenham's chorea or infectious chorea (occurs almost always in children, several weeks after streptococcal throat infection, often accompanied by joint rheumatism or endocarditis. Signs include tiredness, psychic lability, and irritability, ultimately leading to chorea)
- Chorea gravidarum (exhibits the same symptoms as chorea minor, or Sydenham's chorea; afflicted women usually have had chorea minor in childhood)
- Huntington's chorea (an autosomal dominant disorder, chronic and progressive, with onset between 30 and 50 years of age, and resulting in impaired gait and progressive dementia, occasionally unaccompanied by choreiform movements)

- Benign familial chorea (an autosomal dominant disorder appearing in childhood, nonprogressive, and unaccompanied by dementia)
- Senile chorea (nonhereditary, occasionally appearing in the presenile period, progressive)
- Postinfarction chorea (occurs after an infarct that has resulted in hemiparesis or, frequently, hemiballismus [*see below*])
- Rarely chorea has occurred after encephalitis, neurosyphilis, tuberculous meningitis, whooping cough and typhus, acute exanthemas, accompanying polyradiculitis, hypoxic encephalopathy at birth, neonatal jaundice (combined with athetosis); with lupus erythematosus, polycythemia, with acantocythosis (without abeta lipoproteinemia), portocaval encephalopathy, tumor, Hallervorden-Spatz disease, Creutzfeldt-Jakob disease, Lesch-Nyhan syndrome, other metabolic abnormalities like glutamyl dehydrogenase deficiency, thyrotoxicosis, chronic subdural hematoma and, sometimes after aspiration of the hematoma, with Behçet syndrome; with hepatolenticular degeneration, progressive pallidal atrophy (Hunt), carbon monoxide intoxication, manganese intoxication, carbon disulfide intoxication, and use of drugs such as oral contraceptives, amphetamine, neuroleptics, phenytoin, chlorpromazine derivatives, and levodopa
- Paroxysmal choreoathetosis (*see* 2.3.1.1)

Predominantly athetotic movement disorders may have the following causes:

- Most often they result from perinatal damage (the disorder may appear immediately but occasionally follows a latent period of months or years after birth; from the onset it is accom-

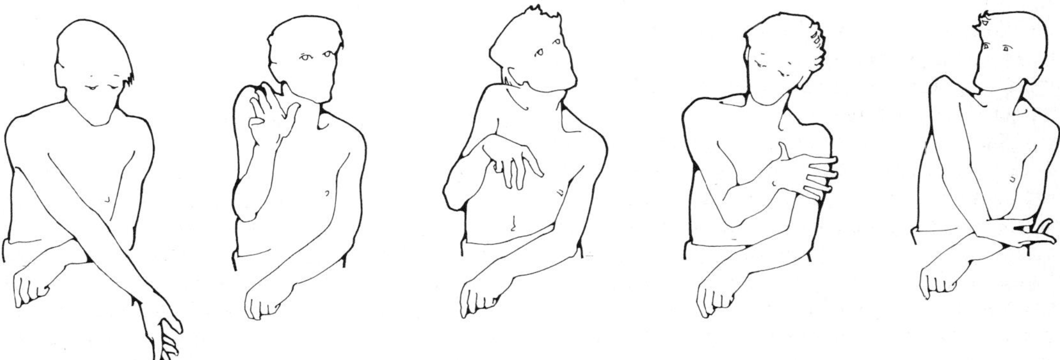

Fig. **48** Various head and arm positions in right-sided hemichorea. Drawing from a movie sequence panied by signs of other cerebral movement disorders). Pathologically there is status marmoratus or status dysmyelinatus (after neonatal icterus gravis)

— Some rare causes mentioned under chorea may also cause athetoid movement or choreoathetoid movement disorders (*see above*)

— Hemiathetosis occurs in rare cases with all the above-named causes and also after a stroke (accompanying hemiparesis or occasionally following a symptom-free interval of weeks or months after a stroke)

2.14.1.9 Ballismus and Hemiballismus

These disorders are characterized by wide-ranging, throwing, lightening-like movements appearing in several limb segments but particularly pronounced proximally. The patient may suffer severe trauma from collisions with obstacles and muscle tears from torsions of the whole body. The basis of this disorder, which affects mostly one body half and is usually accompanied by a motor hemisyndrome, is a lesion primarily of the subthalamic nucleus or damage of the striatum or globus pallidus.

Etiologic factors are those already mentioned in connection with chorea, along with primary vascular insults and local space-occupying processes (which can result in the sudden onset of hemiballismus). The rare hereditary degenerative ballismus is bilateral. Transient recurring episodes of hemiballismus can occur with disordered blood flow of the basilar artery.

2.14.1.10 Torsion Dystonia

The movements in dystonia are slow and carried out against the resistance of antagonist muscles. They therefore appear forced. They often have a rotatory component. With localized dystonic syndromes (*see* 2.14.1.11), only several muscle groups in a circumscribed area of the body are involved, but with the completely developed picture of torsion dystonia, numerous muscles in the trunk and proximal part of the extremity as well as in the distal area are involved in the pathologic movements. Because of this, patients are often grotesquely deformed, and their volitional movement must be forcibly executed against the dystonia. A fixed abnormal posture with strong hypertonia of

several muscle groups that no longer is accompanied by hyperkinesia is known as myostatic torsion dystonia.

Causes of full-blown torsion dystonia (dystonia musculorum deformans) are those mentioned under chorea (*see* 2.14.1.8). The most common is perinatal damage, in particular as a result of kernicterus (the dystonia is present from early childhood, accompanied by other signs of cerebral movement disorders). Intermittent, but eventually continuous, dystonia or choreoathetotic syndromes can be due to certain metabolic disorders — for example, enzymatic defects with disturbed detoxification of glutaric acid or a deficit in β-galactosidase with GM_1 gangliosidosis. An idiopathic (familial) form, in which the illness begins in the first or second year of life with localized dystonia, is frequently but not exclusively found in Jewish families. Symptomatic forms may occur in encephalitis, particularly epidemic encephalitis with hepatolenticular degeneration, in Huntington's chorea (*see* 2.14.1.8), in Hallervorden-Spatz disease, Lesch-Nyhan syndrome, cortical venous thrombosis, in the early stages of ataxia-telangiectasia and with tumors of basal ganglia or angiomas in these locations. A persistent late dystonia may occur after longterm (of varying duration) therapy with antipsychotics or neuroleptics, sometimes this dystonia may be localized e.g. spastic torticollis.

2.14.1.11 Localized Dystonias

Localized dystonic movements that appear spontaneously or are manifest with certain activity may be the initial symptom of generalized dystonia (or of chorea, torsion dystonia, and so on); they may, however, remain localized and may occur in attacks (*see* 2.3.1.1).

Spastic torticollis is characterized by tonic irregular, predominantly twisting movement of the head, always toward a particular side in any individual patient. The sternocleidomastoid, particularly, and other neck muscles visibly contract in irregular spasms against the resistance of the antagonistic muscles. Occasionally the posterior neck muscles are predominantly involved, leading to retrocollis. By touching the skin of the chin on the face in a certain area, the patient can occasionally decrease the abnormal movement or completely abolish it. No specific cause for this disorder is known, but symptomatic forms of spasmodic torticollis sometimes indicate dystonia of a generalized nature (*see above*). Spasmodic torticollis must be distinguished from fixed acute 'rheumatic' torticollis resulting from mechanical lesions of the spinal column (sudden in onset with neck pain and absence of active or passive movements) and from caput obstipum musculare occurring after perinatal trauma to the sternocleidomastoid (with shortening of the muscle due to scar formation). Head tilt may result from trochlear paralysis. Head tilt is also occasionally found in space-occupying lesions in the posterior fossa or the craniocervical junction and in syringomyelia. Intermittent head tilt in children may be a manifestation of labyrinthine disorders, and attacks are ushered in by vomiting.

Writer's cramp occurs only during the act of writing, developing after several words or lines; the fingers become stiff and assume abnormal positions, and the writing becomes increasingly illegible. Occasionally the writer cannot even sign his name. The disorder may be confined to the right hand, but other activities of the hand may proceed quite normally. Rarely there are analogous isolated functional disturbances of the fingers, for example, with typing.

Dystonic posture of the hands occurs with lesions of the thalamus ("thalamic hand"). However, abnormal fixed extreme finger joint position also can occur, in rare cases, with purely mechanical disturbances: With or without rheumatoid arthritis, the extensor tendons may lose the capacity for fixation and may slip beyond the joint so that they come to lie below the point of rotation. This can occur in one or several fingers, which then appear dystonically positioned, but they can be passively replaced in the original normal position by the patient. Similar abnormalities can occur in patients with congenital abnormal flaccidity of joint capsules, in whom increasing stress during life leads to abnormal joint positions.

Isolated dystonic postures of the feet occurring with walking and particularly with stepping are sometimes seen, as is faciobuccolingual dystonia, in which bizarre movements of lips, perioral muscles, and tongue occur spontaneously, especially during speaking. Neck muscles are also occasionally involved, rarely muscles of other body parts. If these movements are accompanied by forced opening and closing of the jaw and blepharospasm (*see* 2.14.1.2), the designation of Brueghel syndrome is appropriate. This syndrome is probably identical to Meige syndrome in its symmetric appearance and intensity of the axial (midline) muscular involvement. Causes are phenothiazine medication, L-dopa therapy (in-

dicated in the history), circulatory disturbances (in elderly individuals with signs of circulatory disorders or risk factors) or causes mentioned above in connection with torsion dystonia. Faulty dental occlusion and nocturnal bruxism may cause dystonic movements of the mouth. These dystonic movements must not be mistaken for oral automatisms in temporal lobe seizures, and if unilateral for hemifacial spasm or aberrant innervation after Bell's palsy. In edentulous subjects orofacial dyskinesias are more frequent then in similar aged individuals with partial dentures. Orofacial dyskinesias have also been described with vascular lesions in the mouth area of the cerebellum.

2.14.1.12 Tics and Tic-like Spontaneous Movements

These spontaneous movements are mostly constant and confined to particular body parts where they reappear at irregular intervals. They are usually quick, but not lightning-like, and they disappear during sleep. All body parts can be affected by tics, but they are particularly common in the muscles of the face and upper extremity. They may be manifest in blepharospasms, twitches of the corner of the mouth, stereotyped gestures, or grunting noises. The majority of tics are psychogenic. To this category also belongs a form of tic found in children (rarely also at later ages), manifest in typical grinding movements of the back of the head on the pillow, which take place when the subject is recumbent — so-called jactatio capitis. The signs and symptoms of psychogenic tics do not readily distinguish them from organic tic-like movement disorders, such as spastic torticollis (in which the stereotyped movements are often greater than tics, gradually increasing with eventual appearance of dystonic symptoms) and many cases of blepharospasm. With organic tic-like disease (Gilles de la Tourette syndrome) there are tic-like twitches in the neck and face with forced activities, echololia, uncontrolled utterances, and coprolalia. The "jumping Frenchman of Maine," a hereditary disease, is associated with sudden jumps and forced activity, often initiated when the patient stretches.

2.14.1.13 Spasmus Nutans

This benign condition appears in the first year of life and usually disappears in the second year. It is characterized by irregular flexion movements and habitual tilting of the head with marked nystagmus in one eye. A similar clinical picture may appear with tumors of the third ventricle and of the chiasm.

2.14.2 Uncontrollable Disturbances of Active Movements

In contrast to the movement disorders described previously, the following conditions do not occur spontaneously and therefore are not present at rest. Instead they are present only when the patient makes a movement, as a disturbance in the consonant flow of the motion. (It must not be forgotten, however, that in many movements disorders that appear spontaneously, the abnormal movements are exaggerated during voluntary effort and may become disabling only during that activity.) Figure 49 gives an overview of disturbances of active movements; the disorders are described in detail below.

Ataxia (Fig. 49a) causes all movements to be disconsonant during the entire range of motion, thus causing deviation of the ideal trajectory. These deviations are, as a rule, not very prominent, but occasionally may become very disabling. Ataxia can be transitory (with diphenylhydantoin and other intoxications) or attack-like and episodic (for example, in certain familial metabolic disorders), but in most cases ataxia is present throughout the illness.

Ataxia is present

— With disturbances of afferents, leading to incomplete information about limb position; this type of ataxia increases with eye closure. Such disturbances occur
  ● with diffuse lesions of peripheral nerves or spinal roots, resulting in predominantly sensory disturbances. These lesions include polyneuropathies (*see* 1.3.5) and polyradiculitis (the same symptoms as in polyneuropathy, but with associated progressive flaccid motor paralysis [*see* 1.3.1])
  ● with posterior column lesions, for example, vitamin B_{12} deficiency, tabes dorsalis, paraneoplastic spinal column degeneration (resulting in gross ataxia, severe joint position sense deficits, and absence of vibration sense, without significant motor weakness or predominantly distal sensory disturbance)

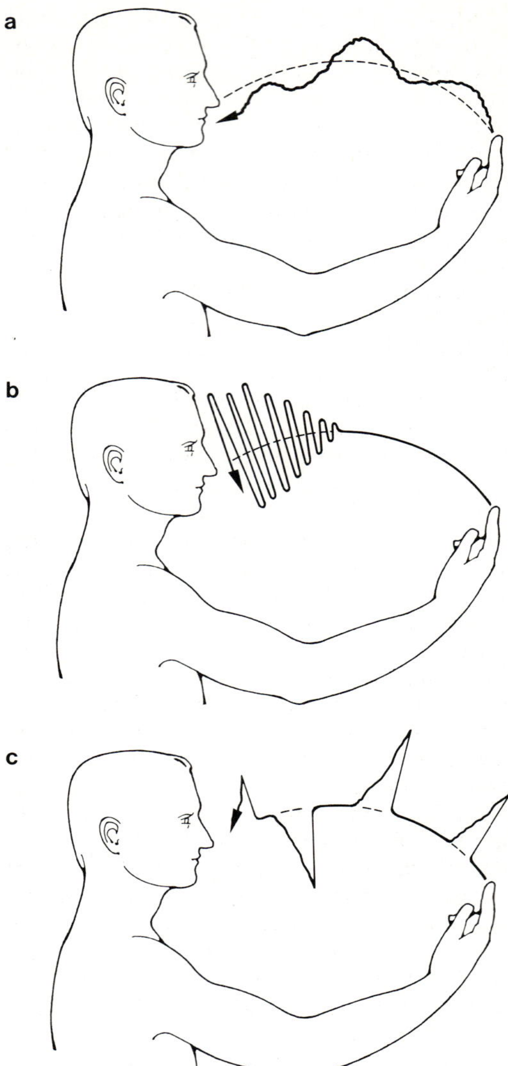

Fig. 49 a–c Various abnormalities indicated by the finger-nose test. **a** Ataxia, the disturbance beginning at the start of movement with deviation from the ideal line. **b** Intention tremor, the disturbance increasing as the target is approached. **c** Action myoclonus with sudden, brief, irregular, superimposed deviation from the ideal line of movement

— With disorders of the cerebellum, disturbing its regulatory influence on movement. Cerebellar ataxia is usually not aggravated by eye closure or darkness (for example, at dusk). (For etiologic factors, *see* 1.1.4)

– With disordered motor afferents. Such ataxia is designated as paretic, and is always accompanied by a motor weakness (*see* 2.13)

The clumsiness of movements after prolonged confinement to bed can resemble ataxia ('bed ataxia'). The same applies to the poor movement coordination in children with discrete cerebral movement disorders ('clumsy child') or with vestibular disturbances (*see* 2.7.1).

In intention tremor (Fig. 49b) the deviation from the ideal line of movement increases or becomes visible as the limb approaches the target. The tremor may become so violent that grasping an object is impossible.

This abnormality is usually related to a lesion of the dentate nucleus or its efferents. Most often this is caused by a focus of multiple sclerosis (earlier examinations will often have revealed neurologic deficits hinting at lesions in other parts of the nervous system). Less common is an intention tremor occurring with vascular brain stem lesions – for example, the ruber syndrome (acute appearance of tremor together with homolateral hemiparesis and oculomotor paresis on the opposite side) – or after skull trauma (occurs only after a comatose state following severe trauma; always associated with other cerebellar or brain stem dysfunction).

In the rather rare action myoclonus (also termed intention myoclonus [Fig. 49c]) a strong nonrhythmic twitching lasting only fractions of seconds occurs at the beginning of movement; it does not increase with the approach of the target. Action myoclonus occurs after anoxic brain damage (indicated by history and by other cerebellar symptoms), but occasionally also with disorders of the cerebellum and as part of myoclonic epilepsy (*see* 2.3.1.1). It is also found in acute uremia and in chronic mercury poisoning. Of diagnostic importance is its characteristic good response to colonazepam.

Other disorders of contraction, and particularly relaxation of muscles, also impede active movement. In this category are the myotonias (myotonic dystrophy and congenital myotonia) and the paramyotonias. In these disorders the strongly contracting muscle at the beginning of movements can only be relaxed slowly. With percussion (particularly of the tongue) there is a visible and long-lasting contraction of the muscle (percussion myotonia) – that disappears only after several seconds. With hypothyroidism, mounding (myoedema) occurs on percussion of muscles with the

reflex hammer, disappearing only after seconds, and ankle jerks are delayed in their relaxation. With the Lambert-Eaton syndrome (a paraneoplastic syndrome, most often seen with carcinoma of the bronchus) the initial muscle contraction is slower and less powerful than the subsequent voluntary one (facilitation). With neuromyotonia, continuous muscle fiber activity results in hard, tight muscles, allowing contraction to occur only slowly and with difficulty. Delayed muscle contraction *see* also hypokinetic gait (2.15.1.3)

2.15 Disturbances of Gait

For humans, walking is the most common motor act that can only be realized optimally when a large number of systems functions normally. In particular, the act must be willed; continuous motor impulses must flow through the pyramidal system; there must be unconscious coordination through the intermediate activity of the extrapyramidal and cerebellar control systems. The continuation of these impulses through the spinal cord and to the appropriate muscles, the sensory feedback from the periphery, and the orientation in space through the optic and vestibular systems must all take place appropriately; also necessary is a sound mechanical structure of bones, joints, and muscles. Finally, the gait must not be impaired through pain.

Because of the large number of structures involved in normal gait, there is a correspondingly large number of causes that may disturb normal ambulation. Each one of the structures involved in gait influences it in a characteristic or even pathognomonic way. Therefore careful observation of the act of walking is often of value in differential diagnosis and should be carried out at the beginning of all neurologic examinations. It should be noted that many patients with a broad variety of disturbances of gait complain of 'dizziness'.

In Figure 50 there is a schematic representation of the most common disturbances of gait. Below, I discuss the symptoms and signs and categorize the various causes of gain disturbances, noting their pathophysiology.

2.15.1 Inhibited (Impaired) Gait

The act of walking is slowed. The feet are pushed forward with evident difficulty, often scraping au-

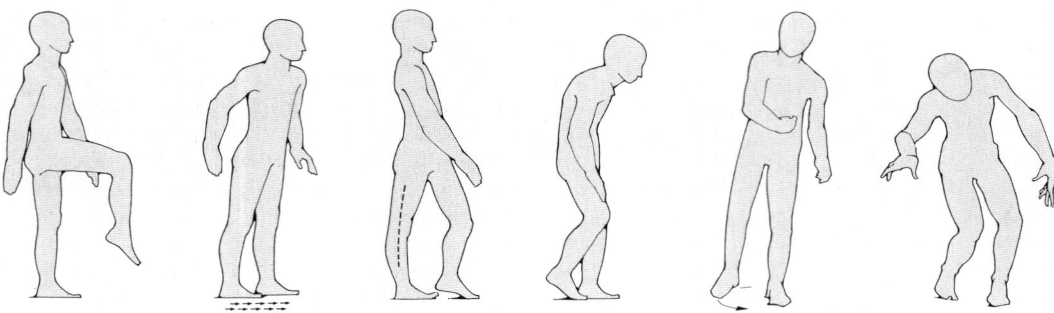

Fig. 50   Some characteristic gait disturbances. Left to right: steppage gait with weakness of foot extensors, resulting in abnormal elevation of legs and repositioning of the foot on the ground toes first; paraspastic gait with dragging of both feet; quadriceps paralysis in which the supporting leg is planted with knee extended; Parkinson's gain (similar to senile gait with lacunar state) posture slightly flexed, knees and elbows continuously flexed and steps small; gait with rightsided hemiparesis in which there is circumduction of the extended leg and slight plantar flexion of the foot, and there is also flexion of the abducted arm; hysterical gait in so-called psychogenic dysbasia with irregular, almost acrobatic, movement without falls

dibly along the floor. The following categories are recognized:

2.15.1.1 Paraspastic Gait

The legs are usually extended. The feet drag audibly along the floor (corresponding wear is evident on the soles of the shoes). Sometimes they are moved in scissors fashion with toes slightly inverted (pigeon toes). This type of gait disturbance is usually the result of a more or less symmetric bilateral lesion of the pyramidal fibers at any level.

The causes of this type of gait are similar to those of the paraspastic increase in tone mentioned above (*see* 2.12.1.1). Paraspastic gait is particularly common in the following circumstances

— In multiple sclerosis (the characteristic spastic atactic gait, also mentioned under other symptoms, *see* 2.13.2.5.1)
— In a lacunar state (in elderly individuals with hypertension or other risk factors for vascular disease; often preceded by evidence of small ischemic vascular insults and accompanied by pseudobulbar symptoms with disturbances of speech and increased perioral reflexes, small stepped [tripping] gait, pyramidal signs)
— After spinal cord trauma (indicated in history, sensory level, disturbances of micturition)
— With Little's disease (a special form of cerebral gait disorder that is present from birth with delayed motor milestones but normal intellectual development; often only selective involve-

ment of the limbs, particularly of the lower extremities, and marked scissors movement with crossing of the legs during walking)
— In familial spastic spinal paralysis (hereditary, appears in the second to third year of life, slowly progressive)
— As a result of rarer, in part reversible, conditions such as hyperthyroidism, portacaval shunt, lathyrism, spinal cord disease (with vitamin B_{12} deficiency or as a paraneoplastic syndrome), adrenoleukodystrophy or malabsortive hydrocephalus (*see* 2.1)

An intermittent paraspastic gait is rare and may occur with vascular insufficiency of the spinal cord accompanying so-called intermittent spinal claudication (*see* 2.15.5)

2.15.1.2 Paraspastic-Ataxic Gait

In this gait disturbance the characteristics of the paraspastic gait are joined by clear ataxic elements such as stamping feet, sudden equilibrating movements of the trunk, and slight retroversion of the knee. This picture is characteristic, almost pathognomonic, of multiple sclerosis.

2.15.1.3 Hypokinetic Gait

This type of gait is characterized by slow nonfluid positioning of the legs with few or no associated movements and with stiff posture.

Common etiologic factors in this type of gait include

- Hypokinetic-hypertonic extrapyramidal syndromes, particularly Parkinson's syndrome (in which the torso is bent slightly forward; the gait is flexed with lack of associated movement of the arms; also marked by rigidity, mask-like facies, monotonous and soft speech; tremor not always present, but cogwheel phenomenon may be found)
- Other hypokinetic extrapyramidal syndromes, among them progressive supranuclear palsy (*see* 2.8.2.2), olivopontocerebellar atrophy (*see* 1.1.4), and orthostatic hypotension. In lacunar states there can also be paraspastic (*see* 2.15.1.1) and pseudobulbar paralysis with difficulty in swallowing (*see* 2.10), speech disorder (*see* 2.11.2), and parkinsonian-like hypokinesia of gait
- In young individuals, torsion dystonia may initially be manifest as a peculiar stiff and inhibited gait
- The designer drug 1-methyl-4 phenyl-1,2,3,6-tetrahydropyridine (MPTP) can cause acute severe akinesia with severe impairment of gait
- The syndrome of continuous muscle fiber activity (*see* 2.12.1.3), most often seen in young patients. The peculiar tension of all muscles, including antagonists, inhibits gait and all other movements
- Depression and catatonia, may be expressed as a hypokinetic inhibited gait. Catatonia may appear apart from dystonia in schizophrenia, and also in a number of somatic disorders. These include metabolic disorders e.g. in hypercalcemia, porphyria, liver and renal failure, intoxications and also the malignant neuroleptic syndrome, encephalitis, hydrocephalus and other encephalopathic disorders. Attacks of catatonia may be part of the semiconscious state of status epilepticus

2.15.2 Dystonic Gait

Movements necessary for normal gait are interrupted in this condition by extraneous, incongruous, irregular movements. The patient must continuously struggle against these disruptions to move purposefully. (For causes of dystonic gait *see* 2.14.1.8 to 2.14.1.11)

Dystonic disturbances of gait are commonly found in chorea, athetosis, ballismus, and torsion dystonia. They are to be distinguished from hysterical gait disturbances (*see* 2.15.6). The early stage of torsion dystonia is often difficult to differentiate from hypokinetic disorders resulting in stiff gait, particularly in children and young individuals. In parkinsonian patients successfully treated with high doses of levodopa, definite dystonia can appear during walking.

2.15.3 Ataxic Gait

The disorder of movement during ataxia (*see* 2.14.2.1 and Table 20) is manifest in abrupt, poorly measured placement of feet, often evident as stamping. Equilibrium is more or less impaired, leading to corrective movements that give the gait an irregular and incongruous character. The gait also becomes broad based as a result of the swaying and uncertain stance.

Causes of ataxic gait are enumerated in 2.14.2.1. In lesions of the cerebellum, particularly affecting the vermis, the gait is very wide based. The patient often sways during walking and even while standing or sitting. In vestibular disturbances (*see* 2.7.1) there is less ataxia but more swaying, particularly at dusk. In posterior column lesions (*see* 1.2.2) the gait is particularly ataxic, with much stamping, and in extreme cases, walking is totally impossible because of the marked loss in deep sensibilities. With marked polyneuropathy (*see* 1.3.5) and polyradiculopathy (*see* 1.3.1), the gait can be ataxic and stamping, resembling that of posterior column lesions (so-called polyneuropathic pseudotabes, diabetic or alcoholic in origin), or it may be characterized by paralysis of the foot extensors. With such paralysis the foot hangs limply when the leg is elevated. Therefore, the leg must be markedly elevated to move the foot forward and set it down toe first. This results in bilateral steppage gait (*see* 2.15.4.2). With intoxication the gait may be atactic as in cerebellar lesions (for example, with diphenylhydantoin intoxication), or it may be marked by gross swaying and reeling (chronic barbiturate intoxication or alcohol intoxication).

2.15.4 Motor Paretic Gait

Paralysis often influences gait in a characteristic way. The paretic leg is exposed to weight bearing for shorter periods than the healthy leg. With central hemiparesis (*see* 2.13.2.5) there is circumduction; the leg is extended at the knee with slight plantar flexion of the foot and is carried with a slight circular outward movement; the homolateral arm loses some of its swing. If a cane is used, it is carried on the healthy side (to which the patient leans and transfers more weight). (For description of the gait of bilateral central paralysis of the legs in paraparesis, *see* 2.15.1.1.) Paralysis (peripheral) of the foot extensors is mostly unilateral, leading to unilateral steppage gait (*see* 2.15.3), evident in unilateral regular slapping of the foot.

A common cause of unilateral foot extensor paralysis is impairment of peroneal nerve function, occasionally a lesion of the roots of L4 and L5, as with disc herniation ('vertebral peroneal paralysis'). Bilateral foot extensor paralysis with bilateral steppage gait is common in polyneuropathies (*see* 1.3.5) (marked by paresthesia, stocking-like sensory impairment, deficient or impaired ankle jerks), but also occurs in peroneal muscular atrophy of Charcot-Marie-Tooth – *see* 2.13.2.4 – hereditary high-arched feet, marked calf atrophy (stork legs), absence of ankle jerks, little or no sensory impairment, with spinal muscular atrophy – *see* 1.2.3 – (in which the paralysis is accompanied by atrophy of other muscles, slowly progressive fasciculation, no sensory impairment) and with certain myopathies (*see* 1.4 and 2.13.2.4), in particular with dystrophia myotonica of Steinert (*see* 2.13.2.4.2).

Paralysis of the knee extensors (quadriceps femoris) results in hyperextension during placement of the leg. When the weakness is bilateral, both legs are hyperextended at the knees during the gait; otherwise the transfer of weight between the legs would cause the knees to buckle. Descent of stairs occurs with the paretic leg first.

Causes of unilateral paralysis include paralysis

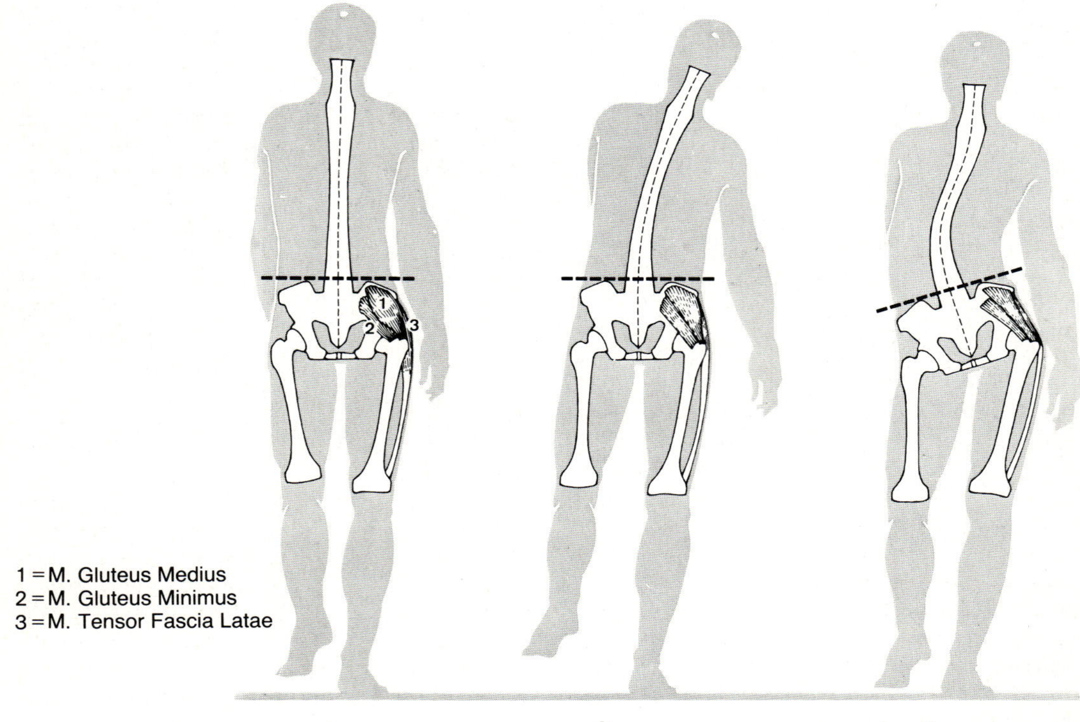

Fig. 51 a–c   Walking when there is weakness of the thigh abductors: **a Normal:** The pelvis is maintained in relation to the supporting leg by the healthy abductors. **b Duchenne limp:** To prevent the slipping of the pelvis on the side of the swinging limb, the center of gravity is transferred by the tilting of the upper body to the right. **c Trendelenburg limp:** With marked weakness of the thigh abductors, the pelvis slips with each step on the side of the swinging leg of the femoral nerve (*see* 1.3.4 [absence of knee jerk, disturbed sensation in the region of the saphenous nerve of the lower leg]) and lumbar plexus paralysis (*see* 1.3.3 [signs are similar to those of femoral nerve damage, but the abductors and the iliopsoas muscles are also involved]); rarely the patellar ligament may rupture, sometimes on both sides. A likely cause of bilateral paralysis is myopathy (*see* 1.4), particularly a limb-girdle form of progressive muscular dystrophy, polymyositis, or, in boys, Duchenne dystrophy.

Paralysis (or mechanical insufficiency) of the hip abductors (gluteus medius, gluteus minimus, and tensor fasciae latae) (Fig. 51) results in incapacity to hold the pelvis horizontal in relation to the weight-bearing leg. If the insufficiency is only partial, then the overextension of the trunk toward the supporting leg can be sufficient to displace the center of gravity and prevent descent of the pelvis. This is the so-called Duchenne limp (Fig. 51 b), which when it occurs bilaterally leads to a peculiar waddling gait. With complete paralysis of the hip abductors the transfer of the center of gravity described above is inadequate, leading, with each step, to descent of the pelvis on the side of the moving leg — the so-called Trendelenburg limp (Fig. 51 c).

Unilateral paralysis or insufficiency of the hip abductors can be caused by a lesion of the superior gluteal nerve, sometimes resulting from intramuscular injection. Even in the recumbent position there is insufficient strength to laterally abduct the affected leg, but there is no sensory loss. The same insufficiency is found in unilateral congenital dislocation of the hip or in post-traumatic or postoperative (prosthesis) approximation of the origin and insertion of the hip abductors, particularly after introduction of a hip prosthesis. Bilateral paresis (or insufficiency) is usually due to myopathy, in particular progressive muscular dystrophy (*see* 1.4), or bilateral congenital dislocation of the hip.

If the hip extensors are involved, particularly the gluteus maximus, ascent of stairs is possible only with the healthy leg first, but descent of stairs is with the involved leg first. Walking on an even flat surface is only impaired as a rule with bilateral weakness of the gluteus maximus; such patients walk with the pelvis tilted ventrally and with exaggerated lumbar lordosis. In unilateral gluteus maximus paralysis the affected leg cannot be elevated dorsally, even in the prone position. Its cause is always a (rare) lesion of the inferior gluteal nerve — for example, due to intramuscular injection.

Bilateral gluteus maximus paralysis is found most often with progressive forms of muscular dystrophy of the pelvic girdle and the Duchenne form.

2.15.5 Pain-Induced Disturbances of Gait

When there is pain during walking, the patient attempts to avoid, modify, or shorten the phase of gait that is most painful. When the pain is unilateral the affected leg bears weight for shorter periods. Pain may occur at particular points during each step, but it can also occur throughout the act of walking, or it may gradually decrease with continued walking.

Intermittent claudication is the term used to denote pain that appears only after walking a specific distance. In a restrictive sense this designation applies to pain arising from arterial insufficiency. This pain regularly appears after a certain distance of walking, gradually arising with increasing intensity and shorter distances. It appears sooner when the patient ascends hills or walks faster. The pain forces the patient to stop walking, but it disappears after a short period of rest even if the patient remains standing. The pain is most often localized in the calf. The typical cause is stenosis or occlusion of blood vessels in the upper area of the thigh (indicated by a typical history, vascular risk factors, absence of pedal pulses, bruits over the proximal blood vessels, absence of other causes of pain, and sometimes stocking-like sensory disturbances). Under similar circumstances there may, in addition, be pain in the saddle area or hips, resulting from occlusion of the pelvic arteries; such pain must be distinguished from sciatica or processes involving the cauda equina, however.

Intermittent claudication of the cauda equina is the term used to denote pain arising from compression of roots and occurring after walking, particularly downhill, for varying distances. The pain is due to the compression of the roots of the cauda equina in the thigh lumbar canal when that tight channel is narrowed even further by spondylotic changes. This pain is therefore found most often in elderly patients, particularly men, but generally it occurs in somewhat younger age groups than the pain due to vascular intermittent claudication. Because of the pathogenesis of this type of pain it is usually bilateral, of radicular character, and therefore predominantly posterior in the saddle area, the upper part of the tight, and the calf. Patients often also have backache and pain on sneezing (Naffziger sign). Pain during walking causes the patient to stop, but it does not usually disappear when the patient stands still. It is more likely to improve when the position of the spinal column is changed — for example, by sitting, bending forward sharply, or even kneeling. Root signs are evident especially after the pain on walking is provoked and also during the other painful phases: There is absence of vascular disease; radiography shows marked reduction of the sagittal diameter in the lumbar spinal column; myelography shows impaired passage of the dye at several levels. Diastomatomyelia in the lumbar region may appear for the first time in older subjects and may on rare occasions manifest itself as intermittent claudication.

Intermittent impairment of gait without pain may result from exercise-dependent ischemia of the spinal cord. This is termed intermittent claudication of the spinal cord (mostly in elderly individuals with vascular risk factors, weakness and/or spasticity after walking a set distance, transient pyramidal signs). Similar symptoms may be caused by an arachnoid cyst due to mechanical compression of the spinal cord. Differential diagnosis is usually possible because of localization of the pain and other characteristics.

Pain in the lumbar region on walking may be a manifestation of spondylosis or disc disease (suggested by a history of acute back pain with sciatic nerve radiation, sometimes by absence of ankle jerks, and by paralysis of the muscles supplied by the nerve). It can be due to spondylolisthesis (partial dislocation of the lumbosacral joints). It can result from ankylosing spondylitis of Bechterew, and so on. Radiographic studies of the lumbar spine are often diagnostic. Pain due to spondylosis and disc disease is often aggravated by prolonged sitting or inappropriate posture and may improve or even disappear with walking.

Pain in the hip region and in the inguinal region is usually the result of arthrosis of the hip. The pain is usually sharper during the first few steps and then decreases with continued ambulation. Occasionally there are pseudoradicular radiations of the pain to the side of the leg, impairing the inward rotation of the hip and resulting in pain and a feeling of pressure deep in the femoral triangle. When a cane is used, it is used on the side opposite the pain with a transfer of weight toward the healthy side (roentgenograms). Pain in the inguinal region during walking or after prolonged standing also occurs because of lesions of the ilioinguinal nerve. Rarely spontaneous, these most often occur after surgical procedures (lumbotomy, appendectomy) in which the nerve trunk has been injured or irritated by compression. This cause is suggested by history of a surgical procedure, improvement when the hip is flexed, pain that is usually most marked in a two-finger-breadth region medial to the anterior superior iliac spine, and sensory impairment in the inguinal region and in the scrotum or labium majus.

Burning pain in the lateral aspect of the thigh is found in meralgia paresthetica (*see* 2.16.2.1).

Local pain in the region of the long bones of the leg occurring on walking should arouse suspicion of a localized tumor, a bone cyst osteoporosis, Paget's disease, a pathologic fracture, and the like. In many of these conditions, which may be evident from palpation, pressure pain, or roentgenograms, there is also back pain. Anterior calf pain can appear during or after a prolonged hike or other abnormal exertion of the lower leg muscles or after an acute vascular occlusive event of the involved leg. It can also occur after surgical procedure on the lower limb. The pain is an expression of arterial insufficiency of the muscles in the anterior compartment, variously known as shin splint and arteriopathic anterior tibialis syndrome (intense increasingly painful swelling and reddening; pain on pressure of the anterior compartment; initially at least, disappearance of the pulse of the dorsalis pedis artery; impairment of sensation on the dorsum of the foot in the distribution of the deep branch of the peroneus nerve; paralysis of the extensor digitorum and extensor hallucis brevis muscles).

Pain in the feet and toes is particularly common. In most cases, the cause lies in deformities of the feet such as flat feet and broad feet. Such pain usually appears after some walking, after standing in shoes with hard soles, or after carrying loads. Even after a short walk, a calcaneal spur may cause pain in the region of the heel and pressure sensitivity on the plantar side of the heel. Chronic Achilles tendonitis shows, apart from the local pain, palpable thickening of the tendon. Pain in the anterior aspect of the foot is seen with Morton's metatarsalgia. This is due to a pseudoneuroma of an interdigital nerve. Pain is initially manifest only after prolonged walking, but later can occur after short distances and even at rest (pain localized distally between metatarsals III/IV or IV/V; also evident when metatarsal heads are compressed or displaced against one another; sensory loss on the contiguous areas of the toes; disappearance of pain after local anesthesia in the proximal intermetatarsal space). Pain in the plantar aspect of the foot severe enough to prevent walking altogether may occur with the tarsal tunnel syndrome (usually associated with antecedent dislocation or fracture of the malleolus; results in pain behind the medial malleolus, paresthesia or sensory loss on the sole of the foot, dry, thin skin and absence of sweating on the sole, and, relative to the opposite foot, inability to abduct the toes).

2.15.6 Irregular Bizarre Gait

There are disturbances of gait that, unlike those described above, do not show consistent characteristics, but constantly show new and unpredictable features. In a certain sense, dystonic disturbances of gait belong in this category (*see* 2.15.2 and what follows), but most of these bizarre anomalies of gait occur with psychogenic disturbances like hysteria. These gait disorders often seem to express imagined falls. In the course of their grotesque, uncoordinated motions, patients seem to lose their equilibrium repeatedly. Nevertheless, they always manage to catch themselves and avoid falling no matter how precarious their positions. When the patient is provided with an audience, these contortions may even become acrobatic feats. This disturbance is designated Camptospasm, and it must be distinguished from other characteristic disorders of gait. Clinical findings must be entirely normal otherwise, and even then it is important to carefully consider the possibility of true dystonic disturbances or cerebellar or vestibular gait disorders. All these may show marked irregular deviations from normal gait without pathologic findings apparent on clinical examination.

2.16 Disorders of Sensations

The anatomic basic of sensation is depicted in Figure 52. From this it can be seen that a sensory disorder may be classified either according to its distribution or according to its quality (*see* 2.16.2). Moreover, disorders can be further subdivided into spontaneous or abnormal sensations or sensory deficits.

2.16.1 Paresthesia and Dysesthesia

Spontaneous sensory disturbance (paresthesia) and disordered feelings of touch (dysesthesia or hyperesthesia) are symptoms. The following varieties are found:

− Symmetric, spontaneous paresthesia. These disturbances are frequently localized to the extremities, in which case they are usually expressions of a polyneuropathy (*see* 1.3.5), but in rare cases, expressions of tetany (*see* 2.3.2) or of an attack of basilar migraine (*see* 2.17.1) the paresthesia accompanies or follows the headache in the same attack or follows it in another, affects either side of the body, and is occasionally associated with disturbances of consciousness and often with epileptic discharges in the EEG). An acute generalized painful dysesthesia, occurring, together with a feeling of numbness, in a *symmetric pattern on the face and the whole body*, has been designated sensory neuromyopathy. This disorder appears after the administration of antibiotics for febrile disorders and has been attributed to an acute dorsal root lesion. Symmetric or, occasionally, unilateral paresthesia of the face can occur with cervical disc lesions. Usually unilateral paresthesia and later sensory defects and trophic disturbances occur with trigeminal neuropathy. Symmetric paresthesia in the perioral area occurs with tetany (*see above*) and (basilar) migraine (*see above*)

− Symmetric paresthesia can occur with certain inducing maneuvers, including the neck flexion sign of Lhermitte: With flexion of the head anteriorly, there are lightning-like electric sensations spreading into both arms, down the back and the sacral area, and occasionally even into both legs. This is a common sign in multiple sclerosis (*see* 2.13.2.5.1), and it can also be seen in arachnoiditis and with tumors of the cervical or thoracic spinal cord before or during atlantoaxial dislocation (usually suggested by objective signs of a high spinal cord lesion, CSF abnormalities, and x-ray findings, particularly on lateral views). After head trauma the Lhermitte sign may appear following a latent period of several months, but, providing clinical and x-ray findings are normal, usually disappears after some time. The Lhermitte sign may also occur after x-radiation. It is occasionally seen as the initial symptom of subacute combined degeneration (Vit. B_{12} deficiency)

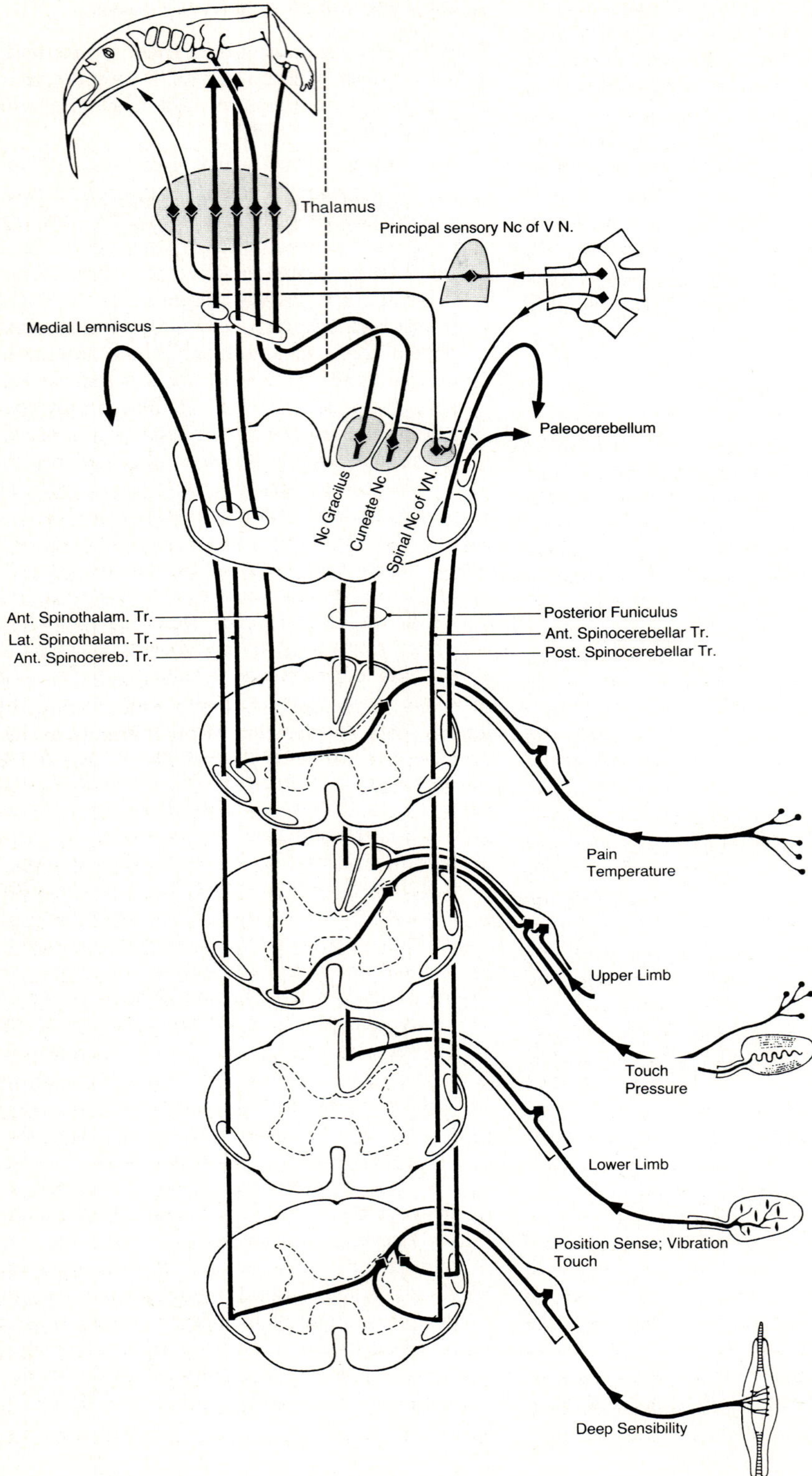

Fig. **52** Sensory pathways from the periphery through the spinal cord to the postcentral gyrus

– Nonsymmetric localized paresthesia can occur spontaneously in various body parts. Paresthesias occurring in attacks, particularly in the extremities and face, are discussed elsewhere: sensory jacksonian fits, migraine accompagnee (*see* 2.3.1.2.1), spontaneous attacks of pain as during tonic brain stem fits (*see* 2.3.2), and others.

Spontaneous, localized, more or less continuous paresthesia occurs as an initial or permanent accompaniment to numerous radicular or peripheral neuropathic sensory deficits. The distribution of these disorders almost always indicates the affected peripheral nerves or roots (*see* 2.16.2.1). However, paresthetic nocturnal brachialgia, usually a manifestation of chronic distal median nerve compression of the hand with the carpal tunnel syndrome (*see* 2.17.2.3) generally extends beyond the normal cutaneous sensory area of the median nerve. The most common spontaneous paresthesia in the lower extremity is meralgia paresthetica on the lateral aspect of the upper thigh (*see* 2.17.5)

Localized paresthesia or pain occasionally results from a specific mechanism. Mechanical irritation of a peripheral nerve can project such sensations to the periphery; their distribution can give a clue to the involved structure. If movement of the head or trunk or pressure or coughing provokes paresthesia, this suggests a mechanical root process: disc herniation (signs include aching of the neck or back, torticollis, or acute lumbago with signs over the vertebral column and radicular dysfunction (*see* 1.3.1) or tumors in the area of the roots (suggested by objective radicular dysfunction and eventually by spinal cord symptoms and destruction or enlargement of intervertebral foramina on x-ray film). If pressure on a peripheral nerve provokes paresthesia, then a (post-traumatic) neuroma or chronic compression, occurring, for example, in an anatomic narrow area (tunnel) or as a result of a scar, is to be suspected. If the pain is initiated by movement of a joint, there may be a ganglion (one example is paresthesia in the peroneus distribution with a ganglion of the tibial fibular joint).

In a separate category is the dysesthesia occurring with thalamic lesions: When the contralateral body part is touched, unpleasant burning sensations appear after a delay and outlast the stimulus. Occasionally there are also spontaneous burning pains on one half of the body (*see* 2.17.6) associated with difficulty in temperature sensation (*see* 2.16.2.2)

2.16.2 Decreased Sensation
(for psychogenic disorders, *see* 2.16.4)

Analysis of the kind and topographic distribution of the deficits gives a clue to the structure involved (Fig. 52).

2.16.2.1 Impairment of All Modalities of Sensation

All modalities of sensation are equally involved only in the case of lesions of peripheral nerves or roots, in transverse syndromes when all columns of the spinal cord are involved to an equal extent, and when all the afferents in the brain stem and hemispheres are equally affected, including the lateral spinothalamic tract and the medial lemniscus. A sensory disturbance of all modalities of sensation in the face is, as a rule, the result of a lesion of the trigeminal nerve and can be accompanied by paralytic keratitis or trophic disorders of skin and mucous membrane. Space-occupying lesions (pain, involvement of other cranial nerves, progression), especially cerebellopontine angle tumor, trigeminal neurinoma, and aneurysm of the carotid artery (affecting the first division of the trigeminal nerve) are common causes. Isolated impairment of sensation in the trigeminal territory has been reported in scleroderma and sarcoidosis. Another cause is trigeminal neuropathy (sudden in onset, a feeling of deafness and paresthesia, trophic disturbances, spontaneous improvement). (For another cause, Raeder's syndrome, *see* 2.8.1.) A rare cause is a lesion of the trigeminal nuclear area, usually following a circulatory disturbance in the caudal part of the pons, sometimes designated Gasperini syndrome (homolateral, trigeminal, facial, abducens and acoustic nerve paresis, contralateral sensory disturbance on the trunk and extremities). Such a lesion may also occur in association with a brain stem glioma or syringobulbia (*see* 2.16.2.2).

A disorder of sensory modalities involving one side of the face, trunk, and extremities occurs only with an extensive contralateral lesion of the lateral spinothalamic tract, including the medial lemniscus in the brain stem (medulla oblongata, pons, and midbrain). The lesion must be situated prior to the entry of the sensory afferents into the posterior ventral nucleus of the thalamus or in this nucleus itself or involve the thalamocortical sensory pathways in the posterior limb of the internal capsule (Fig. 52). Such localized processes never cause complete anesthesia and analgesia; the sensory disturbances they cause are usually accompanied by motor hemisyndromes or, in the case of brain stem lesions, other neurologic deficits. Rare exceptions are isolated thalamus lesions e.g. ischemia in the territory of the anterior choroidal artery.

A spinal cord lesion can affect all sensory modalities only if it is bilateral. It then causes a bilateral deficit of sensation on the trunk and extremities with a sensory level. The height of the sensory level gives a clue to the site of the lesion. It is important to avoid mistaking the natural differences of sensitivity in various areas of the body — for example, the decreased sensory acuity over the clavicle and rib cage — for a sensory level. Only spinal cord processes causing a transverse lesion can, in fact, cause a sensory level; such processes therefore involve other pathways and functions as well causing disturbances of motor function or spasticity or both in the lower limbs. Causes are space-occupying lesions, multiple sclerosis, spondylosis, vascular deficits of the spinal cord, and syringomyelia (*see* 1.2.1, 2.12.1, and 2.13.4).

Loss of all sensation in circumscribed, well-demarcated areas of the trunk or extremities can give hints to the topography of the lesion and a clue to its site in certain roots, plexuses, or peripheral nerves. Details of the arrangements and distribution of various peripheral nerve lesions, explaining the topography of circumscribed areas of anesthesia, are given in Figure 53 and Tables 8 and 9.

— Radicular disturbances often cause changes in sensation that are strip-like in extent on the extremities and form a girdle halfway around the trunk. They are, however, difficult to define objectively, particularly when only one root is affected. The overlap of dermatomes, especially for tactile sensation, is very extensive. Paresthesia, if any, may give a clue to the site of the lesion. An examination of pain sensibility, using a pin, is usually more rewarding because the overlap of pain dermatomes is less extensive

— Sensory disturbances with lesions of peripheral nerves usually accompany peripheral motor paralyses and are not the leading symptoms. An exception is sometimes found with lesions of pure sensory peripheral nerves, the frequency of which is emphasized in Figure 53. The borders of the sensory impairment in peripheral nerve lesions are always sharp and distinct. With complete lesions (for example, pressure palsies) dysesthesias (*see above*) and paresthesias are often found. Among peripheral deficits are the lack of sensory feedback when shaking hands, resulting in inappropriate pressure, that occurs with lesions of the dorsal ramus of the radial nerve or ulnar nerve (injury at the wrist due to tight watchbands or handcuffs); deficits at the radial border of the thumb, designated cheiralgia paresthetica (chronic local pressure due to the use of scissors or other similar instrument); sensory disorders (and pain) in the inguinal region due to lesions of the ilioinguinal nerve, often known as the ilioinguinal syndrome (rarely spontaneous; often due to appendectomy scars, marked by a flexion position of the hip to decrease load and by pain on extension of the hip); burning sensation and feeling of deadness like meralgia paresthetica on the outer, upper aspect of the thigh, due to lesions of the lateral cutaneous nerve of the thigh (usually spontaneous compression syndrome in the inguinal ligament, occasionally due to a scar, for example, after hip replacement); sensory disturbances, sometimes painful dysesthesia in the medial aspect of the knee — the Howship-Romberg syndrome — due to lesions of the obturator nerve (always look for recognizable, though often missed, paralysis of the adductors) at its exit from the pelvis through the obturator foramen (tumor or fracture of the pelvis, obturator hernia); sensory disturbances and dysesthesia below the patella, known as patellar neuropathy or gonalgia paresthetica (chronic compression of the infrapatellar branch, just proximal to the medial femoral condyle); sensory disturbances on the medial aspect of the large toe, particularly when hallux valgus is also present (pressure due to inappropriate footwear)

A distal symmetric disorder of sensation is almost always due to a polyneuropathy (*see* 1.3.5) or a polyradiculopathy (*see* 1.3.1). In addition to the commoner mixed sensory-motor neuropathies there are also pure sensory neuropathies. These may be genetic and progressive or symptomatic. Examples are a beta lipoproteinemia (with low serum cholesterol and triglycerides, acanthocyto-

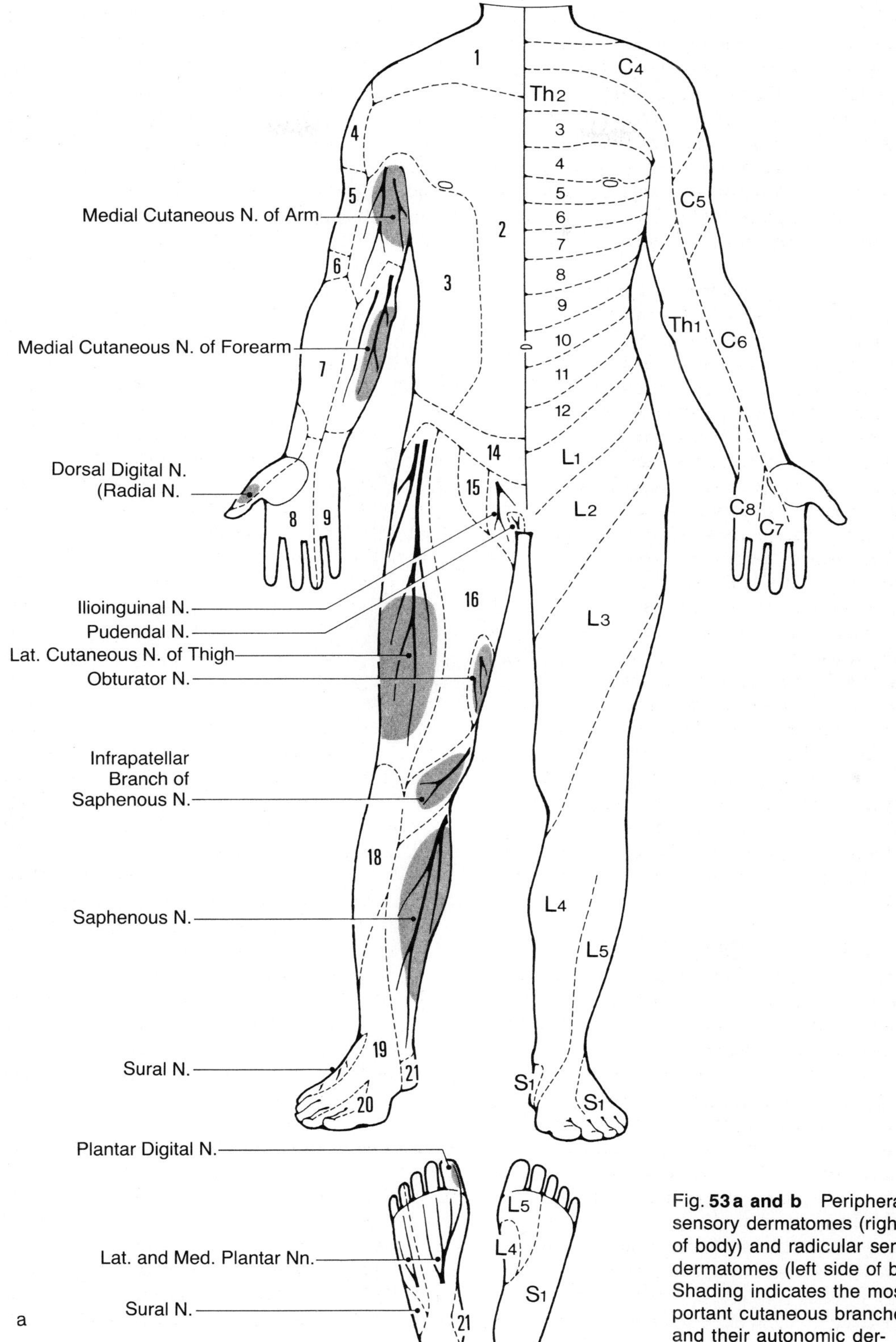

Fig. **53 a and b** Peripheral sensory dermatomes (right side of body) and radicular sensory dermatomes (left side of body). Shading indicates the most important cutaneous branches and their autonomic dermatomes

C4
Th2
C5
1
4
5
Th1
3
10
6
7
L1
11
14
L2
12
L3
13
S4 5 6
S3
L4
C6
C7 C8
S2
17
18
S1
Medial Cutaneous N. of Arm
Medial Cutaneous N. of Forearm
Dorsal Branch of Ulnar N.
Superficial Branch of Radial N.
Lateral Cutaneous N. of Thigh
Saphenous N.
Sural N.
Medial Plantar N.

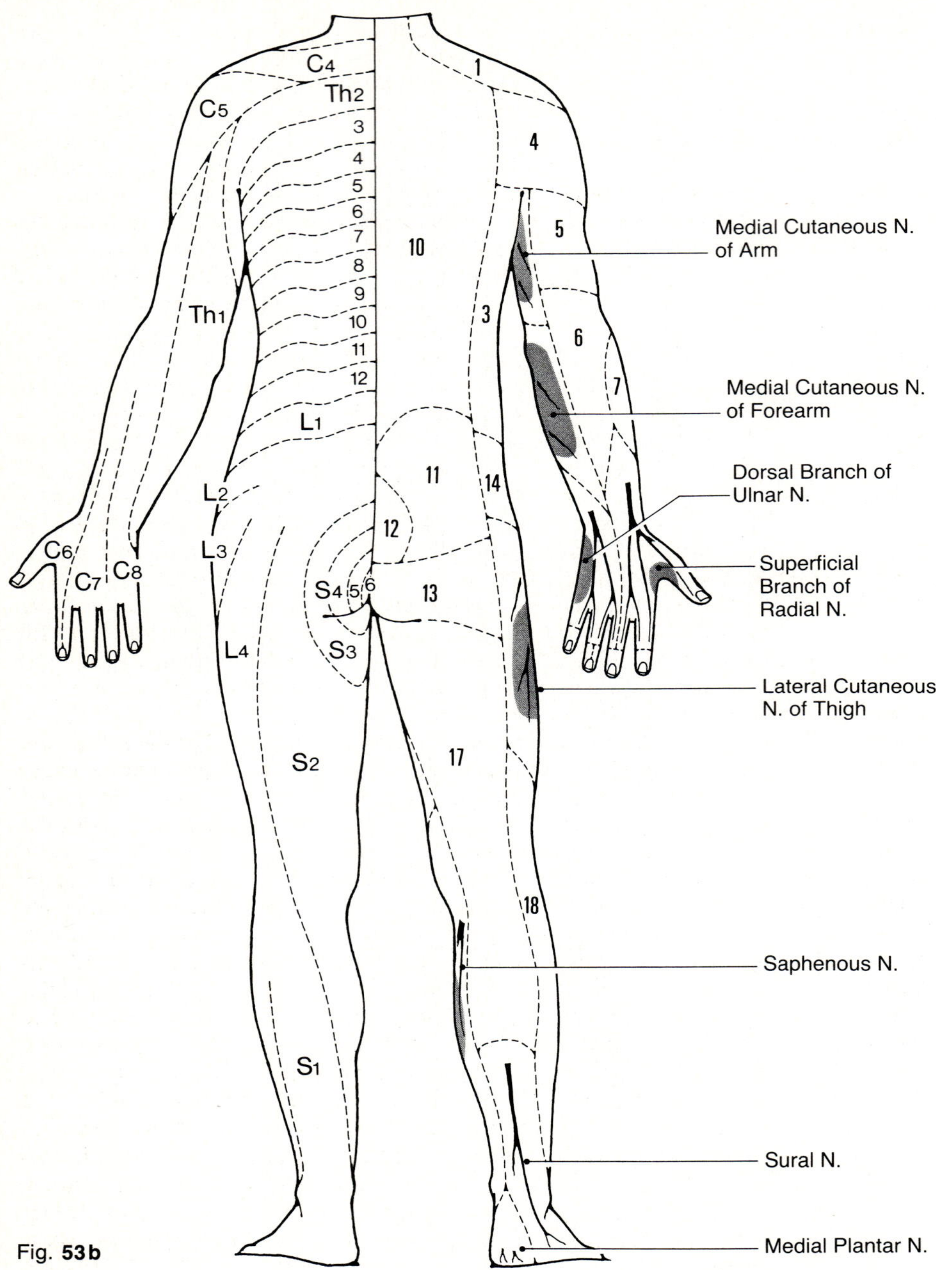

Fig. **53 b**

sis, areflexia, proprioceptive loss and retinitis pigmentosa).

2.16.2.2 Dissociated Disorders of Isolated Sensory Modalities

A disturbance affecting only isolated sensory modalities is known as dissociated sensory loss. This term is also used somewhat inaccurately for an isolated disturbance of pain and temperature sensation. The presence of dissociated sensory disturbance is anatomically traceable to the separate pathways taken by sensory modalities after they enter the posterior root of the spinal cord and before their reunion in the posterior lateral ventral nucleus of the thalamus (Figs. 8, 11, and 53). On this anatomic basis, it is evident that dissociated sensory loss must always be due to a lesion of the spinal cord or brain stem. With congenital insensitivity to pain, sensory radicular neuropathy, and leprosy (*see below*), the absence of pain endings in the skin and changes in spinal ganglia and in peripheral nerves may cause dissociated sensory loss.

A special case is generalized absence of pain sensation. This can occur as familial congenital insensitivity to pain (pain asymbolia). It may be present since earliest childhood and manifest itself in self-mutilation, fever, and, in certain variants, anhidrosis. Self-mutilation is also the leading symptom, along with insensitivity to pain, of the Lesch-Nyhan syndrome (choreoathetotic dystonia, psychomotor retardation with high uric acid levels). The presence of partial insensitivity to pain since birth or early childhood is part of familial dysautonomia (Riley-Day syndrome [*see* 2.20.1.1]). In the autosomal dominantly inherited sensory radicular neuropathy (ulceromutilating acropathy of Thévenard) other symptoms accompany the dissociated sensory loss (*see* 2.20.3). In leprosy, small areas of analgesia and loss of sweating in various parts of the skin are an initial sign. Later there are peripherally caused paralyses of mixed nerves in addition to the anesthesia.

Dissociated loss of pain and temperature sensation in the face can be found with a central lesion in the high cervical spinal cord or medulla oblongata. Such a lesion or process interrupts the nucleus of the descending tract of the trigeminal nerve on the side opposite the ascending crossed fibers of the spinothalamic tract. The sensory loss is usually bilateral. In a lesion ascending from the cervical spinal cord (resulting, for example, from syringomyelia), Figure 54 shows why the occipital region of the head and face is involved first and

most severely, but in a lesion of the medulla oblongata the rostral areas of the face are involved first. If such a lesion is bilateral, the sensory loss occurs in an onionskin distribution, but the corneal reflex remains unimpaired because of its direct connection from the main sensory nucleus of the trigeminal nerve to the facial nucleus.

Common causes of such sensory disturbances include high cervical syringomyelia or syringobulbia (atrophy of neck and shoulder girdle muscles, occasionally tongue atrophy, difficulty in swallowing, dysarthria, and pyramidal signs, with a basilar impression occasionally visible roentgenographically), a brain stem glioma (signs as above, but, in addition, evidence of increased intracranial pressure), and in rare cases a vascular insult due to ischemia in the vertebral artery territory near the most cranial portion of the anterior spinal artery (sudden in onset, usually seen in elderly patients with vascular risk factors; accompanied by other neurologic deficits).

Dissociated sensory loss mainly affecting only one side of the body is due to lesions of the lateral spinothalamic tract of the opposite side. The height of the lesion determines the extent of the loss of pain and temperature sensation. If the lesion is in the cranial-lateral part of the pons, there is, in addition, impairment of pain and temperature sensation in the face. Because the lateral spinothalamic tract is closely associated with the medial lemniscus, which carries other sensory modalities, true dissociated sensory loss alone does not occur with such a lesion, except when the lesion is situated below the medulla oblongata, resulting in dissociated sensory loss primarily affecting the trunk and extremities (Fig. 52). With lesions in the vicinity of the thalamus (usually of vascular origin) the contralateral side of the body can experience spontaneous painful burning sensations (*see* 2.17.6), delayed touch perception, and prolonged longlasting (beyond stimulus) modified sensation induced by contact (*see* 2.16.1). Difficulties with temperature discrimination also are usually found. Frequently an ipsilateral Horner syndrome and disturbed thermoregulatory sweating also occur as manifestations of the affection of descending central sympathetic fibers. Dissociated hemisensory loss, extending from the most cranial cervical segments downward, is due to a lesion in the medulla oblongata. The most common cause is a vascular insult to the brain stem (acute in onset, associated with other neurologic deficits; for details, see Table 18). In rare cases, syringomyelia or syringobulbia (*see below*), a brain

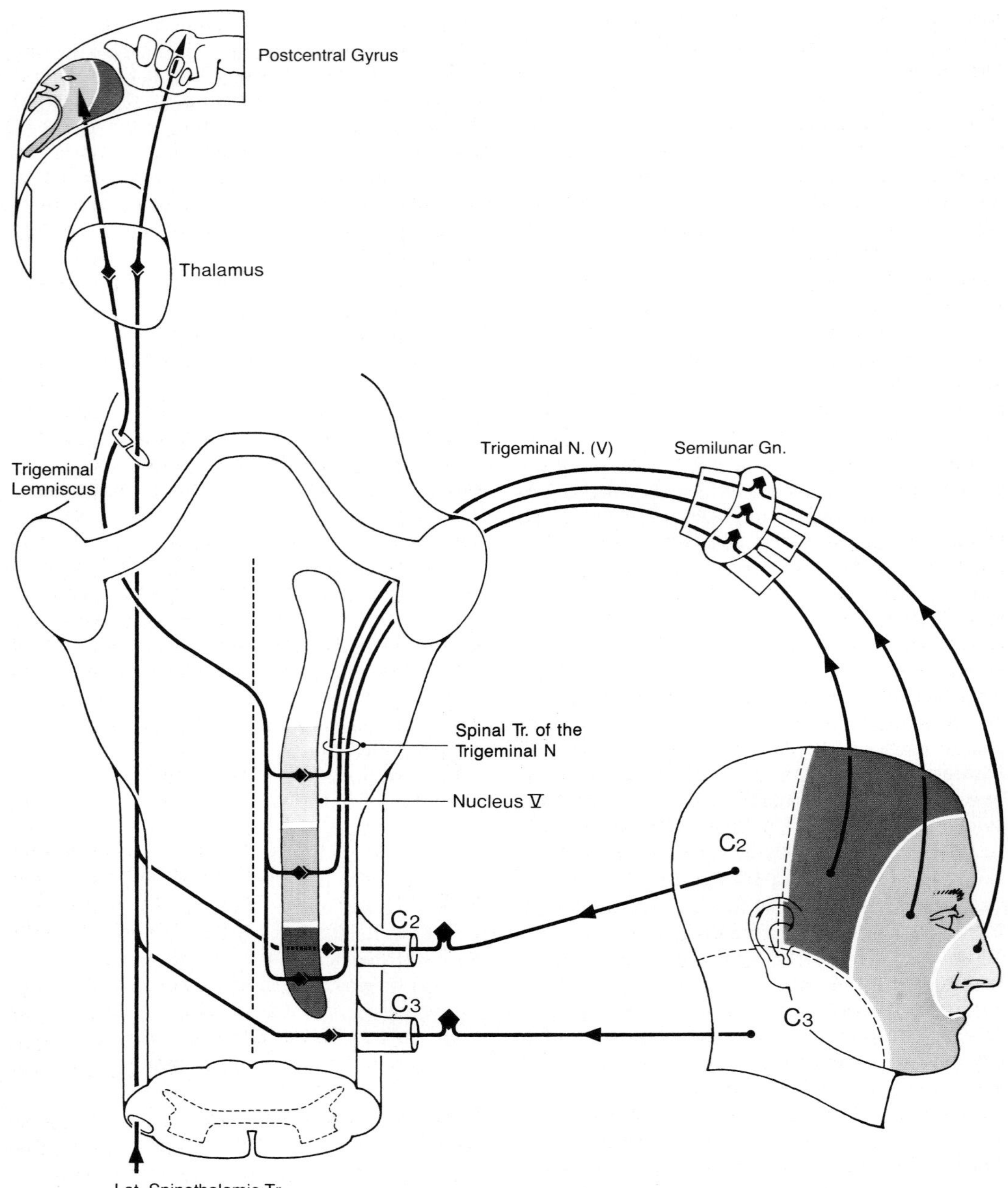

Fig. **54** Anatomic basis of (dissociated) sensory disturbances in the face stem glioma (*see above*), multiple sclerosis (*see above*), or the effects of spinal cord trauma cause this deficit.

If the sensory deficits are evident only on the trunk and extremities, sparing the neck, then the process is within the spinal cord. Causes are trauma (evident from history and deficits that are most marked initially), tumor, or other space-occupying lesions (progressive symptoms, initially pain, and occasionally the Brown-Séquard syndrome [*see* 1.2.1.2]; abnormal findings in the CSF and on myelography), angioma (attacks of deficits, all with similar localization; acute episodes with subarachnoid bleeding), multiple sclerosis (in younger patients, resulting in sudden deficits with remissions, accompanied by other neurologic deficits, CSF findings, and visual evoked potentials), syringomyelia (segmental due to the sensory loss, accompanied by muscle atrophy, due to loss of anterior horn cells, sometimes bilateral and segmental dissociated sensory disturbances on the opposite side; pyramidal signs also are evident).

A symmetric, segmental disturbance of pain and temperature that is not found in the more caudal segments results from lesions of the anterior commissure (Figs. 8 and 13). The most common cause is syringomyelia (marked by very slow progression, muscle atrophy, trophic disturbances in the skin, bones, and joints [*see* Fig. 59], pyramidal signs), or, in rare cases, an anterior spinal artery syndrome (*see* 1.2.1.3 [acute in onset; mostly found in elderly patients with vascular risk factors; accompanied by pyramidal signs and flaccid segmental paralysis with later muscle atrophy, sphincter disturbances]). Segmental sensory disturbances can also appear in younger patients, occasionally in a setting of angioma of the spinal cord, or they can be caused by hematomyelia (acute, usually with pain), either spontaneous (often occurring with angioma) or post-traumatic (check for a history of trauma in the long axis of the body with falls in the sitting position).

Dissociated sensory loss of deep sensibility that spares other sensory modalities is found with lesions of the posterior columns. Position sense is more markedly affected or totally absent, leading to marked ataxia and gait disturbance (*see* 2.7.2). The most frequent causes are diseases of spinal columns, usually with vitamin B_{12} deficiency (found with gastrointestinal disease or deficient nutrition; eventually involves other spinal tracts, giving rise to pyramidal signs; the optic nerve may become affected and polyneuropathy can occur; the onset may be acute and progression rapid; an abnormal Schilling test is found), tabes dorsalis (signs include pupillary abnormalities [*see* 2.8.4.2], areflexia, often deficient pain sensibility, arthropathies, abnormal serologic findings in the CSF; history is unreliable in diagnosis), paraneoplastic syndromes (sometimes the neoplasm has been diagnosed; occasionally it may not yet be manifest; often cerebellar symptoms and polyneuropathy are apparent), and some hereditary spinocerebellar syndromes.

2.16.3 Extinction Phenomena, Neglect and Astereognosis

In extinction phenomena, normal quality and quantity of sensation for all sensory modalities are preserved, but with simultaneous touching of symmetric body sites, the sensation from one site is not registered – it is "extinguished" or neglected. This is a manifestation of a contralateral parietal lobe syndrome (*see* 1.1.2.1) and is sometimes accompanied by visual extinction, apraxia, and disturbed optokinetic nystagmus (*see* 2.7.1). Astereognosis, the inability, in spite of normal touch sensation, to identify an object by touch alone, is discussed in 2.1.

2.16.4 Psychogenic Disturbances of Sensation

Psychogenic sensory disorders almost always affect all sensory modalities. It is rare that an isolated sensory defect is of psychogenic origin. The following are hints of the nonorganic nature of the disturbance.

- The borders of the sensory disturbance do not conform to known anatomic distribution of sensory pathways; ring-like sharply demarcated deficits of a whole extremity are common
- Objective neurologic deficits such as disturbances of tone, reflex disorders, or trophic changes in the skin or muscles are absent

The proof of the psychogenic nature of the disorder lies in contradictory test results on sensory examination and the incompatibility of the sensory loss with the anatomy and function of the nervous system. In diagnosing individual cases, the same principles apply that were discussed with psychogenic motor paralysis (*see* 2.13.3). The following evidence can be definitive:

- When the patient closes his eyes and is touched on body parts previously claimed to be insensitive, he may respond to each touch by saying that he cannot feel anything, showing that he is sensitive to contact. In this test the touch should not be rhythmic, nor should the examiner inquire after each touch. The examiner should also perform movements without touch
- In testing temperature, vibration, or graphesthesia in intelligent patients, all the results will be abnormal, but if the patient reports any sensory input at all, touch sensation is clearly present
- When handling an object with closed eyes, the patient may claim not to recognize it, but its proper manipulation suggests an intact sense of touch. The opening of a buttoned shirt or untying of shoelaces with apparently anesthetic fingers while the eyes are closed is not explicable on an organic basis. In this test it is important not to confuse a psychogenic disturbance with astereognosis, which can be associated with inability to recognize objects that may be handled appropriately. Sensation of touch is normal in such patients (*see* 2.1), but it has been misinterpreted in the past as having a psychogenic basis
- With repeated testing of an area claimed to have a very sharp circumscribed border of sensory loss, that border may be found to vary. By carefully noting landmarks, the examiner can demonstrate that areas once totally insensitive may miraculously have acquired new sensation
- When, in the case of a sensory loss leading to claimed hemianesthesia, the skin is moved over the skeleton, the patient may still refer to the skeletal structure in defining the center of the body, in effect changing the extent of the claimed sensory loss
- With hemianesthesia or unilateral anesthesia of an upper extremity, the patient may be confused about the topographic representation through a variety of tricks: Displacement of the testicles from one side to the other or crossing of the fingers may lead to mistakes in claims of sensory loss
- In isolated loss of pain sensibility with preservation of touch, the suspicion of psychogenic origin is reinforced by the patient's refusal to admit to pain. In such cases the examination is restricted to temperature sensation and its topographic distribution, from which arise clues to the true nature of the symptoms

2.17 Pain Syndromes

Pain may often be the sole or leading symptom of a disorder. The physician must depend for his etiologic diagnostic clues on the pain type alone if objective signs are absent on clinical examination.

Analysis of a pain syndrome must take into account its localization, its temporal profile, the pain quality, factors that precipitate and factors that decrease pain, accompanying signs and symptoms, the effect of the pain, and objective findings on examination.

The discussion that follows concentrates on pain syndromes often seen in a neurologic practice or necessary for differential diagnosis in neurology.

2.17.1 Head and Face Pain

Differential diagnosis of the individual head and face pain syndromes can be made with use of Table 21, in which the pain is grouped according to

- Localization
- The temporal profile of its appearance and disappearance
- Initiating factors
- Clinical findings

From these characteristics one can often — but not always — establish a probable cause for the pain.

2.17.2 Cervical and Shoulder-Arm Pain (Fig. 55)

Pain in the region of the neck is usually due to local causes, most often in the spinal column. When the onset is acute, a likely cause is cervical disc herniation (torticollis, acute stiffness of the neck, coughing, and radicular pain, often radiating into the arm). Herniated disc can result from sudden movement or car collision. Pain that appears over hours to days can also be due to a cervical disc lesion (*see above*). Other causes of such pain include spondylosis (symptoms similar to those of disc herniation, but with less neck stiffness; x-ray findings — not definitive, since similar findings are often seen in symptom-free individuals — and occasionally headache), primary chronic polyarthritis in juveniles, in which the

Table 21 Differential diagnosis of head and face pain according to localization and characteristics

Localization	Temporal Aspects			Quality	Initiating Factors	Accompanying Features	Finding	Diagnosis	Remarks
	Onset	Duration	Characteristics						
	Head (including eyes and temple region, but not face)								
±Diffuse	Sudden: within seconds	Episode(s) day long, but decreasing	Once	Unbearably intense	Pressure	Vomiting, confusion	Meningismus	Subarachnoid hemorrhage	Lumbar puncture
		Minutes to hours	Recurring	Knife-like Very severe	Coughing pressure	–	Normal	Tissive syncope	Occasionally space-occupying lesions in posterior fossa
		Minutes	Recurring	Very severe Fronto-temporal	Intense cold stimulus (ice cream)	–	Normal	Ice cream headache	
		Hours to day	Rare recurrences	Very intense	Coitus	–	Slight meningismus	Coitus headache – meningeal migraine	Differential diagnosis from subarachnoid hemorrhage
	Rapid: within minutes	Minutes to hours	Recurring	Very intense	Change of position, pressure	Vomiting	Increase in intracranial pressure	Intermittent impaired CSF circulation	Sometimes unilateral
		Usually less than 15 min	Within minutes	Very intense	Tyramine-containing foods	Nausea, facial flush	Blood pressure elevation	Attacks of increased blood pressure (pheochromocytoma, hot dog headache, Chinese restaurant syndrome)	Differential diagnosis from hypertensive crisis
			Reaching its maximum intensity	Very intense	–	Vomiting, fits	Changes in fundus High blood pressure		
		Hours to days	Repeatedly	Very intense	–	Vomiting, confusion	Focal symptoms, often increase in blood pressure	Hypertensive crisis Intracerebellar hematoma	Sometimes unilateral
		Days	Increasing intensity Increasing intensity						
	Rapid: minutes to about 1/2 hours	Days	Increasing intensity	Very intense	Pregnancy, birth control pills, infection	Epileptic attacks	Focal symptoms Xanthochromic CSF	Cerebrovenous thrombosis	
		Hours to days	Constant and intense	Intense	–	Acute neurologic dysfunction	Focal signs	Occlusion of large intracranial arteries	Sometimes localized
		Depending on body position	Appearing on sitting or standing and increasing	Increasing Intense	Orthostation, sitting	Nausea	Low CSF pressure on lumbar puncture	Low CSF pressure syndrome	Disappearance on recumbency or pressure on jugular vein
			Often recurring	Boring, deep seated, torturous	Alcohol, stress	–	Normal	Vasomotor headache	Present since childhood Posttraumatic
	Slowly (over hours to days)	Hours to days Hours to days	In morning, decreasing during day	Boring, deep seated, often occipital	–	–	Increased blood pressure	Headache with hypertension	Mostly elderly patients

(continued)

Table 21   (continued)

Localization	Temporal Aspects			Quality	Initiating Factors	Accompanying Features	Finding	Diagnosis	Remarks
	Onset	Duration	Characteristics						
	Head (including eyes and temple region, but not face)								
		Increasing until headache continuous	–	Boring, torturous	–	Generalized illness	Meningismus, fever	Meningitis, malignant meningitis	Lumbar puncture, pathologic findings
		Increasing until headache continuous	–	Boring, torturous	After infectious diseases	–	No meningismus No fever	Postinfectious headache	Lumbar puncture, normal findings
		Increasing until headache continuous	–	Boring, deep	Increasing with pressure	Vomiting, psychogenic syndrome	Focal signs, increased intracranial pressure	Space-occupying intracranial lesion	
		More or less continuous headache	–	Boring, deep	Head trauma	–	Normal	Post-traumatic headache	Increasing with exposure to sun+alcohol intake
		Increasing in frequency until headache continuous	–	Boring	Exogenous toxic	Depending on cause	Depending on cause	Toxic e.g. carbon monoxide, lead, bromine, birth control pills	
Hemicranial	Sudden onset: within seconds	Several days (decreasing)	Once only	Very intense	–	Confusion	Focal signs	Vascular, intracerebral processes e.g. angioma, aneurysm	Compare with subarachnoid hemorrhage
	Very fast: within several minutes	Minutes to hours	Recurring	Very intense	Change of position, pressure	Vomiting	Increased blood pressure	Impaired CSF circulation from one lateral ventricle	
	Fast: minutes to about 1/2 hour	Days	Increasing intensity	Very intense	–	Often vomiting, fits	Focal signs, increased blood pressure	Intracerebral hematoma	
Temporal-retro-orbital, always same side		1/2 to 2 hours	Recurring, periodic increase	Unbearably intense	–	Tearing of eye, rhinorrhea, or blocked nose	Redness of eye and face	Cluster headache	Always unilateral, on same side
Eye and temple, leads to hemicrania		Hours	Usually only once	Temporal and retro-orbital	Mydriatics	Vomiting, unilateral dimness of vision	Large pupil, increased intraocular pressure	Glaucoma	
Temporal, leads to hemicrania (changes sides)	Gradual hours	within hours (rarely days)	Recurring	Boring	Menstruation, stress, change in weather, birth control pills	Vomiting, scintillation	Normal, except with migraine accompagnee	True migraine	Present since youth; changes sides
Neck and occiput, leads to hemicrania	Gradual hours	within hours to days	Recurring	Very intense to sharp	Whiplash injury, occasionally prolonged abnormal head position	Torticollis, brachialgia	Pain in neck, decreased motions	Headache with cervical spondylosis or cervical migraine	Do not overestimate value of radiologic findings

(continued)

Table 21 (continued)

Localization	Temporal Aspects				Quality	Initiating Factors	Accompanying Features	Finding	Diagnosis	Remarks
	Onset	Duration	Characteristics							
Head (including eyes and temple region, but not face)										
Diffuse unilaterally localized	slow (hours to days)	Hours to continuous pain	Symptom-free periods		Dull, boring, deep	Frequently after dental extraction	–	Normal	Atypical facial neuralgia	Often found in women Differential diagnosis from Carotidodynia
Temporal to hemicranial	Slow	Increasing in frequency to continuous pain	Increasing with pressure on temporal artery		Dull, intense	–	Poor general nutrition, feeling of illness	Painful temporal artery	Temporal arteritis	High sedimentation rate Poor general health Always found in elderly patients
Face	Slow	Increasing in frequency to continuous pain	–		Dull, feeling of pressure may be intense	Depending on cause	Depending on cause	Depending on etiology	Otorhinologic or dental pain	Look for precipitating causes
Face	Slow	Increasing in frequency to continuous pain	–		Dull, stabbing	–	–	Sensory impairment	Symptom of facial neuralgia, for example, trigeminal neuralgia	
Preauricular with radiation	Slow (hours to day)	Hours	–		Dull, boring	Chewing or after dental extraction	Dizziness	Malocclusion	Costen syndrome	Usually found in elderly patients Differential diagnosis from auriculotemporal neuralgia
Preauricular with radiation	Very rapid (within minutes)	Minutes	–		Burning	Chewing, acid foods, after diseases of parotid gland	Redness and sweating in preauricular area	Normal	Auriculotemporal neuralgia	Differential diagnosis from Costen syndrome
Upper or lower jaw	Apoplectic (within seconds)	Seconds	Frequent attacks		Ripping, unbearably intense	Chewing, talking, Trigger points	Grimacing of face (tic douloureux)	Normal	Trigeminal neuralgia	Differential diagnosis from hemifacial spasms
Face and Neck										
Inner canthus and eyeball	Apoplectic (within seconds)	Seconds	Frequent attacks, sometimes continuous pain		Ripping, unbearably intense	Chewing, local pressure	Rhinorrhea, redness of eye and forehead	Normal	Nasociliary neuralgia	
Inner canthus and eyeball	Apoplectic (within seconds)	Seconds	Frequent attacks, sometimes continuous pain		Ripping, unbearably intense	Chewing, local pressure	Rhinorrhea, redness of eye and forehead	Sinus infection	Sluder neuralgia	
Throat and base of tongue	Apoplectic (within seconds)	Seconds	Frequent attacks, continuous pain		Ripping, unbearably intense	Swallowing, cold foods	–	Normal	Glossopharyngeal neuralgia	Accompanied by sneezing

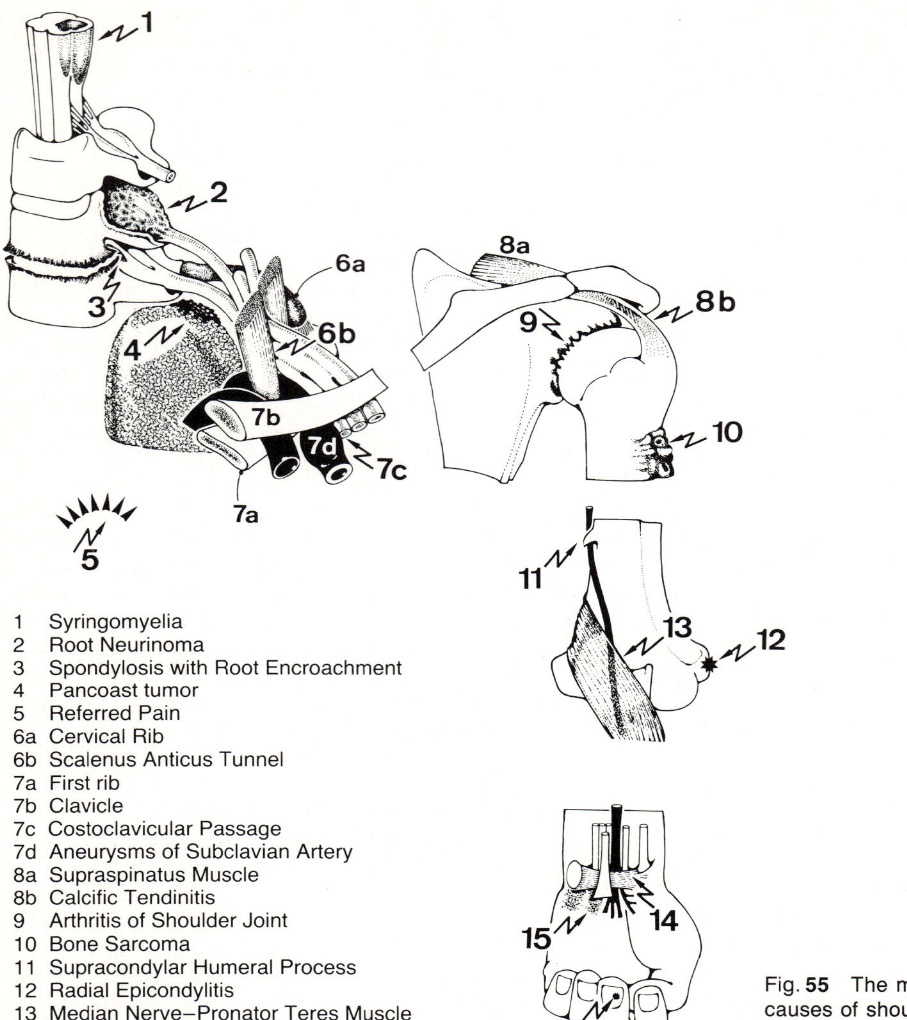

1   Syringomyelia
2   Root Neurinoma
3   Spondylosis with Root Encroachment
4   Pancoast tumor
5   Referred Pain
6a Cervical Rib
6b Scalenus Anticus Tunnel
7a First rib
7b Clavicle
7c Costoclavicular Passage
7d Aneurysms of Subclavian Artery
8a Supraspinatus Muscle
8b Calcific Tendinitis
9   Arthritis of Shoulder Joint
10 Bone Sarcoma
11 Supracondylar Humeral Process
12 Radial Epicondylitis
13 Median Nerve—Pronator Teres Muscle
14 Carpal tunnel syndrome
15 Sudeck
16 Glomus Tumoro

Fig. 55   The most common causes of shoulder-arm pain (M. Mumenthaler: Shoulder-Arm Pain, 2nd ed. Huber, Bern 1982)

pain can be an accompanying symptom on the first manifestation (positive rheumatoid factors, sedimentation rate, x-ray findings [later], and joint manifestations), bacterial spondylitis, although it is rare in the cervical region (signs of inflammation, fever, increasing pain, primary sources of infection, x-ray findings), tumor (in elderly patients, usually metastasis; pain that is continuous and increasingly intense, extreme sensitivity on movement, increased sedimentation rate, x-ray findings), and eventually radicular or medullary symptoms.

Tension headache with continuous contraction of neck muscles can manifest psychologic conflicts or local cervical spine changes. Tension headache is marked by changing intensity, symptom-free periods, and tense, sensitive neck muscles, but no torticollis. Local sensitivity in certain zones of the shoulder or arm is usually the product of a local cause. In rare cases it may be a true radicular or pseudoradicular pain projection. In the shoulder region, pain is usually from humeroscapular periarthritis, which generally lacks initiating causes, but occasionally occurs after direct or indirect trauma (found in elderly patients; marked by pain on movement, particularly while reaching backward, lifting objects with the involved arm, pressure sensitive anterior at the shoulder joint, and occasionally calcification in the rotator cuff, visible on x-ray films). When humeroscapular periarthritis involves the supraspinatus tendon, abduction of the arm is particularly painful in its middle phase; when the region affected is the acromioclavicular joint, the pain is most marked during the last phase of abduction, before the vertical position is reached.

Tumors (evident on roentgenograms) cause continuous pain. Arthritis of the shoulder joint is usually less painful (results in decreased range of motion on abduction of the upper arm and on external rotation of the scapula; evident on x-ray film). Intense continuous pain, acute and usually nocturnal in onset, is often the neuralgic shoulder amyotrophy type (often right-sided, usually found in men, generally younger individuals; leading after several days to proximal muscle paralysis). In rare cases, shoulder pain results from compression of the suprascapular nerve in the incisura of the scapula (accompanied by atrophy of the supraspinous and infraspinous muscles, paralysis of external rotation of the shoulder; pain in the scapular incisura) or from paralysis of the accessory nerve (usually after gland biopsy in the neck) leads to atrophy and paralysis of the upper trapezius portion, low scapula position, weakness of shoulder elevation).

In the region of the elbow, epicondylitis of the lateral or radial humeral head, known as tennis elbow, is the most common cause of pain (local sensitivity to pressure in the region of the radial epicondyle, pain increasing with contraction of the hand and finger extension). Analogous pain of the ulnar side of the elbow, medial humeral epicondylitis or golfer's elbow, is rarer (it must be differentiated from ulnar dislocation). Pain in the region of the elbow also appears with arthritis or chondromatosis of the joint (deformity, impaired range of motion, and eventual stiffness) and with the pronator teres syndrome (the pain usually radiates distally and increases with forced pronation of the forearm).

In the distal region of the forearm or hand, radial styloiditis can cause local pain of the styloid process of the radius (occasionally secondary to a primary pain process in the arm). Acute pain at the root of the hand region appears with fractures of the carpal bones, particularly navicular fractures (difficult to visualize). Pain at the root of the

hand also occurs with lunate malacia and acute gout (chiragra [extremely severe swelling and redness]). Rapidly increasing pain accompanies acute rheumatism of the joints of the hand.

Intense local finger pain occurring on pressure can accompany glomus tumor (strictly local symptoms; exquisite tenderness, mostly at the fingertips and sometimes under the fingernail; sometimes a translucent bluish dot the size of a pinhead; eventually diffuse pain). In the lateral aspect of the thumb a burning painful sensation occurs with cheiralgia paresthetica (the result of chronic pressure due to the use of tools, such as scissors; produces local dysesthesia in the region of the lateral cutaneous branches of the digital nerve).

Diffuse pain in the region of the arm can be due to local causes. Because of the complex functional relationship of various shoulder and arm structures, pain in the arm region is diffuse and only occasionally reveals its local basis. Typical nocturnal arm pain involving the entire upper limb to the shoulder, so-called brachialgia paresthetica nocturna, is pathognomonic of the carpal tunnel syndrome (causes awakening, pain, a feeling of swelling in the fingers and hand, the urge to shake and massage the upper limb; objective findings include pain over the thenar eminence on pressure, atrophy of the lateral thenar muscles, weakness of abduction of the thumb, sensory impairment in the distribution of the medial nerve [Fig. 53]). Pain in the arm due to lesions of roots is usually evident during the day (pain often radiating segmentally into a finger, which is often affected by local paresthesia, increasing with coughing, pressure, and on certain head movements; increased pain on extension of the arm; reflex abnormalities and segmental motor paresis demonstrable on careful search [Fig. 53]). Root lesions due to spinal column spondylosis (or disc herniation) show a cervical syndrome with positive neck compression and a stepwise progression with recurrences; their effects may be bilateral. Further causes of radicular pain syndromes are herpes zoster (occasionally accompanied by paresis and evidence of pustular rash), tick bite (evidence of the bite with surrounding redness, paresis, occasionally myelitic signs), a root tumor (increasing pain, progressive sensory and motor deficits, occasionally enlarged intervertebral foramina with a root neurinoma; visible on roentgenograms of the cervical spine).

Lesions of the brachial plexus cause diffuse arm pain; with the more common lower brachial plexus lesion in the ulnar forearm or ulnar part of the hand, there may be segmental radiation of the pain as well. Etiologically important in this syndrome are compression in the costoclavicular angle, the scalenus anticus syndrome with or without cervical rib (suggested by the dependence of pain on certain positions and on weight bearing, vascular syndrome, bruits in the supraclavicular area, positive Adson maneuver, sensory or motor deficit, muscle atrophy in the hand, and cervical rib occasionally visible in x-ray examination of the neck), Pancoast tumor (very severe continuous pain, cervical sympathetic deficit with Horner syndrome and loss of sweating in the upper body quadrant, and, as a result of lower brachial plexus involvement [*see above*], pathologic clinical and radiologic findings in the lung apex), past radiation therapy (evident from history, radiation dermatitis; continuous pain that increases within months; progressive deficits due to brachial plexus dysfunction). Upper limb pain may also be vascular, due to arterial insufficiency. This can result from a compression syndrome in the shoulder girdle region (*see above*). In this setting, an aneurysm of the subclavian artery can produce emboli (resulting in acute pain in fingers due to occlusion of small hand arteries, Osler's nodes). If the pain appears only with arm exercise, intermittent claudication of the arm is the likely cause. This points to stenosis of the proximal main artery (other signs include decreased pulsation, bruits in the supraclavicular region, pathologic pallor of the hand on making a fist with the arm elevated). If such pain is accompanied by dizziness, a subclavian steal is present. The typical finger changes in Raynaud phenomenon and in "dead finger" syndrome facilitate the diagnosis. With venous occlusion (Paget-von Schroetter syndrome; effort thrombosis) the pain is generally sudden in onset and accompanied by swelling of the arm.

Chronic irritation or compression of peripheral (mixed and sensory) nerves causes diffuse or locally accentuated pain in the arm. Irritation of the ulnar nerve is most commonly found at the elbow in the ulnar sulcus (pain and ache in the sulcus with radiation to the ulnar fingers; possible dislocation of the nerve, causing sensitivity and thickening of the ulnar nerve on palpation; history of chronic compression of the nerve during work; sensory dysfunction in the two ulnar fingers; atrophy of the interosseus muscles with clawhand and presence of the Froment sign). Compression of the median nerve can occur at the supracon-

dylar process of the humerus (situated a handbreadth above the medial border of the elbow, palpable, evident on roentgenograms obtained with the upper arm rotated slightly inward) or below the pronator teres muscle (resulting in local pain and sensitivity distal to the elbow crease, and culminating in the "oath hand" position). The most common cause of brachial pain is irritation of the median nerve in the carpal canal, already mentioned in the discussion of carpal tunnel syndrome (*see above*).

2.17.3 Ventral Trunk Pain

The most common causes of pain localized in the chest and abdomen are the concern of the internist and are not discussed here. However, a few causes, most of them rare, will be mentioned. In the upper thorax, pain may be due to the Tietze syndrome (local painful swelling of the sternocostal cartilage region of the second or third rib); pain also occurs in the region of the sternoclavicular joint with arthritis or excessive loads.

Pain in the costal arch region may be due to numerous disorders; one peculiar cause is excessive mobility of the tenth (or ninth) rib (movement most often occurs when bending or carrying loads; the abnormal mobility is palpable, and such passive movement causes pain). The sternal syndrome refers to pain that centers in the sternum, but radiates laterally and also toward the shoulder and distally to the symphysis. It results from abnormal body position that stems from habit or professional demands. Mondor disease consists of phlebitis of thoracic veins (results in dull superficial pain in the chest and palpable thickening running vertically).

Pain in the abdomen can be caused by numerous affections of interest to internists, but it can also accompany some neurologic disorders. The rectus abdominis syndrome is a mechanical neuropathy of the medial cutaneous rami of the sixth caudal intercostal nerves. They become irritated in their passage through the fascia of the rectus abdominis muscle, yielding sharp burning pain along the muscle, particularly during tension of the muscle. Other indications include local pain on pressure, denervation signs sometimes evident on the electromyogram, and disappearance of pain after local anesthetic infiltration. Severe acute pain of the abdominal wall accompanies rupture of the rectus abdominis muscle, which can occur with chronic coughing, the use of abdominal rollers, or toward the end of pregnancy (acute intense pain, usually localized over the symphysis pubis, increasing with tension of abdominal muscles; local tenderness on pressure, and swelling; later the appearance of a visible hematoma).

Pain in the inguinal region is due to the ilioinguinal syndrome, which occurs, with some delay, after appendectomy and herniography, but can also appear spontaneously (pain in the ilioinguinal region on extension of the hip; occasionally a permanently flexed hip and inability to walk brought on by the decrease of pain during flexion of the joint; sensory impairment in the inguinal region and adjacent genital area; point-pressure sensitivity two fingersbreadth medial to the anterior superior iliac spine; pain on extension of the hip in the sense of an "inverted Lasègue sign"; disappearance of pain with the injection of local anesthetic into the ilioinguinal nerve proximal to the compression site). Pain in the genital region is a consequence of spermatic neuralgia, caused by lesions of the genital branch of the genitofemoral nerve, for example, as a result of herniotomy (intense, recurring ripping pain with sensory impairment in the scrotum or labium majus pudendi; absence of cremasteric reflex). In disorders of the hip joint the pain also is usually projected into the inguinal region (pain is worse at the beginning of movement and exacerbated by exercise; results in protective limping; other signs include pain deep in the femoral triangle occurring with pressure, pain on rotation and abduction of the hip joint).

Girdle-like pain in the trunk, which the patient usually describes by moving a hand forward from the back, points to lesions of the thoracic or high lumbar roots. It suggests a spinal tumor (*see* 2.13.2.4.1), herpes zoster (*see above*), or radiculitis after tick bite.

2.17.4 Back Pain

Back pain most often results from affections of the spinal column or iliosacral joint — disorders that concern the orthopedist or rheumatologist. Among them Scheuermann disease, spondylosis, spondyloarthritis, spondylolisthesis and spondylolysis, Bechterew disease, the Baastrup phenomenon, so-called sacroiliac strain, coccygodynia, television bottom.

Pain predominantly in the upper or middle part of the back can be due to Scheuermann disease, thoracic spondylosis, or Bechterew disease. It can also be the manifestation of excessive muscle activity, a result of the scapulocostal syndrome (dull, periscapular pain with diffuse radiation; pain on pressure of the parascapular and subscapular soft tissues) or a consequence of mechanical neuropathy of the dorsal rami of the spinal nerves (dull pain, sometimes also lumbar perivertebral pain when pressure is applied over the exit of the dorsal rami through the fascia; disappearance of pain with the injection of local anesthetic). Intense intercapular pain can also signal tumors of the spinal column, spondylitis, or epidural hematomas and beginning transverse myelitis.

The causes of pain in the lumbar region are predominantly orthopedic-rheumatologic in nature, such as osteochondrosis, spondylosis, spondylolisthesis and spondylolysis, the Baastrup phenomenon, sacroiliac strain, and coccygodynia. In younger men particularly, Bechterew disease with involvement of the sacroiliac joint (nocturnal pain on lying down) is also common. In women, radiologic signs often are absent but quantitative scintigraphy provides evidence of sacroiliac joint involvement. Neuropathy of the dorsal rami can also be localized in the lumbar region. Here it may result from herniation of fatty tissue through the perforating areas of the fascia where the rami penetrate (*see above*). With deep-seated lumbar pain and pressure sensitivity of the iliac crest, there may be irritation of the posterior rami of the lumbar roots by the intervertebral joints to which they are closely apposed. Infiltration with local anesthetic or excision of the joint capsule may be helpful. Lumbar disc disease is a frequent cause of lumbar pain (signs include acute sciatica, in many cases an evident initiating cause, stiffness of movement, decreased Schober index, irritation of roots, and signs of root dysfunction). Disc disease is also evident from the patient's posture and from a deformity of the lumbar spine (Fig. 56).

Arachnoid cysts may cause chronic pain in the sacral region (evident on a myelogram, with a later film obtained during standing). Sacral pain can also stem from chronic irritation of the periosteum of the ischial tuberosity or from ischial bursitis, caused by prolonged sitting and designated tailor's bottom or television bottom (the history suggests the specific cause; general findings include local pressure sensitivity and pain radiating to the back of the leg). A final cause of sacral pain is the piriform syndrome, associated with trauma to the sacral region (intense gluteal pain radiating toward the sacrum and hip, sometimes along the ischial nerve, increasing with bending and inward rotation of the hip).

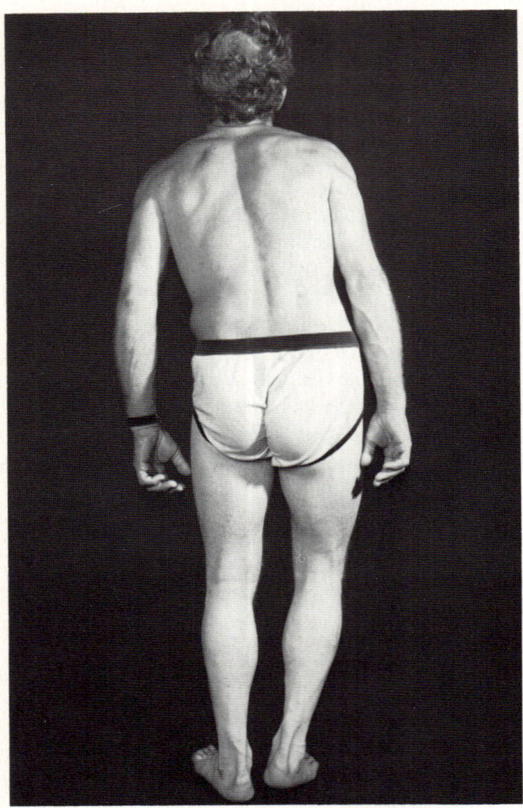

Fig. **56** Typical posture of a patient with right-sided lumbar sciatica due to herniation of the discs between L5 and S1. Note the rightward convexity of the lumbar scoliosis and the flexed position of the right leg

2.17.5 Leg Pain

Orthopedic and rheumatologic disorders often cause leg pain. Nevertheless, neurologists are called upon to diagnose a number of lower-extremity pain syndromes. Pain radiating on the back of the upper aspect of the thigh is mostly caused by irritation of the sciatic nerve or its roots, often as a result of a herniated lumbar disc (*see above*). Lumbosacral root pain resulting, for instance, from chronic adhesive leptomeningitis or tumor does not usually cause a vertebral syndrome but rather a progressive sciatic syndrome with increasing neurologic deficits. Similar considerations apply to lesions of the sacral plexus in the pelvis caused, for example, by retroperitoneal tumors. In contrast to root lesions, a lesion of the

plexus also causes a disorder of sweating (dry skin, abnormal results of sweat tests) as well as leg pain because the sudomotor fibers pass out of the spinal cord above the L2-L3 roots with the anterior roots and reach the plexus via the paravertebral chain. A sweating disorder is also seen with the vascular sciatic neuropathy that occurs in a setting of vasculities and causes sciatic pain. In rare cases, sciatic pain may occur with spinal cord tumors (pain felt at rest, lightning-like shooting pains on bending with head or trunk movement; absense of vertebral and typical radicular symptoms). (For pain resulting from the piriform syndrome and gluteal bursitis, *see above*.) (For intermittent claudication of the cauda equina [one-sided or bilateral], *see* 2.15.5)

Pain on the lateral aspect of the thigh may be due to pseudoradicular radiation caused by diseases of the hip joint ("commanding-general stripes" distribution), and it may even radiate to the lower part of the leg. Such pain can also manifest a high lumbar root lesion as can occur with high lumbar disc herniation (signs include acute lumbago, appropriate vertebral syndromes, weakness of the quadriceps, decreased knee jerks, absence of the Laségue sign, pain on rotation of the extended hip, and a sensory deficit of the fourth lumbar root sometimes extending to the lower inner aspect of leg). Burning pain on the lateral aspect of the thigh with meralgia paresthetica occurs with lesions of the lateral cutaneous nerve of the thigh (possible causes are surgery on the hip joint or removal of bone from the iliac crest or overweight; signs include an area of sensory impairment the size of a hand ventrolateral on the upper aspect of the thigh; exquisite pressure sensitivity over the penetration of the nerve through the inguinal band in an area of several fingerbreadths medial to the anterior superior iliac spine). Irritation of the trochanteric bursa can cause pain centered laterally on the upper part of the thigh, with diffuse radiation toward the knee (local pressure sensitivity, increase of pain with forced abduction of the hip against resistance). Pain over the greater trochanter belt on walking can be an expression of a slipped hip (the slipping of the fascia lata over the major trochanter is detectable on palpation).

Pain radiating ventrally over the thigh occurs predominantly with lesions of the femoral nerve, for example, after hernia operation for neurofibroma and with disease processes in the lower abdomen. Such lesions are accompanied by paresis of the quadriceps muscle, decreased knee jerk, sensory loss on the upper ventral aspect of the thigh and the medial aspect of the calf, and pain on extension and rotation of the hip. The differential diagnosis between a high lumbar root lesion (L3-L4) and a lesion of the lumbar plexus in the pelvis (tumor infiltration) is often difficult. Intense pain in the femoral area with thigh atrophy (*see* 2.20.5) is mostly due to asymmetric proximal neuropathy of diabetes mellitus (the presence of diabetes is sometimes recognizable only from a glucose tolerance test; acute in onset with severe pain and a deficit in the lumbar plexus; spontaneous recovery). Tearing, extremely severe pain in the same region appears together with paresis of the quadriceps in retroperitoneal hematomas, often due to anticoagulant therapy or bleeding disorders. Pain in the region of the knee is commonly due to mechanical disorders or orthopedic rheumatic causes. In juveniles, disease of the patellar cartilage is an especially common cause. Pain on the medial side of the knee may radiate from diseases elsewhere — in the hip, for example. Knee pain also stems from epiphyseal separations and lesions of the obturator nerve roots — so-called Howship-Romberg syndrome (suggested by the presence of a possible underlying cause, such as prostatic carcinoma, pelvic cancer, pelvic ring fracture; results in dysesthesia or sensory impairment of the inner aspect of the knee and weakness of the thigh adductors). Compression of the infrapatellar branch of the saphenous nerve as it penetrates the fascia causes patellar neuropathy, with pain and tenderness on the outer aspect of the patella.

Pain syndromes in the calves may be bilateral. One example is the syndrome of restless legs (anxietas tibiarum); its cause is not clear, although it occasionally is familial, occurs mostly in women (results in a painful unpleasant feeling of restlessness in the calves leading to constant leg movement when the patient lies in bed or sits quietly on a soft chair; also manifested by occasional myoclonic jerks of legs and hypnogogic jerks; normal physical examination). A syndrome resulting in bilateral lightning-like pain (unilateral form *see below*), mainly confined to the lower limbs, but also appearing in other body parts, with fasciculation, cramps, burning sensation and paresthesia, is designated the muscle pain-fasciculation syndrome and is most probably due to chronic polyneuropathy. A similar painful syndrome may be accompanied by "restless toes" (continuous movement, usually a manifestation of polyneuropathy). It may also appear together with alope-

cia and diarrhea and polyposis of the gastrointestinal tract. Intermittent claudication of the cauda equina, resulting in episodic pain, may be unilateral or bilateral (*see* 2.15.5). Intense pain, centered in both calves, but also felt in the upper thigh muscles, appears within 24 to 48 hours after infection of the upper respiratory tract and with acute myositis, most often in children. Usually unilateral are nocturnal cramps of calves (resulting in temporary cramped plantar flexion of the foot and a hard, painful triceps surae muscle). After local trauma to the calf or foot a homolateral restless leg syndrome (*see above*) may develop. There need not be evidence for Sudeck's atrophy. Intermittent claudication with arterial disease of the lower extremity may be unilateral or bilateral and generally causes pain in the calf (sometimes also in the tibial area). A constant claudication distance is suggested by pain that decreases with quiet standing, absence of pedal pulses, bruits over the proximal arteries in some cases, and a pathologic Ratschow test. In pseudoclaudication and in intermittent claudication of the cauda equina with (congenital) narrowing of the lumbar spinal canal, the pain radiates unilaterally or bilaterally from the upper aspect of the thigh down to the calf (other indications are the lack of a constant claudication distance, pain that is more marked on walking uphill, and that is relieved by bending or a change in position of the spinal column but not by stopping and remaining standing; pain that may radiate like sciatica during attacks; a decrease in Achilles tendon reflexes; and x-ray evidence of severe spondylosis and a sagittally narrowed spinal canal). The arterial tibialis anterior compartment syndrome causes intense unilateral pretibial pain (precipitated by exercise, injury, or operation on the lower leg; marked by swelling, redness, and pain in the anterior tibial compartment; often initial absence of the dorsalis pedis pulse; paralysis of the dorsal extensors of the foot and toes; later, contraction of these muscles with claw-like position of the great toe without footdrop).

Pain in the region of the feet is usually due to orthopedic causes: anomalies of the arches, calcaneal spurs, plantar faciitis, Köhler anomaly, sinus tarsi syndrome, hallux valgus, and so on. Bilateral pain in the feet may take the form of a burning paresthesia, which may be the expression of a polyneuropathy (*see* 1.3.5). This may also be a local irritative phenomenon accompanied by erythema of the soles and excessive sweating due to fungicides incorporated in special work footwear. Erythromelalgia, or erythermalgia, is also bilateral and occurs idiopathically; in rare cases it may be the manifestation of heavy metal poisoning, hypertension, or polycythemia vera rubra (signs include a burning, painful sensation in the feet [and hands], increasing on walking and in bed, the heat and redness of the hands decreasing with elevation). Unilateral foot pain may be caused by the tarsal tunnel syndrome: compression of the plantar nerves behind the medial aspect of the malleolus (mostly preceded by local anatomic distortion results in pain in the sole of the foot, increasing in severity with walking; pain on pressure behind the medial malleolus, hypesthesia, and dry skin on the sole of the foot, with unilateral inability to abduct the toes). Another fairly common cause is Morton's metatarsalgia, chronic neuroma of an interdigital nerve between two heads of the metatarsals usually in the third interdigital space (initially pain occurs in the anterior aspect of the foot only with walking; later pain is spontaneous; pain occurs with pressure in the affected interdigital space and with cross-compression of the metatarsal heads; hypesthesia of the apposing sides of the appropriate toes is noted; pain can be eliminated with proximal regional anesthesia of the appropriate interdigital nerve).

2.17.6 Generalized Pain

Pain felt throughout the body is rare. Generalized pain in every extremity is experienced by patients with angiokeratoma corporis diffusum, or Fabry's disease (pain with a burning character that is particularly pronounced in warm surroundings, absence of sweat secretion, typical cutaneous changes present since puberty). With polyradiculitis of the Guillain-Barré type, intense, diffuse pain may accompany the typical paralysis. Diffuse pain can also be an expression of a schizophrenic psychosis. Generalized pain with a burning character on one side of the body with delayed perception of touch and perseverance of the touch sensation is a manifestation of thalamic lesions. Of less serious significance are the generalized pains experienced after infectious diseases. In a few cases, and often long misdiagnosed, diffuse pains are an expression of polymyalgia rheumatica (seen in elderly individuals; accompanied by generalized disability and symptoms of disease such as sweating, loss of weight, fever, and a very high sedimentation rate; responds promptly to corticosteroids). Diffuse muscle pain or confined to a particularly active muscle group is a feature of numerous myopathies: polymyositis, carnitin-palmityl-transferase deficiency, lipid storage myopathies, glycogen storage diseases, phosphorylase deficiency, paroxysmal myoglobinuria and malignant hyperthermia.

2.18 Disturbances of Micturition and Defecation

2.18.1 Anatomy

Descriptions of the major anatomic structures necessary for normal micturition, defecation, and male sexual activities follow. The structures are shown in Figure 57.

- The bladder is a hollow organ, the wall of which is formed by long smooth-muscle fibers — the vesical detrusor. These fibers are so arranged that their contraction causes a decrease in bladder volume. Because they extend into the urethra, detrusor contraction also causes the fibers forming the smooth internal vesical sphincter to open the bladder neck and form an entrance into the urethra
- The function of the bladder, gut, and genital apparatus is regulated primarily by autonomic parasympathetic innervation
  - the bladder wall contains stretch receptors, arranged in series with the smooth muscle cells. Their afferents reach the pelvic nerves and the dorsal roots of S1 and S4 and through them the sacral bladder center situated in the S1 and S2 cord segments
  - there are afferent impulses that pass cranially to the pontine bladder center as well
  - from the sacral bladder center, efferent impulses pass over the anterior roots of S2 to S4 to the cauda equina and reach the pelvic nerves through the appropriate foramina of the sacrum. These preganglionic fibers synapse in the ganglia of the vesical plexus in the bladder wall and onto postganglionic fibers. Stimulation of the pelvic nerves causes powerful contraction of the detrusor muscle
- Various patterns of sympathetic innervation affect the bladder:
  - preganglionic sympathetic neurons lie in the lateral horns at the level of T12, L1, and L2

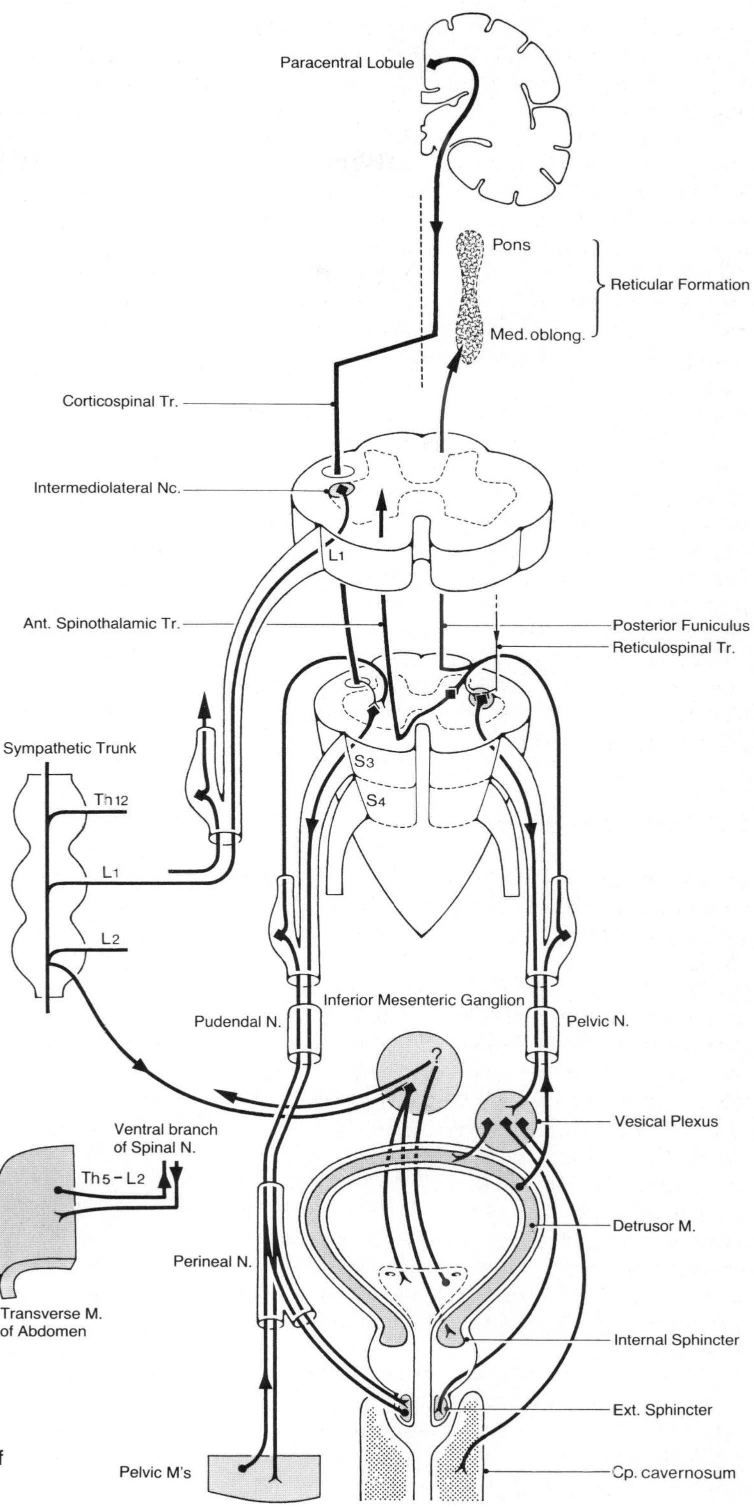

Fig. **57** Neuroanatomic basis of bladder function

- the preganglionic axons pass from the spinal cord through the appropriate anterior roots, reach the sympathetic paravertebral chain without synapsing, then pass via the splanchnic nerves to the sympathetic ganglia in the region of the aortic bifurcation, for example, to the inferior mesenteric ganglion
- after synapsing, the preganglionic fibers form the presacral nerve located bilaterally in the hypogastric plexus and pass to the bladder (particularly the trigonum)
- other postganglionic fibers reach the nervi erigentes in the pelvic nerve and pass to the corpora cavernosa of the penis
- the function of the sympathetic innervation is not quite clear. Stimulation of the sympathetic nerves should inhibit the activity of parasympathetic impulses and thus inhibit bladder contraction. However, the sympathetic innervation has no clinically recognizable influence on bladder function (although this belief is now being challenged), but it certainly has an influence on male potency (*see* 2.19)

- The striated muscles of the pelvic floor, including the external vesical sphincter as well as the muscles of the abdominal wall, play an important role in micturition. Its somatomotor function is regulated as follows:
  - the anterior horn cells innervating the motor neurons of the abdominal muscle lie in the anterior horns of the first and second sacral segments
  - the anterior roots from these segments pass through the cauda equina and through the appropriate foramina of the sacrum and the anterior spinal nerve roots and form the pudendal nerve whose terminal branches, the perineal nerves, pass to the external sphincter and the pelvic floor
  - somatosensory afferents from the gut, penis, and external urethra reach the perineal nerves, the inferior rectal nerves, the dorsalis penis nerve, and the posterior roots of the second and third sacral segments in the conus medullaris

- Supraspinal control is important in normal micturition
  - an important center in the pontine reticular formation (Barrington center) sends facilitating impulses for micturition
  - another center lies in the preoptic region of the midbrain; in animals, when stimulated

it causes micturition, including assumption of the appropriate position
- the cortical representation of the bladder lies in the paracentral lobule in the vicinity of the medial border of the hemisphere; stimulation of this area causes contraction of the bladder. A cortical center in the second frontal gyrus inhibits bladder emptying
- the descending fibers from these centers pass in the vicinity of the corticospinal and reticulospinal tracts in the ventral lateral part of the spinal cord

2.18.2 Physiology of Bladder Emptying and Disorders of Micturition

Fifty milliliters of urine reach the bladder hourly. Bladder pressure increases slowly as its content increases. Only with a content of about 400 ml is a sense of bladder fullness experienced; the micturition reflex may be initiated with a content of 400 to 500 ml of urine. Micturition is initiated by contraction of muscles of the abdominal walls and diaphragm, leading to an increase in intra-abdominal pressure. This leads to extensive impulse traffic from the stretch receptors of the bladder wall and through afferents in the pelvic nerve and the spinal bladder center located in the conus terminalis in the second to the fourth sacral segment. Simultaneously, ascending collateral impulses reach the micturition center in the pontine reticular formation, from which facilitatory impulses pass into the sacral spinal cord. If there are no inhibitory impulses arising in the frontal cortex to block the process, micturition will proceed. Simultaneously with the activation of the spinal parasympathetic bladder centers, both inhibitory and facilitatory impulses pass to the motor neurons in the first and second sacral segments and from there to the pelvic floor muscles. This causes relaxation of the external sphincter and contraction of other pelvic floor muscles as well as those of the abdominal wall.

This anatomic and physiologic arrangement of bladder function determines the organic dysfunction of micturition and its characteristics, summarized in Table 22.

- The cortical uninhibited bladder occurs with lesions of the second frontal convolution. Its hallmarks are

Table 22 Organic (neurologic) disturbances of micturition

Disturbance	Bladder tone	Urge to micturate	Beginning of micturition	End of micturition	Bladder capacity	Residual urine	Complications	Anatomic site of lesion	Causes examples
Cortical uninhibited bladder	Normal	With moderate filling	Uncontrolled	Not voluntary	Normal	None	Uncontrolled micturition	Second frontal convolution	Brain atrophy, tumor, trauma, strokes, cerebral arteriosclerosis
Spinal reflex bladder (neurogenic or automatic bladder)	Spastic	With little filling (urge absent with complete transverse lesions)	Uncontrolled with manipulation (percussion or pinching)	Not voluntary	Small	Small amount or none	Infection: uncontrolled micturition	Spinal cord above S1	Spinal cord trauma, tumor, multiple sclerosis
Denervated, autonomous bladder	Flaccid	None	Not voluntary	Continuous dribbling of urine; overflow incontinence	Very large	Very large amount	Infection	Sacral bladder center (S2 to S4) and its afferent and/or efferent connection to bladder	Conus lesions, cauda equina lesions, lesions in pelvis

- precipitancy of micturition when the bladder is only partly filled with urine
- inability to inhibit micturition even in inappropriate places
- absence of residual urine
— The spinal reflex bladder (neurogenic automatic bladder), caused by interruption of spinal pathways above the sacral segment, is manifested by the following
  - spastic bladder, with emptying occurring with urine volumes of less than 250 ml
  - inability to initiate or terminate the micturition process voluntarily
  - under certain circumstances, autonomic manifestations with bladder fullness, such as sweating, high blood pressure, and increasing spasticity, despite the absence of perception of the urge to micturate or of bladder fullness due to interruption of sensory ascending spinal pathways
  - initiation of micturition by manipulation (for example, percussion or pinching of the thigh)
  - little or no residual urine
— The denervated or automatic bladder, with lesions of the afferent or efferent connections between the bladder and the sacral bladder center or with lesions of the sacral center, is marked by
  - a flaccid distended bladder
  - perception of bladder fullness
  - overflow incontinence, leading to continuous dribbling of urine
  - considerable residual urine and great risk of infection
  - depending on the site of the lesion, other appropriate neurologic deficits

2.18.3 Clinical Importance of Disturbances of Micturition

Primary enuresis is the uncontrollable emptying of large quantities of urine in children who have remained untrained since their earliest childhood. Almost always this is of psychologic origin (indicated by behavioral abnormalities, neurotic disturbances, absence of residual urine, in very rare cases incontinence of feces, absence of urologic or neurologic abnormalities). To rule out organic causes the neurologist will in such cases look for spina bifida or other abnormalities in the lumbosacral region (tufts of hair over the sacrum, rachischisis, x-ray findings, pes equinus, absence of ankle jerk, abnormal anal sphincter tone).

Secondary enuresis in children also is often of psychologic origin and only rarely organic in nature (*see below*). In adults, however, its cause is always organic.

The occasional loss of several drops of urine (dribbling) is almost always due to mechanical or urologic causes (descent of the urethra in elderly women or mothers of several children; such dribbling may be accompanied by incontinence or occur only occasionally, during lifting or laughing or coughing; it can also occur with sphincter insufficiency in elderly men).

Uncontrollable loss of large quantities of urine can be the expression of cortical disinhibition of the bladder (*see* 2.18.2) and occurs, for example, in vascular cerebral insults, tumor of the frontal lobes, parasagittal meningioma, aneurysm of the anterior communicating artery, and presenile dementia with focal frontal atrophy. A rarer cause of this form of incontinence is multiple sclerosis, in which pathognomonic precipitancy of urination is sometimes found: the patient feels an intense, almost continuous urge to pass urine, which occasionally can no longer be controlled.

Overflow incontinence (*see* 2.18.2), that is, frequent uncontrolled dribbling of small quantities of urine, is the most common initial manifestation of a neurogenic bladder disturbance. An organic cause is likely when this disorder is accompanied by an enlarged full bladder and large amounts of residual urine after micturition. Rarely a similar disorder of micturition results from psychogenic causes.

One organic basis is an early stage of an acute spinal cord lesion, such as trauma, transverse myelitis, or space-occupying lesions (indicated in history, symptoms of transverse myelitis, and in the signs of spasticity that soon appear). In the later stages of acute and chronic spinal cord lesions, spastic automatic bladder may be present instead (*see* 2.12.1.1).

Overflow incontinence is a typical disturbance of micturition in the following disorders:

— Destruction of the sacral bladder center itself by trauma, tumor, medial high disc herniation, ischemia, occasionally lumbosacral syringomyelia. Important localizing symptoms include decrease in tone of the external anal spincter, absence of bulbocavernous reflex (S3 to 4), sometimes absence of anal reflex (S5), a feeling of deadness and sensory impairment in

the perigenital and perianal regions, fecal incontinence, and, in men, impotence
- Lesions of the cauda equina with appropriate objective signs (*see* 1.3.1), caused, for example, by tumor (lipoma, dermoid, neurinoma, ependymoma), spina bifida, medial lumbar disc herniation (suggested by acute onset of symptoms of pain, previous episodes of trauma, pain in the lumbar region). Sudden incontinence is rarely the only symptom of medial disc herniation
- Polyradiculitis (rarely in a setting of the Guillain-Barré syndrome [*see* 1.3.1])
- Polyneuropathies, particularly those accompanied by marked autonomic involvement (for general symptoms *see* 1.3.5), such as diabetic polyneuropathy, primary amyloidosis, and paraproteinemia. Such polyneuropathies can also cause extensive paralysis of the gastrointestinal tract with paralytic ileus
- Multiple or diffuse lesions of the nerves in the pelvis, supplying the bladder, for example, as seen with retroperitoneal extension of tumors (rectal carcinoma, carcinoma of the prostate, and, in women, genital carcinoma), and after extensive surgical intervention in the pelvis
- Some disorders in which the pathogenesis of bladder dysfunction is not clear − for example, spinal column disease, vitamin B_{12} deficiency (for symptoms, *see* 1.2.2), tabes dorsalis (areflexia, impairment of deep sensibility and pain perception, arthropathy, and pupillary function disturbances), and orthostatic hypotension of Shy-Drager and other syndromes with pronounced dysautonomia (*see* 2.20.1)

Acute retention of urine with a painful sensation of fullness of the bladder and the necessity for catheterization may occur as a result of mechanical obstruction of outflow (prostatic hypertrophy or an intravesical process), or with transverse myelitis or lumbar disc herniation, and after a disc operation or myelography. It may also have a psychogenic basis.

2.19 Impaired Potency in Men

In principle, in both men and women the anatomy of the innervation of the sexual organs both centrally and peripherally is analogous and controlling influences are similar. Organic dysfunction, however, is more frequently evident in men and

therefore is likely to be referred to the neurologist. Therefore only the differential diagnosis of disturbances of potency in men will be discussed.

2.19.1 Anatomic and Physiologic Substrates of Sexual Potency in Men

From the word *potency* is understood the capacity to obtain erection of the penis, which is necessary for emission. Excitation of the centers situated in the hypothalamus, probably in the preoptic and interseptal regions, and in the limbic system (amygdala?) is important in erection. In these areas there is convergence of endocrine influences (a certain level of sexual hormones is necessary for libido)

- Impulses from the hypothalamic centers pass bilaterally to reflex centers for erection and ejaculation situated in the anterior lateral quadrants of the spinal cord

The following structures and mechanisms are involved in erection (Fig. 57)

- The sacral segments (S2 and S4) contain the parasympathetic center for erection
  - this center contains somatic afferents from the skin of the genital and perigenital region (which pass via the pudendal nerve [S2 to S3] through the perineal nerve and scrotal nerves, including the dorsal nerves of the penis). Visceral afferents from the bladder reach this cord center
  - from this center of erection, efferent impulses pass via parasympathetic fibers in the S2 to S4 roots to the pelvic nerves (nervi erigentes). After synapsing, particularly in the prostatic plexus, the postganglionic fibers pass to the prostate and, more importantly, to the blood vessels of the corpora cavernosa (*see below*)
  - the sacral center for erection is under the influence of hypothalamic centers
- Through the pudendal nerve, the somatic motor efferents from segments S2 to S4 reach the sphincter urethrae and the striated bulbocavernosus and ischiocavernosus muscles.
- The sympathetic innervation of the genital organs
  - apparently originates in the thoracolumbar region of the spinal cord
  - extends through its efferents from T12 to L2 to the paravertebral sympathetic chain

- continues from there through the splanchnic nerves to the hypogastric plexus and then to the inferior mesenteric ganglion

There, after synapsing, the sympathetic postganglionic fibers reach the hypogastric nerves via the pelvic plexus and supply the smooth muscles of the seminal vesicles, the vas deferens, and the ejaculatory ducts in the prostate.

— The corpora cavernosa of the penis are not normally filled with blood. The arterial inflow through the arteria profunda of the penis does not pass through the cavernosus arteries because their lumina are normally obstructed by muscular cushions, but instead reaches via the anastomotic arteries to the superficial vein. During erection, however, the muscular cushions, which normally inhibit arterial inflow, relax under parasympathetic influence, the blood fills the venous lakes of the corpora cavernosa, and contraction of the venous side of the circulation along with the mechanical effect of the fibrous tissue in the corpora cavernosa, helps to retain the blood in these structures and maintain erection.

2.19.2 The Male Sexual Act

The above description of the anatomic substrate includes the structures involved in sexual activity and suggests the neurogenic and other causes of disturbed sexual function:

— In psychogenic erection, psychic (exogenous and endogenous) influences, the product of hormonally influenced libido, cause impulses from the hypothalamic centers to pass over the spinal cord to the sacral center for erection. Reflex erection, however, can also be achieved independently of central stimuli through segmental afferents from the genital region
— In both types of erection, parasympathetic efferent impulses from the sacral center for erection pass through the roots of S2 to S4 and influence the blood flow to the corpora cavernosa and cause tumescence
— Ejaculation is achieved through
  - sympathetic activity, which causes secretion of prostatic and seminal fluid and peristaltic movement, by contraction of the smooth muscle of the seminal vesicles, vas deferens, and the ejaculatory ducts, and contraction of the internal vesical sphinc-

ter, which prevents reflux of semen into the bladder
  - somatosensory efferents, which cause rhythmic contractions of the striated muscles of the pelvic floor — the bulbocavernosus and ischiocavernosus — during orgasm, contributing to ejaculation, and also cause rhythmic contractions of other muscles of the pelvis and upper aspect of the thigh
— Detumescence, which ensues soon after orgasm, results from inhibition of parasympathetic impulses and through sympathic reduction of the blood supply to the corpora cavernosa

2.19.3 Clinical Consideration and Differential Diagnosis in Impairment of Potency and Other Disturbances of Male Sexuality

The causes of disturbances of potency in men can lie at any level of the anatomic mechanisms described above

— The most common cause is, however, psychogenic. The following considerations suggest psychogenic impotence
  - local genital examination normal
  - general examination, particularly of endocrine function and autonomic activity (search for diabetes), normal
  - vascular findings, particularly in the lower aspects of the thigh and body, normal
  - neurologic examination normal
— Further support for this diagnosis includes
  - the presence of nocturnal or early morning tumescence
  - the presence of erection under special circumstances
  - evidence of psychic conflicts, depression, marital problems, and the like
— Disturbances of potency with endocrine diseases are accompanied sooner or later by signs of endocrine dysfunction. The abnormal appearance of the skin, growth of hair on the face and body, and secondary hypothyroidism all indicate such dysfunction. With tumor of the pituitary, impotence may be accompanied by field defect, but it may be years before other neurologic dysfunction is evident. The presence of an endocrine psychic syndrome, with disturbed energy and drive, also suggests an endocrine basis for the impotence

- Disorders of potency with hypothalamic (or other cerebral) lesions are usually accompanied by other signs of central nervous system dysfunction: disorders in water and electrolyte homeostasis, blood pressure regulation, sleep, and hunger. Disorders of potency may also accompany lesions of the temporal lobe
- Disturbances of potency can be due to anticholinergic drugs, alpha-methyldopa, barbiturates, phenothiazine, tricyclic antidepressives, monoamine oxidase inhibitors, amphetamine, heroin, cocaine, and alcohol
- Lesions of the spinal cord above the spinal center for erection or ejaculation cause a disorder of the psychogenic phase of erection, but preservation of reflex erection and, therefore, preservation of potency under certain circumstances. Even in traumatic transverse lesions of the spinal cord the majority of patients retain reflex erection (and ejaculation). Such partial disturbances of potency in multiple sclerosis are due to lesions of the spinal cord caused by the disease, as are the disorders of potency in amyotrophic lateral sclerosis and tabes dorsalis. Disorders of potency may be early manifestations of spinal cord tumors and can occur after bilateral cordotomy. Under these circumstances, other signs of spinal cord lesions, evident on neurologic examination, and often related disorders of micturition also (*see* 2.18.3) accompany the disturbance of potency
- Direct bilateral and total destruction of the sacral center for erection (resulting from tumor or vascular disorder) leads to complete impotence. Disorders of micturition (and of defecation) are always present as well, and objective neurologic signs point to a lesion of the conus medularis or an epiconus syndrome (*see* 1.2.1.1). With partial lesions of the distal spinal cord, as after trauma, reflex erection may be absent, but psychogenic erection can still be achieved
- A bilateral lesion of the sacral roots or the pelvic nerves also causes impotence. This can occur after trauma or tumor of the cauda equina (when it is accompanied by disturbance of micturition and saddle anesthesia), after fractures of the pelvis with rupture of the posterior urethra, after extensive operations in the pelvis — for example, resection of the rectum, after perineal prostatectomy and the like.

Disorders of perineal and genital sensory function and related reflex disturbances always accompany the lesions of the pelvis
- Lesions of the sympathetic nerves in the region of the lower thoracic sympathetic chain, of upper lumbar efferents in the region of the paravertebral chain, or of the peripheral sympathetic fibers can sometimes cause disturbed function, but only when they are bilateral. Potency may remain undisturbed, however, even with bilateral lumbar sympathectomy. Bilateral disorders do affect the ejaculatory mechanism
- Probably as a result of lesions of the parasympathetic and sympathetic efferents, there are usually disturbances of potency in certain neuropathies. Such disturbances occur in younger men with diabetes mellitus, in patients with the Shy-Drager syndrome (*see* 2.20.1.1), and in those with acute pandysautonomia
- Vascular disease of the pelvic or penile arteries can cause impairment of the filling mechanism of the corpora cavernosa, resulting in impotence. Thrombosis can occur at the bifurcation of the iliac arteries (Leriche syndrome) or in the distal pelvic arteries after fracture of the pelvis. The penile arteries themselves can, for example, be occluded in diabetes or arteriosclerosis (suggested by history, findings on palpation and auscultation of the blood vessels, and risk factors; occasionally selective arteriography can be useful)
- Lesions of the anatomic structures of the penis itself that cause impotence are easily recognized from the history and clinical examination: plastic induration of the penile skin, priapism, and severe trauma
- Preservation of potency and orgasm without ejaculation can be an initial sign of impending general impotence. However, it usually results from retrograde ejaculation into the bladder, due to impaired closure of the internal vesical sphincter during ejaculation. Neuropathies, particularly in diabetes mellitus or transverse lesion of the spinal cord, are the most common cause, and the disorder is often accompanied by disturbance of bladder function
- The cause of priapism can be a (high) spinal cord lesion in addition to the well-known local causes
- For disturbed sexual behavior with central nervous system diseases, *see* 1.1.2.1 and 1.1.3.2.

2.20 Disorders of Trophic and Vegetative Function

(without disorders of micturition or potency [for these, *see* 2.18 and 2.19])

The notion of trophic function encompasses diverse aspects of body tissues, including their volume, consistency, moisture, and surface structure. Trophic function is mainly a product of functional demands on the organs (compare "inactivity atrophy"), but is also influenced by endocrine factors and exogenous and other endogenous influences of the somatic or autonomic innervation. Autonomic disturbances, however, are not only manifest by trophic disorders, but also have other effects, such as disturbances of blood pressure. In what follows, I confine myself to disorders of trophic and certain autonomic functions that are the leading symptoms or the overwhelming symptoms of neurologic disease, and are important in its differential diagnosis

2.20.1 Disorders of Sweating

Figure 58 shows the anatomy of sweat secretion, comprised of the following structures and anatomic relations:

— A center for sweating in the hypothalamus (the exact location of which is not known) is under the influence of central structures that control it through the contralateral cortex. Endocrine and autonomic reflex functions (for example, thermoregulatory activity) also affect the center
— From this hypothalamic center, fibers pass caudally in the uncrossed central sympathetic pathways. They lie in the brain close to the aqueduct and in the pons below the floor of the fourth ventricle. In the medulla oblongata they pass in the dorsolateral part, and in the spinal cord, in the lateral columns
— This central sympathetic pathway ends in the ganglion cells of the lateral horns of the spinal cord (located in the intermedial lateral nucleus)
— From the cells of this nucleus that lie in the first thoracic to the second lumbar spinal segments, the preganglionic fibers reach the paravertebral sympathetic chain through the anterior roots and the white rami communicantes

— The fibers for sweat secretion passing to the glands synapse in the paravertebral ganglia, and the unmyelinated postganglionic fibers join the mixed peripheral spinal roots via the gray rami communicantes
— The fibers innervating sweat glands reach the trunk and extremities with the sensory branches to the skin
— The sympathetic fibers for the face pass in the paravertebral chain to the superior cervical ganglion and then, after synapsing, along the external carotid artery in a plexus to the head and face, where they innervate the sweat glands, blood vessels, and smooth muscles of the hair follicles
— The sudomotor fibers — unlike most of the sympathetic nervous system — are cholinergic rather than noradrenergic. Therefore, administration of parasympathomimetic drugs (neostigmine, pilocarpine, methacholine) causes sweating
— Absence of sweat secretion in response to thermal loads (induced by a heating chamber or drinking hot tea) and after pilocarpine administration suggests a lesion in or peripheral to the paravertebral sympathetic ganglia
— If there is a simple disturbance of thermoregulatory sweating, however, with preservation of sweating after pilocarpine administration, the cause lies in a disorder of central sympathetic pathways
— The sweat glands on the palms and soles are probably older phylogenetically. They do not serve a thermoregulatory function, but react predominantly to emotional stimuli.

2.20.1.1 Differential Diagnosis of Sweating Disorders

Excessive generalized sweating has little neurologic significance. Its causes are usually general internal diseases (like fever, tuberculosis, Hodgkin's disease) or, more commonly, neurovegetative overreactivity. In familial dysautonomia (Riley-Day syndrome [an autosomal recessively inherited disorder almost always found in Jewish children and evident in the neonatal period; marked by attacks of fever, orthostatic hypotension, ataxia, defective lacrimation, difficulty in swallowing, decrease in sensitivity to pain, and psychic lability]) there is generalized abnormal sweating. Excessive localized sweating may be paroxysmal and is then of diagnostic importance. This may occur after par-

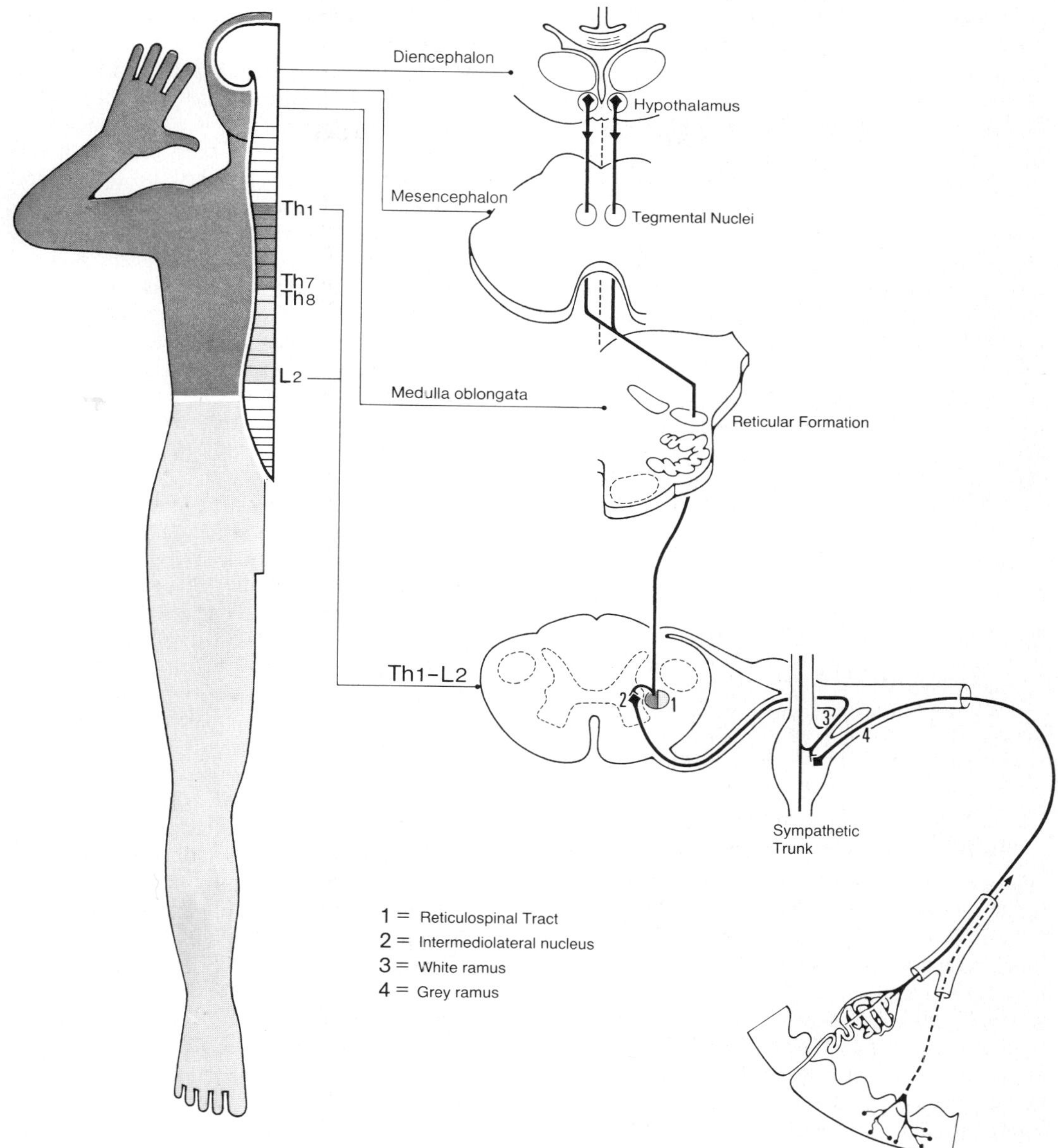

Fig. **58**   Neuroanatomic basis of sweating. Note that in the spinal cord the vegetative neurons are situated only in the portion of the intermediolateral nucleus between T1 and L2. The appropriate efferent pathways leave the spinal cord only from those segments and then are distributed via the sympathetic paravertebral chain to the entire body surface

tial sympathetic denervation due to disease or surgery and can be found in spinal cord disease e.g. syringomyelia, tabes dorsalis, tumors of the spinal cord and trauma to the cord as well as in le- sions of the hypothalamus. Localized excessive sweating has been described in peripheral nerve le- sions; examples are: cervical ribs, osteomas of the spinal column, bronchial carcinoma, pleural endotheliomas, testicular teratomas and in the so-called sudoriparous naevus. There is a rare idiopathic form without obvious cause.

The neurologist is sometimes asked about the therapy for hyperhidrosis: general drug regimens are usually unsuccessful; local application of lotions containing resorcinol or methenamine, and x-irradiation of the axilla may be helpful. With very severe and disturbing axillary and hand sweating a thoracoscopic instrument can be used to divide the paravertebral sympathetic chain at the level of the third thoracic ganglion, interrupting the sudomotor fibers to the arm.

Anhidrosis is significant in differential diagnosis in neurology, giving a clue to the site of the lesion. Unilateral anhidrosis of the face is most often found with lesions of the carotid plexus. The most common cause is tumor or injury in the region of the neck. Unilateral anhidrosis on the face, neck, shoulder, and arm can occur with lesions of the paravertebral sympathetic chain in the following sites:

- Directly below the stellate ganglion of the paravertebral sympathetic chain (never accompanied by Horner syndrome)
- Within the stellate ganglion (always accompanied by Horner syndrome)
- Isolated Horner syndrome without disturbances of sweating can be due to lesions of the roots of C8 to T2 proximal to and not involving the paravertebral sympathetic chain

Tumor in the apex of the lung and paravertebral tumor are the most common causes. Disturbances of sweating, pain, and deficits due to lower brachial plexus involvement usually are present also. Local anhidrosis on the trunk and extremities without accompanying sensory loss points to a lesion of the sympathetic paravertebral chain. The affected areas of the skin are dry and initially also warm because of the accompanying vasodilatation. Localized anhidrosis of the hand or trunk may be due to paravertebral tumor, but local paravertebral processes such as lymphogranuloma, also marked by loss of sweating of the feet, are more commonly the cause. Retroperitoneal tumor, rectal carcinoma, and gynecologic tumor in the pelvis can also result in localized anhidrosis. In eczemas of the palms and soles with hyperkeratosis there may be hypohidrosis of these areas, though this is usually preceded by an hyperhidrotic phase. Local anhidrosis accompanied by similarly localized disturbance of sensation may be due to

- A lesion in the region of the spinal roots of T1 to L2:
  - when it is preganglionic and involves the appropriate spinal roots, pilocarpine-induced sweat secretion is also impaired
  - when it is postganglionic, that is, in the peripheral nerve, sweating is absent also after pilocarpine administration
  - the segmental distribution of the deficits provides a clue to the site of the lesion
- A lesion in the region of the spinal roots of C1 to C8 or L3 to the coccygeal roots and in the cervical brachial plexus or lumbosacral plexus results in special deficits. There are no special segmental sweat fibers that leave the spinal cord with the appropriate roots (Fig. 58). The fibers for sweat secretion in these segments reach their destination through the thoracic and two cranial lumbar segments passing to the paravertebral sympathetic chain, and then only do they participate in the formation of peripheral nerves. From this, it is clear that
  - in these areas of the body, sensory loss that is accompanied by disturbance of sweating does not have a radicular cause but
  - is almost always due to damage of the plexus or one of the peripheral nerves arising from it
  - footdrop with a disorder of sweating therefore cannot be due to a local disc herniation but must be the result of a lesion of the lumbar plexus, sciatic nerve, or peroneal nerve
- A lesion of central sympathetic pathways in the spinal cord results in impairment of sweating on the entire hemibody or on both sides of the body with an upper level. In such patients sweating can be induced with pilocarpine. Almost always there are also other signs of spinal cord damage. With intramedullary processes (for example, syringomyelia) isolated dysfunction of sweating, segmental in extent, may occur as an early sign of the disease. It is due to lesions of the lateral horns
- Disease of the autonomic nervous system, in which a general disturbance of sweating is an accompanying symptom:
  - acute pandysautonomia (subacute in onset with duration to remission of several months; accompanied by orthostatic hypotension with fixed heart rate, absence of tear secretion, impotence, hypotonic bladder, and nonreactive pupils; cause unknown)

- orthostatic hypotension of Shy-Drager (found in middle-age or older groups, progressive; marked by hypotension with orthostatism, leading to collapse without cardiac acceleration, impotence, incontinence of urine, Parkinson's syndrome, fasciculation, and paralysis of extraocular muscles). A newer classification refers to this disorder as multiple system atrophy (MSA)
- other rare diseases with congenital insensitivity to pain may be accompanied by anhidrosis
- a chronic idiopathic anhidrosis in part pre- and also post-ganglionic sudomotor impairment and without other autonomic deficits has been described
- anhidrosis with diffuse pain is found in angioteratoma corporis diffusum (Fabry's disease *see* 2.17.6)
- a variety of intoxications, particularly with drugs, that impair cholinergic transmission are accompanied by a decrease in sweating – for example, botulism or intoxication with atropine

2.20.2 Disorders of Trophic Function of the Skin and Its Appendages and the Subcutaneous Tissues

The trophic integrity of the skin can be affected by a number of diseases not specifically neurologic, for example, scleroderma and endocrinopathies with peripheral disturbances of blood flow. Hemiatrophy of the facial skin along with the underlying tissues and bones and occasionally the brain is called facial progressive hemiatrophy (Romberg disease). Abnormally thin, smooth skin with decreased papillary patterns and creasing is usually seen with lesions of the peripheral nerves. Such abnormalities are confined to the territory of the involved nerve; in polyneuropathy they are generalized and symmetric. In diabetic polyneuropathy, particularly in women, there is painless, circumscribed, reddish yellow atrophy of the skin – necrobiosis lipoidica diabeticorum. The many neurocutaneous syndromes are not discussed in this book.

The subcutaneous fat may be the site of lesions. Generalized disappearance of fatty tissue is found in progeria and in muscular atrophies. Disappearance of subcutaneous fat in the upper half of the body with a skull-like appearance of the face is known as progressive lipodystrophy (Morgagni-Barraquer-Simons disease). This may begin as atrophy of Bichat's fat-ball. Localized disappearance of subcutaneous fat can also occur; it is found, for example, in the upper thigh in diabetics as a result of insulin injection and in persons who habitually bump against obstacles or furniture or who lean against objects with their upper thigh. Infection with *Borrelia burgdorferi* (tick-bite, Lyme disease) can cause cutaneous changes e.g. dermatitis atrophicans Herxheimer and perhaps also morphea. Localized fatty atrophy may accompany focal interstitial myositis.

A localized increase in fatty tissue appears with lipoma; fatty masses can be numerous and painful in Dercum disease, so-called adiposis dolorosa, and occur symmetrically on the neck in Madelung fatty neck. Other changes in tissue include abnormal calcification of the subcutaneous tissues in scleroderma and of subfascial muscle in calcinosis universalis (particularly common in girls and young women; marked by initial muscle weakness, muscle pain, and generalized malaise). Trophic changes in nails and hair are found only in association with neurologic disease; abnormally rapid growth of nails, often with brittleness, accompanies irritated lesions of the appropriate peripheral nerves. On the other hand, complete interruption of conduction in a peripheral nerve slows growth of the appropriate nails and increases the convexity of the nailbed. In such cases the skin of the nailbed is also thickened and pulled forward (Alföldi sign). Transverse ridges or transverse white lines in the nail found in polyneuropathy, for example in the case of arsenic or thallium poisoning, are designated Mees lines. With such poisoning there is also loss of hair. Nails are also abnormal in a number of rare neurologic syndromes, such as the Sjögren-Larsson syndrome (oligophrenia, paraspasticity, and ichthyosis). Among trophic changes in progeria is abnormal early graying of the hair, which accompanies the weakness. The combination of congenital abnormalities of the hair together with neurologic symptoms is termed *neurotrichosis trichorrhexis nodosa* (broken hair shafts with brush-like ends) can occur after mechanical trauma but also in Menke's disease (copper deficiency) and in arginin-succinic aciduria and biotin deficiency. *Pili torti* (kinki-hair) is found in Menke's disease. *Monilethrix*, characterized by knot-like swellings of the hair shaft, is a feature of many metabolic disorders of childhood.

2.20.3 Ulcers

Ulcers can be superficial and involve only the skin. They can, however, also be deep and reach the underlying bone. They are due to a combination of the following:

— Impairment of blood supply to the appropriate tissue (for example, with vascular gangrene)
— Disease of the tissue (which is often accompanied by a local vascular disorder [for example, rat-bite-like ulcers of the fingertips in scleroderma]) due to constant long-lasting local pressure occurring with protracted immobility (for example, decubitus ulcers in paraplegia or prolonged unconsciousness)
— A lesion, located in either the spinal cord or peripheral nerves, of the sympathetic fibers important for trophic function of a tissue

In neurologic disease, ulcers can be of value in differential diagnosis. They can be analyzed according to their site:
— In the region of the head and face, they can occur with lesions of the trigeminal complex (*see* 2.16.2.1). Such ulcers may occur on the scalp, the nasal septum (including perforation) or the palate. An objective sensory loss always accompanies the ulceration. Causes are trigeminal tumor (for example, neurinoma) or trigeminal neuropathy. Ulcers also occur in ophthalmic zoster, producing transient pains, and, following the pain, the typical pustular eruption. These neurogenic face ulcers are to be distinguished from ulceration due to arteritides (particularly giant cell arteritis or temporal arteritis), granulomatous processes (Wegener's granulomatosis), or neoplastic disorders, none of which causes sensory loss in the region of the ulcer
— Ulcers on the hands and fingers are particularly common. When they are accompanied by (a dissociated) sensory disturbance and loss of pain sensitivity the causes are
  - syringomyelia (*see* 2.16.2.2) or a sensory radicular neuropathy (*see below*)
  - neuritis with leprosy (symptoms include nodular thickening of nerve trunks, peripheral paresis, and, early in the course of the disease, signs of whitish analgesic areas in the skin)
  - self-mutilation in children (evident from history) as with congenital insensitivity to pain or the Lesch-Nyhan syndrome

In the differential diagnosis of hand and finger ulcers with impaired sensibility, vascular causes and collagen disease (scleroderma) must also be considered.

— Ulceration of the feet is found in syringomyelia and other diseases that also cause ulceration of the hand. Ulcers in the feet, however, are more commonly due to the following:
  - sensory radicular neuropathy (ulceromutilating acropathy of Thévenard and acrodystrophic neuropathy) (found in children and up to the 40th year of life; marked by dissociated sensory loss, pain, absence of tendon reflexes, and muscle atrophy)
  - diastomyelia, often associated with other spinal anomalies or abnormalities of the spinal cord (often high arched feet and later disorders of micturition)
  - syphilis, particularly tabes dorsalis, when ulceration is often associated with trophic changes in the joint (*see below*)
  - certain polyneuropathies, particularly with diabetes amyloidosis (also due to vascular involvement) and hereditary sensory neuropathy
  - lesions of peripheral nerves, particularly of the peroneal nerve (on the big toe or the lateral aspect of the foot) or the tibial nerve (particularly on the heel); when the peroneal palsy mimics arterial anterior tibial syndrome, differentiation of the resulting ulcers from those due to vascular disorder is difficult (*see* 2.15.5)

2.20.4 Disorders of Trophic Function of Bones and Joints

With prolonged immobilization in patients with central paralysis (for example, after cerebral anoxia, with spinal cord lesions), frozen joints with calcification of muscles can occur (neurogenic myositis ossificans; *see also* 2.20.5.3). Painless destruction of large joints, particularly of the shoulder, elbow, and knees, is characteristic of syringomyelia (Fig. 59) and of tabes dorsalis (marked by hypotonia areflexia, decreased sensitivity to pain, excessive extensibility of joints, deformity of knees, ataxia, and pupillary abnormalities [*see* 2.8.4.2]).

Destruction of small distal joints is also found in the central affections mentioned above, but is predominantly seen in certain polyneuropathies.

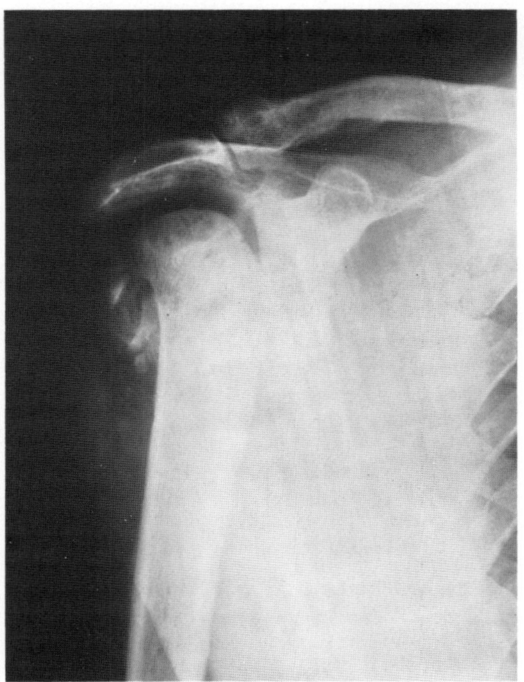

Fig. **59** A 59-year-old patient with syringomyelia and severe deforming arthropathy, resulting in painless deformity and impaired mobility of the right shoulder. Several bone fragments protrude laterally from the head of the humerus. There is periosteal calcification of the shaft of the humerus (Roentgenogram courtesy of Central Radiologic Institute of the University of Bern. Director Prof. W. A. Fuchs. [M. Mumenthaler: Shoulder-Arm Pain, 2nd ed. Huber, Bern 1982])

It is particularly prominent with osteolytic lesions, resulting in destruction of the tarsometatarsal, tibiotarsal, and distal toe joints. The neurologic deficits that always are present permit differentiation from rheumatologic and arthritic degenerative processes. Sudeck's algodystrophy with severe patchy osteoporosis can be due to trauma, but can also occur after myocardial infarction, in central paresis, or following a peripheral nerve lesion.

2.20.5 Disorders of Trophic Aspect of Muscles

Muscles can decrease in volume — that is, become atrophic; they can also become hypertrophic or show other peculiarities. Muscle atrophy is often a significant leading symptom of neurologic disease. Generalized atrophy can be present without evident weakness. It can be mimicked by extreme thinness (in anorexia nervosa, Russell syndrome of children, and progressive lipodystrophy). In progeria the muscle atrophy may be accompanied by weakness. In children, generalized hypoplasia of muscles (Krabbe) has been described. Prolonged inactivity (for example, lying in bed) may cause atrophy of muscles. If more or less generalized atrophy of muscles is accompanied by weakness, the weakness is usually the leading symptom. If there are no sensory disorders, myopathy (*see* 1.4, 2.12.2 and 2.13.1) or spinal muscular atrophy (*see* 1.2.3 and 2.13.1.1) is usually present.

Symmetric distal atrophy of muscles of extremities, especially of the forearm and hands and calves and feet, is particularly prominent. The atrophy is accompanied by motor weakness, which in many cases can be demonstrated only by a neurologic examination; thus the atrophy is the usual reason for consultation. If there is no sensory loss, distal or distally more prominent myopathy may be present: for example, myotonic dystrophy of Steinert (*see* 1.4 and 2.13.2.4); more rarely, myopathy such as scapuloperoneal syndrome or late distal myopathy of Welander (an autosomal dominantly inherited disorder occurring in adults, very slowly progressive); nonhereditary unilateral or bilateral juvenile distal atrophy of forearm and hand muscles (with spinal causes?); or localized distal hereditary juvenile myopathy of Biemond. The adult type of Aran-Duchenne spinal muscular atrophy may be predominantly distal for long periods (marked by fasciculation, progression, absence of reflexes, and typical electromyogram). Apart from common idiopathic forms there are rare symptomatic cases e.g. in hexosaminidase-A deficiency, acid-maltase deficiency, Waldenström's macroglobulinemia (sometimes with polyneuropathy) also in other gammopathies in lymphomas and in other malignancies. Rarely, an atrophy of small hand muscles is seen in multiple sclerosis.

On careful examination, localized muscle atrophies are found to be accompanied by motor deficits, but these may not be permanent or disturbing to the patient.

Some local atrophies appear without accompanying sensory loss

— Muscle aplasia affects the pectoralis major muscle most often and the thenar muscle more rarely. Perinatal trauma to the sternocleido-

mastoid causes malposition of the head (caput obstipum musculare) and atrophy of muscle
- Arthrogenic atrophy of muscles with lesions (and chronic protective spasm) of a joint is particularly common in the quadriceps femoris
- A symmetric predominantly proximal atrophy of the extremities is found in chronic alcoholism and endocrine disorders e.g. Cushing's disease
- Ischemic muscle atrophy of forearm flexors (Volkmann's contracture) may occur. Rarely this may involve extensor muscles (tibialis anterior syndrome, *see below*)
- Rarely ischemic atrophy of facial muscles may occur after combined effects of beta blockade and cold exposure
- Disuse atrophy appears after immobilization in a cast but may also be found after chronic pain
- A form of neurogenic atrophy is monomelic amyotrophy which involves isolated muscle groups of an extremity and may remain unchanged for decades
- Even in the initial stages of myopathy isolated asymmetric muscle weakness is rarely found (for exception, *see above*) but in nuclear lesions muscle atrophy may remain localized for considerable periods, particularly in the small muscles of the hand. Spinal muscular atrophy may remain localized to a specific muscle group for many years without obvious progression. Bilateral atrophy of the tongue margin can occur with tumors of the clivus
- Pure motor lesions of a peripheral nerve also cause local atrophy:
  - atrophy of the upper trapezius with lesions of the accessory nerve
  - atrophy of the supraspinatus and infraspinatus with lesions of the suprascapular nerve
  - atrophy of the serratus muscles and winging of the scapula with lesions of the long thoracic nerve
  - atrophy of the biceps with lesions of the musculocutaneous nerve
  - atrophy of extensor muscles on the dorsum of the forearm with isolated lesions of the penetrating deep branch of the radial nerve (supinator canal syndrome)
  - marked atrophy of the dorsal interossei of the hand causing clawhand, but without atrophy of the hypothenar eminence, with lesions of the deep branch of the ulnar

nerve at the root of the hand (the result of pressure or a ganglion)
  - atrophy of the lateral aspect of the thenar eminence (the abductor pollicis brevis muscle) with lesions of the median nerve in the carpal canal (accompanied by some disturbances of sensation that are discrete and difficult to find)
  - atrophy of the muscles of the lower extremity without paresis or sensory changes with a very distal lesion of the deep peroneal nerve at the ankle, resulting in atrophy of the short toe extensors on the dorsum of the foot (extensor hallucis brevis and extensor digitorum brevis); compare with the opposite foot

Ischemic muscle atrophy may occur in the lower limbs, particularly in the call extensors, in the anterior tibial syndrome.

- Localized muscle atrophy can also be mimicked by changes in the subcutaneous tissues: for example, with scleroderma and with semicircular lipoatrophy or atrophy of the subcutaneous tissue, due to chronic local pressure (as that occurring in the upper and anterior aspects of the thigh as a result of tight clothing or prolonged leaning on sharp borders of furniture or other supports)

Local muscle atrophy accompanied by sensory disturbances is usually due to lesions of a mixed peripheral nerve, the plexus, or nerve root, or, in rare cases, to an intramedullary spinal cord lesion. All these can be identified from the accompanying neurologic deficits.

Muscle hypertrophy is considerably rarer. Somewhat generalized muscle hypertrophy can occur in athletic individuals and with certain kinds of training (body building). It can follow the administration of anabolic steroids. Congenital generalized muscle hypertrophy may occur in association with extrapyramidal rigidity, mental disability, abnormalities of teeth, and disorders of motor function in Cornelia de Lange syndrome. The same abnormalities are also part of the Berardinelli and the Seip-Lawrence syndromes. In children, congenital hypothyroidism may be associated with so-called myxedematous infantilism (Kocher-Debré-Sémélaigne syndrome), resulting in hypertrophy of the muscles of the extremities, which may be weak or retain normal power. In myotonia congenita of Thomsen, patients often have an athletic habitus. Generalized muscle hypertrophy is found in chondrodystrophy with myotonia, in centronuclear myopathy and in excess growth hormone secretion (or exogenous administration of the human recombinant variety). Diffuse muscle hypertrophy is also found in myeloma, sarcoidosis, cysticercosis and amyloidosis. Occasionally it has been described in familial ataxia. There is also a true non-pathologic hypertrophy of muscles. Lastly the exogenous administration of steroids to various athletes causes muscle hypertrophy and increased strength.

Localized hypertrophy of a single muscle may follow unilateral intense activity of the muscle. A symmetric hypertrophy of the masseter can be constitutional, due to bruxism, or a manifestation of the rare branchial myopathy. Unilateral hypertrophy of the masseter (which may accompany lockjaw) can mimic muscle tumor; primary muscle tumor, in turn, can be confused with hypertrophy of other muscles. Symmetric hypertrophy of the calf is a manifestation of Duchenne muscular dystrophy. This symmetric hypertrophy is (rarely) observed in carriers of Duchenne disease. It is seen rarely in spinal muscular atrophy, and may occasionally mislead examiners of patients with that disorder. In Isaac's syndrome (continuous muscle fiber activity) muscle hypertrophy may occur and may be particularly prominent in the calves (*see* 2.12.1). Unilateral calf hypertrophy may rarely be due to lesions of S_1 root or other causes of denervation. Isolated hypertrophy of other muscles may result from chronic denervation. There is spontaneous activity in the EMG and clinically fasciculations may be recognizable. Painful acute swelling of muscles is found in ischemic muscle necrosis (for example, in the anterior tibial compartment in the syndrome of that name) or with paroxysmal rhabdomyolysis and myoglobinuria.

Other trophic peculiarities of muscles must be mentioned

- With progressive muscular dystrophy zones of preserved muscle fibers may remain in otherwise markedly atrophic muscle, standing out as knots (*boules musculaires*). They are not to be confused with the bunching of the short head of the biceps in the upper arm
- Changes in connective tissue lead to shortening and contractures of finger muscles. Such changes are found in myopathies, particularly in dystrophic processes after muscle ischemia (Volkmann contracture of the flexors of the forearm; retraction of the foot with extension

of toes in the anterior tibial syndrome) and after repeated injection (quadriceps contracture in children, particularly after deep injection of antibiotic)
- Calcification of muscles is found in calcinosis universalis (*see* 2.20.2.2), diffuse trichinosis, extensively in myositis "neurotica", and with mechanical irritation — for example, so-called rider's bones found in the upper adductors of the thigh, in horseback riders

2.20.6 Hyper- and Hypotrophy of Body Parts

In these disorders there is either an enlargement or a diminution in size of body parts.

2.20.6.1 Abnormalities in Head Size

2.20.6.1.1 Macrocephaly (Megalencephaly)

In *children*:

- *Primary megalencephaly.* Large head and brain but normal CSF pathways and ventricules. No neurologic deficits and normal intellect. Often familial
- *Macrocephaly in childhood internal hydrocephalus* (protuberant forehead, setting-sun phenomenon of the eyes. Open or enlarged fontanelles in the first two years of life. Psychomotor retardation eventually neurologic deficits).

In *adults*:

- Megalencephaly or hydrocephalus since childhood
- Paget's disease (leonine facies, Paget's deformities of other bones)
- Acromegaly (includes large hands and feet)

2.20.6.1.2 Microcephaly

This is congenital and may be the only symptom, again often familial or associated with complex neurologic abnormalities. In severe cases there is mental impairment (there are, however, microcephalics of normal intelligence).

2.20.6.2 Abnormalities in Extremity Size

Macromelia occurs in

- Congenital lymphangioma
- As part of the Klippel-Trenaunay syndrome with a segmental flat angioma of the affected extremity and varicose venous ectasia (both these signs may be absent)
- Enlargement of a body half or a quadrant as part of the "hemi-3-syndrome" (hypertrophy areflexia, impaired temperature sensation and scoliosis without syringomyelia). There is a hint of familial impairment of neural crest closure. In this condition the scoliosis alone is progressive

Micromelia is found

- As congenital abnormality
- As a consequence of congenital or early childhood lesions to the contralateral parietal lobe
- After poliomyelitis

2.20.7 Cardiovascular Disorders

2.20.7.1 Cardiac Dysrhythmias

2.20.7.1.1 Autonomic Cardiopathy

Autonomic cardiac neuropathy is found in a number of disorders

- In various polyneuropathies (diabetes mellitus, especially type I, amyloidosis, diphtheria, lupus erythematosus, scleroderma, sarcoidosis)
- With some metabolic disorders and endocrinopathies (uremia, cirrhosis of the liver, toxoplasmosis, hyper- and hypothyroidism, drug-induced).

Various neuromuscular diseases:

- Myopathies (progressive hypertrophic muscular dystrophy [Duchenne], myotonic dystrophy [Steinert], X-linked humeroperoneal muscular dystrophy, Kearns-Sayre syndrome, myasthenia gravis)
- Other neurologic disorders (Friedreich's ataxia, Roussy-Levy syndrome, Kugelberg-Welander syndrome)
- Isolated cardiac ganglionitis (possibly induced by viral infection, with lymphocytic infiltrates)

2.20.7.2 Disturbances of Blood Pressure Control

These disturbances can be manifest by orthostatic hypotension and even loss of consciousness. Disturbances of blood pressure control can result from lesions in three different systems but as a rule are only a part of a complex symptomatology of autonomic failure. These disorders of blood pressure control occur in lesions of

- *Peripheral autonomic fibers,* in polyneuropathy (diabetes mellitus, alcoholic neuropathy, beri-beri). (In familial dysautonomia [Riley-Day syndrome] *see* 2.20.1.1 in acquired acute pandysautonomia [*see* 2.20.1.1])
- *Central autonomic structures,* e.g. orthostatic hypotension in Shy-Drager syndrome (now termed multiple system atrophy) (*see* 2.20.1.1) or in high spinal cord transection
- These disturbances also characterize a number of functional disorders of blood pressure regulation e.g. vasovagal syncope (*see* 2.3.3)

3. References

Aita, J. A.: Neurologic Manifestations of General Diseases. Thomas, Springfield (Ill.) 3rd Reprint 1975

Aita, J. A.: Neurocutaneous Diseases. Thomas, Springfield (Ill.) 1966

Appenzeller, O.: The Autonomic Nervous System. An Introduction to Basic and Clinical Concepts, 4th Ed. Elsevier, Amsterdam 1990

Birnberger, K., R. Maurach: Neurologische Manifestationen interner Erkrankungen. Urban & Schwarzenberg, München 1981

Bodechtel, G.: Differentialdiagnose neurologischer Krankheitsbilder, 3. Aufl. Thieme, Stuttgart 1974

Bradley, W. G.: Disorders of Peripheral Nerves. Blackwell, Oxford 1974

Brain, Lord, F. H. Norris: The Remote Effects of Cancer on the Nervous System. Contemporary Neurology Symposia, Vol. I. Grune & Stratton, New York 1965

Calne, D. B.: Parkinsonism: Physiology, Pharmacology and Treatment. Arnold, London 1970

Chusid, J. G.: Correlative Neuroanatomy and Functional Neurology, 19th Ed. Lange Medical Publication. Los Altos, Calif. 1985

Claussen, C.-F.: Differential Diagnosis of Vertigo. De Gruyter, Berlin 1980

Duus, P.: Neurologisch-topische Diagnostik. Anatomie. Physiologie. Klinik, 2. Aufl. Thieme, Stuttgart 1980

Feneis, H.: Anatomisches Bildwörterbuch. Thieme, Stuttgart 1982

Ford, F. R.: Diseases of the Nervous System in Infancy, Childhood and Adolescence, 4th Ed. Thomas, Springfield (Ill.) 1960

Greenfield, J. G.: The Spino-Cerebellar Degenerations. Blackwell, Oxford 1954

Grote, W.: Neurochirurgie. Thieme, Stuttgart 1976

Herman, E. J., A. Prusinski: Neurologische Syndrome bei inneren Krankheiten. Schattauer, Stuttgart 1977

Hertel, G., S. Kramer, E. Placzek: Die Syringomyelie. Klinische Verlaufsbeobachtungen bei 323 Patienten. Nervenarzt 44 (1973) 1 – 13

Janz, D.: Die Epilepsien. Thieme, Stuttgart 1969

Janzen, R., H. A. Kühn (Hrsg.): Neurologische Leit- und Warnsymptome bei inneren Erkrankungen. Thieme, Stuttgart 1982

Jerusalem, F.: Muskelerkrankungen. Klinik – Therapie – Pathologie. Thieme, Stuttgart 1979

Krayenbühl, H., G. Yasargil: Das Hirnaneurysma. Docum. chir. Geigy 4, 1958

Leischner, A.: Aphasien und Sprachentwicklungsstörungen. Thieme, Stuttgart 1979

Matthews, W. B., E. D. Acheson, J. R. Batchelor, R. O. Weller: McAlpine's multiple sclerosis. 2nd ed. Churchill-Livingstone, Edinburgh 1990

Menkes, J. H.: Textbook of Child Neurology, 2nd Ed. Lea & Febiger, Philadelphia 1980

Mumenthaler, M.: Der Schulter-Arm-Schmerz, 2. Aufl. Huber, Bern 1982

Mumenthaler, M. (Hrsg.): Synkopen und Sturzanfälle. Diagnostik, Differentialdiagnostik und Therapie für die Praxis. Thieme, Stuttgart 1984

Mumenthaler, M., H. Schliack: Läsionen peripherer Nerven, 5. Aufl. Thieme, Stuttgart 1987

Patten, J.: Neurological Differential Diagnosis. An Illustrated Approach. Springer, Berlin 1977

Peele, T. L.: The Neuroanatomic Basis for Clinical Neurology, 3rd Ed. McGraw-Hill, New York 1977

Plum, F., J. B. Posner: The Diagnosis of Stupor and Coma, 3rd Ed. Davis, Philadelphia 1980

Rabending, G. et al.: Epilepsien. Leitfaden für die Praxis. VEB Thieme, Leipzig 1981

Schirmer, M.: Einführung in die Neurochirurgie, 5. Aufl. Urban & Schwarzenberg, München 1982

Sunderland, S.: Nerves and Nerve Injuries, Churchill-Livingstone, Edinburgh 2nd Ed. 1978

Toole, J. F., A. N. Patel: Zerebrovaskuläre Störungen. Übersetzt und bearbeitet von M. Mumenthaler und Josefa Caffi. Springer, Berlin 1980

Walsh, F. et al.: Clinical Neuro-ophthalmology, 4th Ed. Williams & Wilkins, Baltimore 1982

Walton, J. N.: Disorders of Voluntary Muscle, 4th Ed. Churchill-Livingstone, London 1981

Willis, W. D., R. G. Grossman: Medical Neurobiology. Neuroanatomical and Neurophysiological Principles Basic to Clinical Neuroscience, 3rd Ed. Mosby, St. Louis 1981

4. Index

Boldface page numbers refer to sections in which the concept is discussed in greater detail.